Textbook of Sociology for Nursing Students

Textbook of Sociology for Nursing Students

KP Neeraja
BSc BSc(N) BPR MSc(N) MA PhD
Principal
Navodaya College of Nursing
Mantralayam Road
Raichur, Karnataka

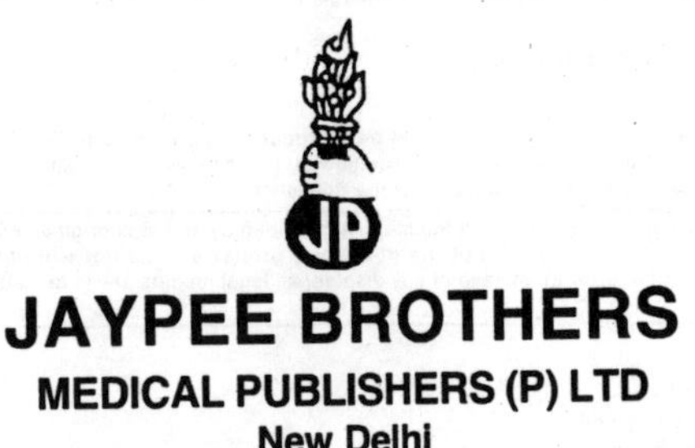

JAYPEE BROTHERS
MEDICAL PUBLISHERS (P) LTD
New Delhi

Published by

Jitendar P Vij
Jaypee Brothers Medical Publishers (P) Ltd

Corporate Office
4838/24, Ansari Road, Daryaganj, **New Delhi** 110 002, India. Phone: +91-11-43574357
Fax: +91-11-43574314

Registered Office
B-3, EMCA House, 23/23B Ansari Road, Daryaganj, **New Delhi** 110 002, India
Phones: +91-11-23272143, +91-11-23272703, +91-11-23282021, +91-11-23245672
Rel: +91-11-32558559 Fax: +91-11-23276490, +91-11-23245683
e-mail: jaypee@jaypeebrothers.com Website: www.jaypeebrothers.com

Branches

- 2/B, Akruti Society, Jodhpur Gam Road Satellite
  Ahmedabad 380 015 Phones: +91-79-26926233, Rel: +91-79-32988717
  Fax: +91-79-26927094 e-mail: ahmedabad@jaypeebrothers.com
- 202 Batavia Chambers, 8 Kumara Krupa Road, Kumara Park East
  Bengaluru 560 001 Phones: +91-80-22285971, +91-80-22382956 +91-80-22372664,
  Rel: +91-80-32714073 Fax: +91-80-22281761 e-mail: bangalore@jaypeebrothers.com
- 282 IIIrd Floor, Khaleel Shirazi Estate, Fountain Plaza, Pantheon Road
  Chennai 600 008 Phones: +91-44-28193265, +91-44-28194897
  Rel: +91-44-32972089 Fax: +91-44-28193231 e-mail: chennai@jaypeebrothers.com
- 4-2-1067/1-3, 1st Floor, Balaji Building, Ramkote Cross Road
  Hyderabad 500 095 Phones: +91-40-66610020 +91-40-24758498, Rel:+91-40-32940929
  Fax:+91-40-24758499, e-mail: hyderabad@jaypeebrothers.com
- No. 41/3098, B & B1, Kuruvi Building, St. Vincent Road
  Kochi 682 018, Kerala Phones: +91-484-4036109, +91-484-2395739
  +91-484-2395740 e-mail: kochi@jaypeebrothers.com
- 1-A Indian Mirror Street, Wellington Square
  Kolkata 700 013 Phones: +91-33-22651926, +91-33-22276404, +91-33-22276415
  Fax: +91-33-22656075 e-mail: kolkata@jaypeebrothers.com
- Lekhraj Market III, B-2, Sector-4, Faizabad Road, Indira Nagar
  Lucknow 226 016 Phones: +91-522-3040553, +91-522-3040554
  e-mail: lucknow@jaypeebrothers.com
- 106 Amit Industrial Estate, 61 Dr SS Rao Road, Near MGM Hospital, Parel
  Mumbai 400012 Phones: +91-22-24124863, +91-22-24104532
  Rel: +91-22-32926896 Fax: +91-22-24160828, e-mail: mumbai@jaypeebrothers.com
- "KAMALPUSHPA" 38, Reshimbag, Opp. Mohota Science College, Umred Road
  Nagpur 440 009 (MS) Phone: Rel: +91-712-3245220
  Fax: +91-712-2704275 e-mail: nagpur@jaypeebrothers.com

North America Office
1745, Pheasant Run Drive, Maryland Heights (Missouri), MO 63043, USA Ph: 001-636-6279734
e-mail: jaypee@jaypeebrothers.com, anjulav@jaypeebrothers.com

Central America Office
Jaypee-Highlights Medical Publishers Inc., City of Knowledge, Bld. 237, Clayton, Panama City, Panama
Ph: 507-317-0160

Textbook of Sociology for Nursing Students

First Edition: **2005**
Reprint: 2006
ISBN 978-81-8061-476-7
Typeset at JPBMP typesetting unit
Printed at Sanat Printers, Kundli

Dedicated to
My beloved parents
Sri Kurudi Padmanabaiah
&
Smt Parvathavardhini

FOREWORD

The author deserves to be congratulated for preparing 'Text book of Sociology for Nursing Students'. I have immense pleasure in presenting the foreword to this book for professional students broughtout by my student, Dr KP Neeraja. The increased application of Sociology in the health profession has necessiated a right kind of textbook applied to the profession and the author has made an attempt to fulfil such a need.

A practicing sociologist with the credit of authorizing several books, Dr KP Neeraja has brought this book various practical points not only in dealing with client, his family and social factors related to client, his family and community as well, to provide total client care with the knowledge of sociology.

This book is aimed at the students of Nursing in under graduation courses, who are studying in various colleges in the country, since it conforms to the syllabus of undergraduates, I am confident that this book would benefit them to acquire knowledge and skills in a broader social outlook.

Dr KP Neeraja's vast knowledge and rich experience in the profession of Nursing and Teaching are definitely an asset in writing this textbook. It comprehensively covers the basic and introductory concepts of sociology as related to the health care profession and help the students to understand the subject in an easy manner. I am delighted that this book is published at a right time when the student need it most. It is of great value in its own right and should guide the student to develop greater insight into the sociological concepts.

I am confident that this book will go through many more editions in future.

Dr K Sreenivasa Reddy
[Social Scientist]

PREFACE

During my long tenure of sixteen years as a teacher in nursing, I observed that there is no comprehensive textbook on Sociology written with an eye on the syllabus and need of the nursing students; hence it motivated me to conceive this text book.

I hope this book will fulfil the felt needs of the students and help them to develop better understanding and insight into the subject of sociology. An attempt is made to make the abstract science of society viz., sociology interesting to the reader. My effort is to stimulate the thinking process and motivate the students to provide holistic care with due consideration to social factors. The contents of this book are carefully planned and compiled keeping in view of the syllabi of graduation in Nursing and Post Basic Nursing courses of different universities and Diploma in General Nursing and Midwifery course. I hope definitely this book will help the students and teachers in Nursing Profession.

KP Neeraja

ACKNOWLEDGEMENTS

I am immensely thankful to my beloved teacher and eminent mentor Dr K Sreenivasa Reddy, Social Scientist, Kurnool who kindly honoured me by writing the foreword.

I am thankful to Mrs Ghousia Begum for assisting me in gathering some related material. I am indebted to Mrs Sundarambal Narayanan for providing conducive environment to accomplish this greatest achievement.

My sincere thanks to Sri Jitendar P Vij, Chairman and Managing Director and other staff of M/s Jaypee Brothers Medical Publishers (P) Ltd, New Delhi, who made it possible to publish the book within short span of time. I am indebted specially to Mr Ravi Kumar, staff of Jaypee, Bangalore branch for motivating me to take up the task.

CONTENTS

CHAPTER ONE

Introduction to Sociology

Introduction

Sociology is the youngest of all social sciences. The history of sociology is as old as society. Systematic studies of society started long back in Greece, i.e. in 427–347 BC. Plato and his disciple Aristotle (384–322) laid foundation for systematic study.

In India, king Manu laid foundation for sociology. He divided people into four varnas. Epics in India reflect the behaviour and various aspects how to live in a society. Manu referred to customs, social affairs in his book, 'Manu Smruthi'.

In 1839, Auguste Comte, a French Philosopher, (1798-1857) coined the term, 'Sociology'. He is considered as, 'Father of Sociology'. Sociology is derived from two words, 'societus' means society, (Latin word) and 'logos' (Greek word) means study of.

Definition

- 'The science of social phenomenon subjected to natural laws, the discovery of which is the objective of investigations'. —Auguste Comte

- 'The scientific study of society' —Gidding and Gidding
- 'Study of relationship between man and his environment' —HP Fair Child
- 'The study of interactions arising from the association of living beings' —Gillin and Gillin
- 'The study of human interactions and interrelations, their conditions and consequences' —M Ginsberg
- 'The science which attempts the interpretive understandings of social being' —Maxweber
- 'The scientific study of social relationships, their variety, their forms whatever affects them and whatever they affect'
- 'Sociology is the scientific study of patterns of human behaviour as they emerge and crystallise out of the interactions of human beings in the groups, which comprise the society'— George Shankar
- 'It is the study of social aggregates and groups in their institutional organisation and the causes and the consequences of changes in institutions and social organisation' —International Encyclopedia of social sciences
- 'It is an academic discipline that utilises the scientific method in accumulating knowledge about man's social behaviour. It studies the patterned, shared human behaviour, the way in which people act towards one another —Prasad, 1977.

The above definitions are based on the following factors

- Human beings have a propensity to organise their behaviour in groups in order to satisfy their needs and wants to fulfill necessary social function
- Human beings have the capacity to know how to organise their behaviour in a wide range of groups
- The behaviours, thoughts and attitudes of human beings are determined to a large extent by the quality of the learned ways of interacting in groups
- The social interaction in which one person influence the attitudes, thoughts, opinions and behaviour of another

- Interaction pattern occurs within the large social systems in societies, groups, crowds, social classes, social institutions, neighbourhood and community.

From all the definitions of sociology, we can list out the following views:

- The sociology is science of society
- It studies the social relationships
- It is the study of social life
- It is the study of human behaviour in group situation
- It deals with social actions
- It studies social systems.

NATURE OF SOCIOLOGY

Sociology as a Science

It emerged as a special discipline among the social sciences, considered as sciences of society. The concept was first developed by Emile Durkheim as it uses scientific methods, investigation, and different bodies of knowledge.

1. *It studies social phenomenon:* It is known as, 'Mother of all social sciences'.

   It uses scientific method. It is a systematic way of dealing with ideas, careful observation and recording of the factual data, and which is classified, analysed and organised in a systematic fashion by logical basis through which generalisations can be made.
2. *Sociology is factual:* It deals with facts only, uses scientific principles to solve the problems.
3. *Sociology frames laws and attempts to predict:* Science can make prediction on the basis of universal and valued laws relating to the problem solving approach.
4. *Principles of sociology are universal:* The laws of sociology proved to be true at all times and places, as long as the conditions do not vary. The laws are devoid of any exceptions.

5. *It discovers the cause and effect relationship:* It structures for the cause and effect relationship in its subject matter and in this connection, it provides universal and valid laws.
6. *Sociological principles are veridical:* The laws of sociology prove true at every verification and re-verification. Any one can examine their validity.

Opposite Views about the Nature of Sociology

Some critics who deny sociology to be regarded as science, sociology is a social science it cannot be regarded as science.

1. It lacks experimentation: Sociology deals with human relationship, which can be neither measured, weighted nor see or analyse.
2. Lack of objectivity: The sociologists cannot maintain complete its objectivity in order to understand its external action.
3. Lack of exactivity: The laws and conclusions cannot be expressed in precise terms. The prediction might not be true. Findings are often limited in time and space.
4. Inability to measure subject matter.
5. It lacks perfect exactness.
6. It cannot make predictions correctly.

Scope of Sociology

There is no one opinion about the scope of sociology. *Calberten* describes, since sociology is an elastic science it is difficult to determine just where its boundaries begin and ends. It is impossible to divide as it studies human interactions, interrelations, their conditions and consequences.

There are two main schools of thoughts: One group of sociologists headed by *Simmel* formulated specialistic or Formalistic School. They thought that it is pure science and systematic one. It is independent science.

I. SPECIALISTIC/FORMALISTIC SCHOOL

Simmel's view

It classifies, analyses and delimits the forms of social relationships.

Small's view

It does not understand to study all the actions of society. It studies genetic forms of social relationship behaviour and activities.

Verkendent's view

It is a specialised branch of knowledge concerned with ultimate forms of psychic relationship, which link men to men in the society.

Maxweber's view

It studies interpretation and understanding of behaviour and it is concerned with analysis and classification and types of social relationship.

Vonwiese's view

The sociology studies all forms of social relationship.

Tonnie's view

He has differentiated the society and the community on the basis of forms of social relationship.

Criticism

- It has narrowed the scope of sociology
- Abstract form is separate from concrete form
- The construction of pure sociology is impractical
- Sociology alone does not study social relationship

II SYNTHETIC SCHOOL

Durkem's View

Sociology was divided into 3 branches.

Social Morphology

Concerned with geographical basis of the life, its relationship to types of social organisation and the problems of population.

Social Physiology

It is divided into number of branches like sociology of religion, sociology of morals. Sociology of laws, sociology of economic life, sociology of language etc.

General Sociology

It discovers the social facts.

Hobhouse's View

The interconnections of social relations and the results; social life as a whole will be studied.

Karl Mannheim's View

Sociology is divided into systematic and general sociology. It describes how the individual will react social changes in a given society.

Ginsberg's View

It studies the types and forms of social relationship. It determines the relation between different factors of social life, social change, persistence and to discover sociological principles governing social life.

Thus the scope of sociology is very wide. It studies the various aspects of society, e.g: Social processes, traditions, morphology, social control and social pathology.

Field of Sociology

In 1902, *Emile Durkheim* has classified sociology into:

- General sociology
- Juridical sociology
- Moral sociology
- Criminal sociology
- Religious sociology
- Economic sociology
- Social morphology.

Sub-fields of sociology

- Industrial sociology
- Family sociology
- Educational sociology
- Medical/health sociology.

The functions of sociology/importance of sociology

- It is a scientific study of society
- It studies the role of institutions, through the knowledge of sociology the individual can understand and establish relationship with the social environment like family, religion, school, governmental policies and working situations
- The study of sociology is indispensable for understanding and planning of society
- It helps in solvation of social problems
- It draws our attention to the institutional worth and dignity of men
- It contributes to understand human culture, to make good citizens
- It keeps us update information on modern institutions
- It adds to the knowledge of society
- It identifies good government with community
- Technical function: To construct society by observing existing problems, customs, traditions, institutions, etc. it can make the people to understand the changing situations.

- Introductory function: It supplies the information about the elements of social system to facilitate the introduction of any desirable changes. It explains different methods, which can introduce this change into various parts of it.
- Informative function: It possesses some important information based on theoretical knowledge with practical experience. It makes the individual to organise society by solving certain social problems. It provides guidance in practical reforms.
- Tolerative function: In India, each individual comes across different religions and cultures. We have to understand all the social institutions to develop a feeling of universal brotherhood.
- Democratic function: To develop a selfless tendency and understands the society in a well-planned manner.

Relationship of Sociology with Nursing

- Nursing plays a vital role in healthcare profession. Nurses are the key persons who have significant influence over the group members within the society. Nurses have to work for maintenance of healthier life styles and high standards of living
- Nurses will be in close association with healthcare team members and they will work in coordination with various agencies in the community for betterment of living and to inculcate healthier habits among the community. The social institutions like family, religion, state, political group, governmental agencies will play dominant role over the societal life. In coordination with primary, secondary groups and social institutions nurses have to work cooperatively in implementation of healthcare activity and implement other national health programme activities to attain 'Health For All'.
- To provide total patient care in a comprehensive manner and render tender loving care to meet the total needs of the clients either in the hospitals or in the community

- To understand and meet the needs of the individual, family and societal needs in a holistic manner thereby nation's development can be achieved
- To broaden the view of nursing students to understand human behaviour in relation to the society. Relationship through good social interaction and thereby good human interpersonal relationship will be formed with the clients in the society
- To understand the cause and meaning of many kinds of patient behaviour to make them comfortable and treat them all alike for improvement of client care
- To understand the problems of clients
- To suggest the ways to work with families, community agencies and groups of persons to provide health counselling in planning for continuity of care
- To provide right motivation, treatment and physical, medical, vocational, psychosocial rehabilitation basing on attitudes and responses of others by understanding their behaviour through good interpersonal relationship
- To understand the emotional reaction pattern, (e.g: Level of perception, attitudes of people towards medical care, barriers of communication, individual differences, social distance, prejudice, change, emotional interpersonal components of disease process, the growth and decline of population in a specified area, socio-psychological factors, etc.) to understand herself and others and the nurse has to make more effective use of her professional skills
- The nurse is having close association and continuous contact with the clients than any other health team member, she has to understand the problems of clients in crucial way
- To gain greater insight into the human problems as related to the illness
- Good observation, communication, guidance skills are essential to understand clients' behaviour
- Nurses need to assume the responsibility for the provision of first level care in the community and thus acting as a

changing agent in bringing about good quality of life to the people at large
- The nurse has to be sensitive to the health needs of the people in the context of broader social change.

Educator

- In the context of overall social development of health for all, the primary role of nurse is to take up the health education activities in community along with the participation and involvement of local people in planning and implementing health care programmes for their attainment of good quality of life, prevention of disease and disability and promotion of health
- Nurse has to impart this knowledge of new focus of nursing care with inputs from behavioural sciences to health and related functionaries in order to sensitise them to the needs of people.

Manager and Supervisor

Nurse should act as a community organiser and leader in planning, organising, and implementing health services through community participation.

Planner

- Nurse should be able to make a diagnosis of people's belief and practices to various diseases
- Identify some of the socio-cultural barriers and promotes the activities related to treatment, prevention of diseases and promotion of health
- Identify available community resources for implementation of the activity to attain the purpose
- Select suitable health education methods
- Develop a plan of operation by involving local people and others engaged in community development keeping in mind the social realities

- It also requires supportive supervision on the part of the community health nurse.

Researcher

- Updating of skills and knowledge, monitoring and evaluating activities
- Analysing health conditions of people and bringing about changes and innovation in health care based on research.

Social Scientist

Man has to be understood as a member of society and his behaviour is dynamic, which has tendency to act and react equally within his dynamic socio-cultural environment, the nurse has to clearly understand the needs of each segment of the society.

Nurse has to study the broader issues of community involvement in health service development requiring the knowledge of:

- Cultural aspects of health services, health institutions, health problems, health practices prevailing
- Modes of prediction
- Social structure
- Distribution of power
- Political organisations
- Mobilisation of resources and pattern of their uses within the community in the context of cultural perception and cultural meaning of the health problems.

Changing Agent

- Examination of individual and social values, effective communication skills, critical evaluation technique and accurate observation skills are most crucial
- Emotional soundness, maturity in dealing with situations and accepting the challenges as required
- Developing work habits to increase efficiency and effectivity

- Nurse should not only understand the client, should be sensitive, responsive, warmth but also intuitive to anticipate and meet the emotional needs of the client
- The nurse has to work with many people like superiors, subordinates, class IV employees, clients, students, visitors, etc. should plan social interactions and establish good interpersonal relationships
- To study the social problems related to behaviour and suggest preventive, remedial approach to tackle the problematic situations in the community in efficient manner
- The knowledge of sociology helps the nurses to identify and analyse different social situations, which are responsible for the incidence and prevalence of morbidity and mortality conditions of the individuals
- To understand the cultural aspects and differences based on clients background, beliefs, and values. Effective motivation can be possible to meet the total needs of the client
- It provides the educational opportunity in the provision of psychological support in a worthy manner by understanding their ideas, emotions in a perspective manner
- It helps in clinical practice and clinical teaching and aid for new discoveries and inventions that will produce an extra dimension to improve the client care
- To demonstrate the practicability and significance of social sciences to understand the behaviour of individual and to establish implications of such knowledge for diagnosis, treatment of conditions. It provides conducive environment to understand the rights of individual and to meet the welfare of the community. To integrate the principles of other social sciences in the nursing curriculum
- Nurses will formulate significant rules, which will have bearing effect upon the patients' responses or resistance for treatment
- Nurse will act as an effective liaison between the client and the health team members

- Nurse will develop discipline sensitivity that gives the meaning of compassion and understanding in order to study the stress in social relationship
- To recognise the sociological factors as intervening variables in the disease patterns.

Relationship of Sociology with Nursing

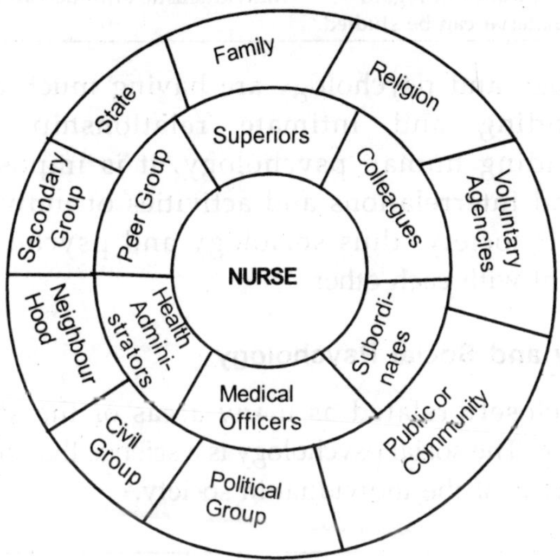

Relationship of sociology with other social sciences

The knowledge of human behaviour with an interdisciplinary approach to understand the human needs in the context of wider social problems. It is a total system approach to understand human behaviour views man as a product of socio-psychological and cultural factors. It analyses man's behaviour in relation to psychological framework, interpersonal orientation and group influence. It helps to find solutions to problems, which are arising due to man's complex nature.

Sociology	*Psychology*
Society is the basic unit.	Individual is the basic unit.
It studies the relationship of individual to the society.	It is a science of human experience and behaviour.
It studies man as a part of societal system and social institutions and social processes will be used in social interaction.	It studies man as an individual and his interaction with heredity and environment. • The psychic and mental processes will be studied
Difference of attitudes in regard to common material can be studied.	Individualistic attitude can be studied.

Sociology and psychology are having much common understanding and intimate relationship without understanding human psychology, it is impossible to understand interrelations and activities of individual in relation to society, thus sociology and psychology are complement with each other.

Sociology and Social Psychology

Both are closely related as many areas of the study are overlapping. The social psychology is a science that deals with the behaviour of the individual in society.

Social Psychology	*Sociology*
It studies the behaviour of an individual in society	Group behaviour can be studied
It studies the mental processes of the individual	It studies social processes, social laws or values related to attitudes
It is the study of individual attitude towards cultural and social values and the laws related to these attitudes	Sociology discuss concrete form of society, its structure and functions
It analyses the frame work of social relationships	It studies the interaction of the human being with the environment

Sociology and Economics

Economics	*Sociology*
It is the study of man's activity devoted in obtaining the material, means for the satisfaction of his wants and restricted ways of behaviour of the individual	Comprehensive and studies the whole society in its scope
It studies economic relationship and activities in economic point of view only	It studies social relationship from societal point of view
The unit is the individual with economic activity	Individual behaviour in relation to the group and environment
Mainly it deals with production, distribution and uses addition, subtraction, induction, deduction as the methods of study	The social relationships can be studied by various methods eg: interview, observation, questionnaire
The scope is restricted	It comprehends the whole society in its scope

Sociology and Anthropology

Sociology	*Anthropology*
It studies modern communities and social problems and suggest solutions	It studies ancient communities and the problems existed
It studies various aspects and problems of society and guides for change	It studies as a whole
It studies social relationship	It studies anatomical characteristics and its influence upon the behavioural change
It makes suggestions concerning to the future	It is pure understanding and past relationship
It makes use of documents, surveys	It makes use of functional method

History and Sociology

History	*Sociology*
It studies past and it is concrete	It is abstract, deals with present, past and future
It presents a chronological description of incidence of events and its culture principles	It studies the human experience and human nature. It attempts to discover their causes and general
It studies those incidence which are peculiar or unusual	It studies those incidence which are frequently repeated

Contd...

Contd...

It describes incidence taking place at a definite place and time. It emphasizes the doings of the individual	It studies to discover universal laws and is not related to particular incidence. Social groups is the unit of sociological study

Sociology and Political Sociology

Sociology	*Political sociology*
It is science of society	It is the science of government off political society, its structure and processes
It studies social point of view	It studies attitude of authority, policy formulation and execution
Studies both organised and disorganised communities	Studies purely organised community
Studies all kinds of social relationship and forms of society	Studies all forms of societies and its laws, economy and the higher powers mainly related to political relationship in political society

Biology and Sociology

Biology	*Sociology*
To understand organisation, nature and progress Describes anatomical, developmental, sexual, personal peculiarities and formulates principles for the adjustments to the environment	The knowledge of the efforts of hereditary and environment upon man is studied

Role of Social Factors in Health

Social situations and social environment will have influence on the occurrence of disease, prevention of illness and health maintenance. Unhealthy life styles and high-risk behaviour predisposes sicknesses such as cancer, AIDS and heart disease. For healthier life maintenance modification of life style is required. Societies have to organise their resources to cope with health hazards and deliver medical care to the population. Individual and societies tend to respond to health problems in a manner consistent with their culture, norms and values. Factors like social, cultural, political, and economic, etc. will have definite influence over health maintenance. It is the responsibility of health care professionals to arrange IEC campaigns through mass media activities emphasising the public on healthy life style and individual responsibility for health care. The high-risk behaviour includes poor diet, lack of exercise, smoking, alcoholism, drug abuse, stress and exposure to STD. Adverse social conditions like poverty reduces life expectancy and creates health problems.

Public health in an applied technology resting on the joint pillars of natural science and social science until these pillars are strong, the arch of the public health will not be firm. The health care professionals use the knowledge of social sciences in implementation of medical and health care activities.

Role of Social Factors in Disease

Deviation in the normal functioning of the body produces discomfort or adversely affects the individual's health status. Every society has certain norms, values, ideals in regard to health and disease, deviation from which is treated as an aberration or a disease. Diseases occurs due to various factors such as invasion by microbes or other pathogenic agents which disturbs the haemostatic balance and results in malfunctioning of organs, low standards of living, poor environmental sanitation, poor housing, bad habits like smoking and alcoholism, inadequate nutrition, low economy, poverty, contamination of food, water with industrial effluents, air pollution, poor urban planning, deprived of family relationships, inadequate physical activities, defective lifestyle, sexual harassment, unemployment, rapid economic growth, over population, job strain, occupational maladjustment, migration and healthy comparisons, illiteracy, discrimination, misunderstandings, stress, large gaps in income, inadequate access to healthy foods, isolation, etc. In the sociological context disease is associated with a particular way of life, vulnerability for diseases are common among the people who are facing certain problems like isolation, geographic or social mobility, inability to fulfill role expectations, changing inconsistency in status, inadequate social support, blocked aspirations, lack of consistency or uncertainty in outcome of vital events, value polymorphism and rapid social changes.

Social factors affects diseases at three levels:

1. *Physical level:* The social class, environment, nutrition, housing, etc. are responsible for occurrence of disease.
2. *Psycho-social level:* Diseases occur due to prevalence of mental stress and strain resulting from specific environmental factors.
3. *Cultural level:* Social milieu, attitudes, beliefs psychosomatic factors, etc. affects the disease pattern and in implementation of preventive and therapeutic modalities. Social environment affects different attitudes among various cultural groups about seeking medical and health care.

The basis of epidemiology was broadened from the study of distribution of communicable diseases among the population in relation to epidemiological triad (agent, host, environment). The multiplication of disease is related to social factors, community involvement is essential in organising health education campaigns to bring health awareness, social and cultural factors similarly affects our ability to stay well. Social support is essential and plays a crucial role in our physical and mental health, through its health sustaining and stress-buffering functions with social ties live longer and have better health. Rapid industrialisation, urbanisation and technological advancement made the social environment giving rise to stress and strain, which leads to chronic and degenerative disease.

Sociological Investigation

'Critical examination into a situation to discover new facts about a particular or specified social phenomenon to discover intellectual and practical answers to problems through the application of scientific methods in the universe' is called social investigation. It is a careful, critical enquiry or examination in seeking facts or principles diligent investigation in order to ascertain something. It is a critical in the light of newly discovered facts. It is the study of activities undertaken to search a solution for the social problems. The society has to march on its present form with the help of constant research and investigation. Long march from Stone Age to computer age has been the result of research. Today society is facing several social problems of formidable in nature. They demand solutions and any attempt to solve the problems must be through scientific enquiry. It aims at increasing our knowledge about society and strategies involved solvation of social problems.

Definition

- 'Systematic investigation to gain knowledge about social phenomena and social problems'—*Moses. C A*
- 'It is the investigation of the underlying process operating in the lives of persons who are in association'—*Bogardus. E*
- 'It is a study of human group relationships'—*Whitney. F L*
- 'It is the systematic study of discovering the new facts or verifying old facts, their sequences, interrelationship, casual explanations and the natural laws, which govern them'—*PV Young*
- 'Systematised effort to gain new knowledge or new mode or orientation of new knowledge'—*Redman and Money*
- 'The manipulation of things, concepts or symbols for the purpose of generalising to extend, correct or verify knowledge; whether that knowledge aids in construction of theory or in the practice of an art'—*M Stephen*

From the above definitions, it is clear that it is concerned with pure social phenomena, answering meaningful questions and finding out the old or new facts through scientific method, which is based on logic and systematic means. To collect and analyses the data more or less within the exiting framework and establishes the exploration techniques. Theoretically, social investigations aims at finding solutions of a problem as a part of social system and behaviour of the individuals under different situations and on utilitarian aspect, it helps in reducing social conflicts and tensions as well as in rectification and removal of social evils. Social phenomena are complex. Therefore different methods and approaches have to be followed to study the social aspects of the individuals. Social phenomena can be indirectly studied through observation of traditions, customs, values and vested interests, which are prevailed in the society. To have the objectivity in studying social phenomena is difficult. The scope of social investigation depends upon several factors such as money, time available to the investigator, availability of the sample, accessibility of thee investigator to the respondents, the amount of time the respondent can spare for these investigation, etc.

METHODS OF SOCIAL INVESTIGATIONS

Social Survey Approach

It is a common method used to diagnose and solve the social problem. The survey design is the non-experimental type of research in which, the researcher investigates a community or a group of people. The researcher gathers the data from a relatively large number of cases at a particular time. It involves clearly defined problem or objectives. It requires expert, imaginative planning, careful analysis, interpretation of data gathered, logical and skillful reporting of the findings.

It may be done by:

- By questioning
- Interview
- Observation

Social survey is one of the important methods of social investigation and helps in solving the group problems. The researcher investigates new situation, organisation or a group and be clear about the nature of enquiry, objectives, nature and scope of study. Researcher formulates questions for the larger study and pursues general overall description of the situation.

Definition

- 'It is a process by which qualitative facts are collected about the social aspects of a community composition and activities' —*Mark Abram*
- 'Collection of data concerning the living and working conditions, broadly speaking the people in a given community'—*Bogardus ES*
- 'It is the scientific study of conditions and needs of a community for the purpose of presenting a constructive programme and social advance' —E*W Burgers*
- 'It is a process by which quantitative facts are collected about the social aspects of a community, composition and activities' —*SM Harison*
- 'Fact finding study dealing chiefly with working class and with the nature and problems of community'—*AF Wells*

Social survey are connected with

- The formation of constructive programme of social reform and amelioration of social problem
- 'Current or immediate conditions of social pathological nature which have definite geographic limits and definite social implications and significance'—*PV Young*

Characteristics

- Done in a large scale and gains a lot of material
- To find out the basic facts of life
- Quality is maintained
- Scientific and well planned
- Conducted regularly e.g.: Census, market survey, etc.
- Costly affair, needs both human as well as economic resources to complete
- Unnecessary data should not be collected

- Trained personnel are required to collect the information and capable of adjusting themselves to the nature of work
- To collect the detailed information about a social problem under investigation or social aspect of community
- To test hypothesis
- Practical and utilitarian view point.

Subject Matter of Social Survey

- Demographic characteristics
- Social environment
- Activities of community members
- Opinions and attitudes.

Uses of Survey Method

- To obtain demographic data, information about people's behaviour (attitudes, opinions, interests)
- To discover casual relationship in a specific area or precise qualitative description of some phase of the universe.

Advantages of Survey Approach

- It can give information about the possibilities of understanding different types of research methods
- It provides an insight into a situation, suggests kinds of questions to ask and the methods to adapt
- It provides hypothesis and helps to test the hypothesis
- Provides data about present situation
- It studies the problems thoroughly and deeply in all aspects
- Guides the researcher about confounding, intervening, independent and dependent variables
- Useful for policy makers and administrators to make a decision
- Specific goals will be obtained
- Changes in society, pressures of public opinion can be obtained

- Provides an opportunity to use researcher's creativity
- Factual information related to life experiences will be gathered
- It has high degree of representation in the reality
- Broad generalisation can be done
- Greater deal of information will be obtained
- Easy, less time consuming.

Disadvantages

- To get resources both human (trained investigators, field workers) and economic (huge fund is required) is problem
- Low degree of control over extraneous variables
- No uniformity in data collection
- Lack of manipulation of independent variables
- Each researcher will try to use their own bias in the study
- One cannot progressively investigate one aspect after another of the independent variable to get closer to the real world
- Time consuming
- Statistical devices are not always able to separate the effects of several independent variables.

Types of Survey

Descriptive Survey

Simplest survey with in the social discipline. To describe objectively the nature of the situation under study and conclusions also drawn.

Evaluation Survey

The researcher looks back to see what has been accomplished with a critical eye and evaluates the results. The researcher is interested in finding out the results of some procedure or methods already in operation. This method is used on small sample atleast initially. To find, if this method in operation meets the criteria stated in the purpose of the original project. It should not be done by the investigators, who have a particular benefit or gain to be made from the results.

Comparative Survey

When two different groups or techniques are compared this technique is used. It should be based on important professional problem, so the resulting data will be significant to the profession. Significant elements will be considered, each element is representative within itself.

Activity Analysis

The analysis of the activities or processes that an individual is called upon to perform. This method may yield information that would prove useful in establishing:

- The requirements for a particular job or position
- A program for the preparation or training of individuals for various jobs or positions
- An in-service program for improvement in job competence
- Equitable wage or salary schedules for various jobs or positions.

Trend Studies

It is based upon a longitudinal consideration of recorded data indicating what has been happening in the past, what the present situation reveals and on the basis of these data, what is likely to happen in the future.

Short-term Survey

Data is collected over short time (days to months) no control over the sample.

Long-term Survey

Data is collected more than five years.

Exploratory Survey

Oriented towards the discovery of relationships between variables where phenomena of interest, but pursues the question: What factor or factors influence, affect, cause or relate to this phenomena? When a new area or topic is being studied it is useful to estimate the feasibility and cost of undertaking.

Developmental Studies

a. Longitudinal studies
   Short-term
   Long-term
b. Trend studies
   Cohort studies
   Panel studies
   Follow-up studies

Psychologists, anthropologists many times uses this method. The researcher repeatedly collects data on the same group of individuals over a period of time. He makes repeated observations on the same group of subjects.

- To understand any stage of life in terms of his developmental origin
- It provides useful perspective of the orderly and coherent developmental sequence and the elements of both change and continuity that human development involves
- It serves as a data collection device, source of hypothesis.

Trend Studies

Sample from a general population are studied over time with respect to some phenomenon. Different samples are selected at repeated intervals, but the samples are always drawn from the same population. To examine patterns and rates of change over time and to make predictions about future directions.

Cohort Studies

Specific populations are examined over a period of time. Different samples are selected at different points in time, but the samples are drawn from specific sub-groups that are often age related.

Panel Studies

The same subjects are used to supply the data at two or more points in time. Panel is used in the longitudinal survey projects, refers to the sample of subjects involved in the study. In this the investigator reveals pattern of change and reasons for the change. Since the same individuals are contacted at two or more points in time, the researcher can identify the subjects who did and did not change and then isolate the characteristics of the sub-groups in which changes occurred.

Follow-up Investigations

To determine the subsequent development of individuals with a specified condition or who have received a specified intervention to ascertain long-term effects of the intervention.

Cross Sectional Studies

It involves the collection of data at one point in time or it observes at only one point in time. The phenomena under investigation are captured as they manifest themselves during the one static time period of data collection. They are easy to manage and are economically advantageous, majority of nursing studies are cross-sectional.

Regular or Adhoc Survey

When a body or an individual organisation conducts the same survey at regular intervals, e.g: Economic survey of RBI; census survey. The survey is conducted with a view to find out some information required for a particular purpose.

Official Survey

Which will be conducted by the Government to find out certain facts for official or philanthropic purpose.

Non-official Survey

Individuals without the help of official agencies will be conducting survey to collect the data for research purpose.

Direct Survey (Personal/Primary Survey)

The researcher himself will collect the data by means of observation or interview for research purpose.

Indirect Survey/Secondary Survey

The collected information will be analysed, the researcher does not start the survey but spends on the work, which has already been done by somebody else.

Postal Survey

Through mailed questionnaire the researcher will obtain the information.

Initial Survey

When a survey is carried out in a particular area or particular subject for the first time.

Repetitive Survey

The researcher carries out the work several times on the same sample.

Open Survey

When the nature and result of survey are open to the public or organisation is called 'open survey'.

Confidential Survey

The results or information gathered through survey are kept confidential.

Comprehensive Survey

The survey covers vast field, variety information and wide range is covered.

Limited Survey

The field covered is comparatively limited.

The process of survey research

- Statement of research problem
- Determination that the problem is appropriate for the survey approach
- Selection of appropriate type of survey
- Objectives, hypothesis, delimitations should be formulated
- Select sampling technique, identification of sources of information
- Plan for data collection
- Examination of all documentary sources; field work
- Coding, recording, analyses and reporting the project, interpretation of findings
- Communicating the findings with the help of graphs.

CASE STUDY

Introduction

The case study is a way of organising social data for the purpose of viewing social reality. It examines a social unit as a whole. The unit may be a person, a family, a social institution or a community. It is often used for descriptive research. It is a longitudinal approach showing development over a period of time.

It studies or understands life cycle or an important part of the life cycle of the unit. It is in-depth, investigation of social unit. It tests hypothesis but not directed towards broad generalisation. The method can be used to analyse the interaction between factors bringing about change usually over a period of time. Consent must be taken from the social unit to get cooperation. Researcher may use past history or may report on current events. Verbal description between interviewer and client or may use artifacts, records, questionnaires. In nursing and medical professions case studies will be used more often.

Evaluation and Scope

The case study method is a widely used systematic field research technique in these days. The credit for introducing this method in the field of social investigation goes to *Frederic Le Play*, who used it as a handmaiden statistics in his studies of family budgets. *Herbert Spencer* was first used case material in his comparative study of different cultures. *Dr William Healy* resorted to this method considered it as a better method over and alone the mere use of statistical data. Similarly, anthropologists, historians, novelists and dramatists have used this method concerning problems pertaining to their areas of interests. Even management experts use case study methods for getting clues to several management problems.

Objects of Case Study

Individuals suffering with social problems like drug addicts, alcoholics, juvenile delinquents, interested events.

Definition

- 'It is a form of qualitative analysis involving very careful and complete observation of a person, a situation or an institution'—*Biesanz and Biesanz*

- 'All inclusive and intensive study of an individual, in which the investigator brings to bear all his skill and methods or as a systematic gathering of enough information about a person to pursue one to understand how he or she functions as a unit of society'—*Young*
- 'It is a way of organising social data so as to preserve the unitary character of the social object being studied'—*Goode and Hat*
- 'It is a technique by which individual factor whether it is an institution or just an episode in the life of an individual or a group is analysed in the relationship to any other in the group'—*H Odum*
- 'A comprehensive study of a social unit'—*PV Young*

Meaning

It is a form of qualitative analysis where in careful and complete observation of an individual or a social situation or a social unit. It is an in depth study. It analyses limited number of events or conditions and their interrelations. It is an intensive investigation of a particular unit under consideration.

Characteristics of Case Study Method

- The researcher can take single social unit for their study purpose
- Intensive study of selected unit covering all facets
- Qualitative approach
- It deepens the perception and gives a clear insight in life
- It studies mutual interrelationship of casual factors
- Generalisation may not be possible.

Methods of Data Collection

- Observation
- Interviews
- Questionnaires

- Government, voluntary or private agencies
- Co-opinionaires
- Psychological tests and inventories
- Recorded data.

Assumptions

The case study method is based on several factors:

1. The assumption of uniformity in the basic human nature inspite of the fact that human behaviour may vary according to situations
2. Assumption of studying the natural history of the unit concerned
3. Assumption of comprehensive study of the unit concerned.

Phases involved in case study

1. Recognition and determination of the status of the phenomenon to be investigated or the unit of attention.
2. Collection of data, examination and history of the given phenomenon
3. Diagnosis and identification of casual factors as in basis for residual or developmental treatment
4. Application of remedial measures like treatment and therapy
5. Follow-up programmes to determine effectiveness of the treatment given.

Advantages

- It enables us to understand total behaviour pattern of the concerned unit, as case study method is exhaustive
- Researcher can obtain real record of personal experience, which would reveal man's inner strivings, tensions, motivations that drive them to action or to adopt certain pattern of behaviour

- Natural history of social unit and its relationship with the social factors and the forces involved in its surrounding environment is possible
- Formulation of relevant hypothesis is possible
- Facilitates intensive study of social unit
- Enhance the experience of the researcher, which in turn increases analysing ability and skills
- To study social change
- Useful for therapeutic and administrative purposes; to take decisions regarding management problems
- Critical and reflective thinking will be promoted
- Researcher may begin or stop at any time
- Detail information will be obtained
- More suitable to nursing and medical profession
- Perceives whole situations
- Opportunity of having an intimate knowledge of subject's conditions, thought, feelings, actions, intentions and environment
- Great number of interesting insights can be observed.

Disadvantages

- Limited approach
- Generalisation and comparison may not possible
- Expensive
- Time consuming
- Subjective biased
- Difficult to check accuracy and objectivity.

OPINION POLL METHOD

To gather the information about a specific social phenomenon from a huge sample at a given time in different areas of a region, opinion poll method of survey is used. Public awareness of a specified event will be collected through this poll. The researcher will take assistance from field investigators, structured questionnaire is formulated to gather the data. The survey conducting areas usually be a common meeting/gathering place of the public.

For example: At the time of election, opinion poll is conducted to know the public view about who will win the election and form the Government.

QUESTIONNAIRE

A good deal of information can be gathered by direct questioning of sample, who have specified characteristics through the use of formal instrument (i.e. questionnaire). If the informants are spread over a vast or in accessible areas, the information is sought with the help of questionnaire.

Definition

Questionnaire (Survey Instrument)

'Any written document, which is used to instruct one or more readers or listeners to answer one or more questions'.

A list of questions/items are compiled by the researcher based on different aspects of the problem. Certain times mailed questionnaires will be sent to the respondents to give the reply. In structured interview with the help of structured questionnaire.

Items

Questions in the questionnaire.

Respondents

The person who answers the items in a questionnaire.

Interviewer

A person who conducts the study, who is having training in interviewing techniques and administering the questionnaire in the study projects.

Characteristics of questionnaire

The heart of the questionnaire method is 'question' itself. It acts as an effective stimuli. It is a device securing answers to questions using a form, which the respondent fills.

Analytical questions

Questions should be capable of analysing the entire problem.

Clarity and Concise/Precise

Items should be clear, complete; questions should be worded simply, as possible to provide an opportunity for easy, accurate and unambiguous responses. Questions should be in limited number to avoid disinterest, tiredness and boring. It should be free from suggestions or leading.

Linguistic, Completeness and Grammatical Consistency

- It is a verbal interaction between researcher and respondent and care should be taken to the linguistic quality of question unit
- Phrases, which are not commonly understood by the respondents, have to be avoided
- Singleness of purpose
- Avoid emotional questions
- Questions should be present in good psychological order to organise their own way of thinking
- Proper planning and listing of questions are done
- Encourage inter-validated questions
- Physical form of questions attracts, encourages and stimulates the respondents; proper spacing, clarity and sequence in the arrangement of the questions then only the respondent will be encouraged to come out with correct answers
- Questions should be objective in nature. Logical in order

- Advisable to pre-construct, a tabulation sheet anticipating how the data will be tabulated and interpreted before the final form of the questions is decided upon to avoid ambiguity in question form
- Questions should be relevant, diplomatically worded
- The length of the question be pertained to collect essential data
- General to specific logical manner be followed in arranging items in questions
- Carefully worded questions, so that the ego of the respondent is not injured in any manner.

Steps in questionnaire construction

- Based on objectives the needed information will be assessed
- Break up the whole information into sub-areas
- In each area, clear the mind and decide what question to ask, identify major area where information has to be gathered
- Read out the questions to experts and consultants
- Pre-test the questions for validity and reliability
- Administer the tool to the reference population
- Apply statistical tests for reliability and validity
- Internal consistency and internal coordination.

Introduction/Instruction

The interviewer read the introductory comments in face-to-face interview or in telephonic interview; the cover letter contains introductory letter. It used to introduce the study the potential respondent and should not exceed one page, thus each sentence should serve a distinct purpose.

The content of letter will be divided into four paragraphs:

1st Paragraph

- Explain the purpose of the study
- Convince the respondent that the study is useful
- Avoid any hint of bias.

2nd Paragraph

- Make respondent to feel the importance to the success of the study.

3rd Paragraph

- The confidentiality and anonymity of respondents will be maintained.

4th Paragraph

- Re-emphasise the basic justification for study
- Availability of study results, offering a copy of it to the respondent
- Introduce each section to the respondent with a brief preface to clarify them, why the questions are being asked.

Elements of questioning method

- Content of the questioning
- The question
- Provision for answering.

Content of questioning

- It is useful to develop a blue print of various aspects of situation about which questions might be asked
- Researcher should decide how much time is allotted for every item
- The selection of content is based on researcher's knowledge of situation, the literature available in the proble m area; objectives of study and needs of the researcher
- Facts about the respondent, behaviour, persons known to the respondent, events and conditions known to the patient
- Beliefs, attitudes, feelings, opinion of respondents
- Reasons for or influences of other person's behaviour
- Level of knowledge about policies, practices, conditions or situations
- Intention for future action.

Order/Sequence of questions

- Open ended questions should be written first to provide an opportunity to conceptualise the issues in their own words rather than formulating their answers based on the responses they have seen in the closed ended questionnaires
- The general questions should be placed first followed by specific questions to avoid putting ideas into people's heads
- The schedule begin with questions that arouse the respondent's interest and motivation to cooperate
- Personal, sensitive, threatening nature questions should not be placed at the beginning as it arouse suspicious about the purpose of the study
- The items bearing on one issue or topic should be in close proximate
- Don't formulate too many questions in the small space
- Every item in the question should relate to the topic under the study
- Logical progression in the question order is necessary
- Identify the information by factual data and subject matter of the survey
- Scrutinisation of question during pretest.

Colleagues, experts assess how well the question will accomplish the study objectives.

Potential users of the information for accuracy, back of bias and ignorance of items.

Problems in construction of questionnaire

1. Problem with clarity of question
   - Clarify in the mind regarding what information is to be obtained for that question
   - Avoid long sentences or phrases double barreled questions; non-specific items;
   - State the questions in affirmative order than negative.
2. Ability of respondents to give response: Use simple language, short statements.

3. Memory: The researcher should not take for granted that the respondents will be able to recall the events, situations or previous activities.
4. Bias: Avoid leading questions that suggest a particular kind of answer. State a range of alternatives within the question itself.
5. Handling a sensitive or personal information: Politeness and encouragement helps to motivate the respondent to cooperate
6. Response alternatives: Significant alternatives should be used. Mutually should be there in ordering of questions and responses. Avoid too long questions.

Advantages of questionnaire

- Simple method of obtaining data
- Items can be constructed easily by beginning researchers
- Less time is consumed in using this method of gathering information thus it saves time, energy and money. Thus it is more economical and sufficient
- Able to gather data from a widely scattered sample in a limited period
- Provides an opportunity to establish rapport to explain the purpose of the study and the items which are not clear
- Reduces interaction between research and respondent
- Provides sufficient time to the respondent to think and give his response
- Complete anonymity of the respondent will be maintained
- Ensures anonymity and kept the information confidential.

Disadvantages

- It lacks depth: to ensure rate of response from questions is difficult as it depends upon the method of administration
- The researcher may omit or disregard any item without giving any explanation

- Some items may force the subject to select responses that are not actual choice
- Respondent may take their own time, which may hamper the research progress
- Creates artificial situation as researcher is asking for verbal response, not for action
- Mailed questions are limited to literate respondents and to get good response from them only when they have research conscious.

TYPES

Structured Question

The items which pose definite, concrete and pre-ordained questions i.e. prepared in advance and not constructed on the spot during the question period.

Pictorial Question

To promote interests in answering the questions; this type will be used to study the social attitudes, prejudices and for studies related to children.

Open ended question

- Calls for a free response in the respondent's own words
- Provides a greater depth of response
- Respondents reveal their frame of reference and possibly the reasons for their responses since it requires greater effort on the part of the respondents
- Involves the respondent's attitudes or feelings expressed in their own words
- Respondents must create their own answers and state them in their own words.

Advantages

- Stimulates free thought, solicit suggestions
- Probe respondent's memories.

Disadvantages

- Respondent must recall past experience, create and articulate new answers
- Difficult to construct responses
- Illegible hand writing pose difficult in mail questions.

Closed ended question

The respondent's answer is limited to the choices offered, short in form, limited responses. They provide chance for marking alternatives. It is easy to fill out, requires little time, objective, fairly easy to tabulate and analyse. Close-ended questions offer a number of alternative replies from which the respondents must choose closely approximate answer.

Difficulties

- Difficult to construct but easy to administer
- Possibility of neglecting or over-looking the important responses, the omission possible alternatives can lead to inadequate understanding of the issues
- If the area of the research is completely new, this type is not advisable
- Pre-testing of the schedule is immensely helpful
- Too superficial questions may be considered.

Types of Closed Questionnaire

Dichotomous Items

It requires the respondent to make a choice between two alternatives. Too restrictive, the respondents may be forced to say within two alternatives, e.g: Do you like to have: (a) Coffee (b) Tea.

Multiple-choice Questions

A range of alternatives provides more information; one can measure intensity of feeling and direction. Most commonly offer 3 or 5 alternatives, e.g: Psychosocial aspect. Liking sweets: (a) with every meal (b) once a while (c) always.

Cafeteria Questions

Which is put forth to the respondents to select a response that most adequately states their view, used in qualitative surveys.

Closed Ended with Ordered Choice or Objective Type

Answer choices are provided; each is a graduation of a single dimension of some thought or behaviour, e.g: How did you get along with the doctor in the emergency room? (a) strongly agree (b) mildly agree (c) neither agree nor disagree (d) mildly disagree (e) strongly disagree.

Closed Ended with Unordered Response Choices

Answer choices are provided but no single dimension underlines them. The respondent must choose discrete, unordered categories by independently evaluate each choice and select the one that best reflects the situation, e.g: The food item I like best (a) samosa (b) sandwich (c) dosa (d) idly.

Partially Closed Ended Questions

It provides a compromise response although answer choices are provided; respondents have to option of creating their own response. Unordered or ordered choices are seen within this structure, e.g: Which of the following areas of expenditures do you want to have the highest priority for improvement in this hospital? (a) emergency dept (b) X-ray dept (c) laboratories (d) others (please specify).

Step Ladder/Rank Order Questions

Questions to rank order their responses along a continum from most favourable to least favourable can be useful; carefully handled because respondents often misunderstand them, e.g: Attitude of job preferences of nursing students after course completion. (a) working in PHN (b) teacher (c) staff nurse (d) mid-wife. The respondents should rank the answers in the order of preference.

Checklist or Matrix Questions

It encompasses several questions on a topic and requires the same response format.

Graphic Rating Scale

It assigns numerical score in order to place the individual along a continuum with respect to the attribute being measured. Respondents are asked to give a judgment of something along an ordered dimension. The specified two opposite ends of a continuum is referred as bi-polar in nature, e.g: How friendly are you with your classmates?

Least friendly 1 2 3 4 5 Most friendly

Direct Vs Indirect Approach or Coming in front door Vs Coming in back door

A check can be made as to the value of the responses by asking a direct or indirect question and then comparing the answers, e.g: Nursing education in India. (a) high image (b) low image (c) no image (d) cheap image.

OBSERVATION

It is one of the basic and oldest research methods to gather data. It is a normal part of daily life and becomes a research method if it is systematically planned and recorded and checked for their validity and reliability. The basis for observation is curiosity.

Meaning

Planned, methodical watching that involves constraints to improve accuracy.

Definition

'It is a technique used for collecting all the data or acquiring information through occurrences that can be observed through senses with or without mechanical devices'.

- 'Systematic viewing coupled with consideration of social phenomena'—*PV Young*
- 'Accurate watching of social phenomena as they occur in nature with regard to cause and effect relationship or natural relationship'—*Oxford Dictionary*

It involves interpretation of phenomena in the environment. Two process are involved

1. Someone is observing—Observer
2. Something to observe—Observed

Observation can be done in natural setting (field research) or in laboratory setting.

Four broad questions that confront the researcher

- What should be observed?
- How should observation be recorded?
- What procedures should be used to try to assure the accuracy of observation?
- What relationship should exist between the observer and the observed and how can such relationship be established.

Features

- It is an eye affair. Observer has to observe the situation very closely and clearly. Observation implies the use of eyes rather than that of ears and voice

- Observation should be definite aim. It is clearly determined (for scientific enquiry) before starting the process
- Proper planning is required, before starting observation necessary equipment and instrument have to be arranged
- After observatory process the events has to be noted down
- Cause and effect relationship will make the whole study useful and purposeful.

Phenomena Amenable to Observation

- Characteristics and conditions of individuals, e.g: Physiological conditions and characteristics through sense or aided by observation apparatus, e.g: Effect of yoga on lung function of patients with pleural effusion (*M Prakasamma*, 1981) using spirometer several readings of FEV_1, FVC, MVV, X-ray chest is used to see lung expansion before giving treatment
- Verbal communication behaviour; (a) Linguistic behaviour (b) Content and structure of people's conversation (c) Social interaction, e.g: Interaction pattern between teachers and students in clinical setting using Flanders's interaction analysis category system (*Vasta*, 1978, *Madanlal*, 1980)
- Non-verbal communication behaviour, e.g: Facial expression, touch, posture, gesture, body movements, extra linguistic behaviour.
- Activities (overt state of an individual many activities can be observed), e.g: Physical and mental functioning of an individual.
- Skill attainment and performance, e.g: Aseptic techniques used by nursing students during nursing procedures.
- Environmental characteristics, e.g: Noise level, cleanliness, ventilation, odour, water supply, mosquito breeding places.

Units of Observation

1. *Molar approach*: Observation of large units of behaviour and treating them as a whole.

2. *Molecular approach*: Observation of small and highly specific behaviour. For example: Each movement, gesture, action.

Steps in Observation Schedule

1. *Selecting the aspect of behaviour to be observed*: To carry out systematic observations; one must select certain aspects or categories of behaviour to be observed.
2. Defining the behaviour that fall within a category.
3. *Training observer:* Observational methods are more vulnerable to perceptual errors than any other data collection. To minimise the bias and maximize the accuracy and objectivity of the observation, training of observer is essential. Observer's manual with detailed instructions can be used. Training sessions are useful for clarifying doubts. Once the observers are fully oriented with the instrument, they should use the observation schedule on a group that demonstrates the same phenomena as under study. Their difficulties can be resolved through discussions and practice sessions.

Quantifying Observation

When the behaviours specified have to provide certain measurement then some form of quantification is required. The qualification usually takes the form of counting. The count may be of number of times that a subject shows a particular form of behaviour during a period of observation. Here observer should be sure of when one act ends, and the next begin. Break the period of observation into short segments and observer can then watch occurrence or non-occurrence of particular behaviour under specified category.

Recording

To have adequate account of what was observed during observation, recording is needed, e.g: Motion pictures, films, video tapes.

Testing

To ascertain the adequacy of content being put to measure the variable under study.

Interrater Reliability

Two or more raters observing the same behaviour/events and their percentage of agreement obtained establishes the reliability of the schedule.

Intrarater Reliability

When a rater observes same behaviour/events on two or more occasions. Multiple observations extending over days/weeks/years.

Advantages

- Important technique for studying human behaviour specially where interventions are used
- Provides variety and depth of information
- Researcher is not dependent on subjects who consent to answer, all subjects are potential respondents
- Subjects are usually available
- It allows view of complete situation, first hand and sequence of events
- All the data obtained by the observation are usable
- Open to use of recording devices, e.g: Tape recorders and cameras
- May be stopped and begin at any time
- May be recorded at the time of occurrence, eliminating bias during recall
- Inexpensive
- Useful in healthcare profession.

Disadvantages

- Observation and interpretation is a demanding task which requires attention, sensation, perception, conception

- Lack of consent to being observed
- Time and duration of event can't be predicted usually observer may wait until an event happens
- Data obtained is vulnerable to many distortions and bias, e.g: Cultural background, personal interpretation, and influence
- Lack of qualified, trained observer
- Chances of wrong interpretation.

Aids to Observation

- Checklist
- Rating scale
- Score cards
- Observation sheets
- Photographs
- Line diagram
- Sketches

Observational Sampling

a. *Time sampling method:* It involves the selection of time periods during which the observations will take place.
b. *Event sampling method:* It selects integral behaviour or events of a pre-specified type for observation

Observational Methods

Unstructured Observation

Participant observation: It is a technique where researcher participates in the functioning of the social group that is under investigation. The researcher will not interpret their views and meaning into the social situations under observation. It provides deep understanding of human behaviour. Observer usually has three types of records:

a. *Logos:* It is a record of events and conversations usually maintained on a daily basis by field worker.

b. *Field notes:* It is much broader, more analytic, more interpretation and represents participants observer's effort to record, inform, synthesis and understands the data.
c. *Anecdotes:* It focuses on behaviour of particular interest. It selects specific kind of events and behaviour for observation before hand. The observer objectively and accurately records the observation.

Structured Observation

It involves indicates of presence or absence of pre-specified behaviour or attributes.

Checklists: Phenomena are recorded by putting a tally against a particular behaviour, event or characteristics depending upon its presence or absence. Researcher must list all the expected behaviour related to the variable being measured, so that all relevant behaviour in the subjects will correctly be identified.

Basic format of observation checklist contains
Sign system: List categories of behaviours that may or may not be manifested by the subjects. The observer watch for instances of the behaviour on the list and puts a check off beside the appropriate behaviour when it occurs. Researcher identifies the occurrence and frequency of particular behaviour.

Analysis of ongoing and discrete elements of behaviour
The observer places behaviour in only one category for each unit of behaviour.

Rating scales: Observation can also be rated in terms of qualitative points along a descriptive continuum. It usually is quantified during the subsequent analysis of the observation data. Here either the observer is required to make ratings of behaviour or events at frequent intervals throughout the observational period or he may make use of rating scale to summarise an entire event or transaction after the observation is completed where a more descriptive method has been used for maintaining observation record.

Category system: Construction of category system to which observed behaviours or characteristics could be assigned.

Types

Non-concealment and Participant

The observer will not attempt to alter the social setting, i.e, being studied and does not make the observation covertly. The observer is a part of the social setting. The subjects are aware of researcher's presence but may or may not be aware of the underlying motive.

Drawback: The interaction between the observer and the observed alters the behaviour of the subject. Ethical issues, as observer will not take consent of subjects.

Concealment and Participant

The observer observes the behaviour of people in their natural setting, where the observed are unaware of being observed; passive role will be maintained with minimum intervention and records.

Concealment and Non-participant

Observer makes the observation from the peripherally of a social setting and does not interact with others.

Non-concealment and Non-participant

The researcher is interested in observing the effects of some specific intervention introduced for scientific purpose. The subjects are aware of their participation in the study. This method is very much useful in nursing research studies.

INTERVIEW

The interview is an oral questionnaire, the interviewee gives the needed information verbally in a face-to-face relationship.

It is an important method of data collection where one can know the views and ideas of other persons. The interviewer gains rapport or establishes a friendly, secure relationship with the subject and obtains some confidential information that the subject might be reluctant to put in writing. The interviewer can explain the purpose of the investigation and can explain more clearly just what information he or she wants.

Definition

- 'The interview is not only the conversation between an investigator and informant but also interviewer will try to understand the gestures, glances, facial expressions and reveals subtle feelings' —*PV Young*
- 'It is a fundamental process of social interaction'—*Goode and Hatt*
- 'It is face-to-face interpersonal situation in which one person, the interviewer asks a person being interviewed and the respondent will answer or gives the responses; the items are designed to obtain answers pertinent to research problem'—*Fred N Kerlinger*

Characteristics

- Close contact or interaction between two or more persons
- Define object to know the views and ideas of others
- Face-to-face relationship between individuals
- Data will be collected related social problem.

Objectives

- Information will be obtained from unknown facts through face-to-face interaction
- Investigator and respondent has to know each other by means of research needs and requirements
- Gives an opportunity to formulate hypothesis, which are based on personal and social behaviour

- Collecting additional information about different situations in qualitative facts, e.g: Ideas, feelings, views, faith and conclusion etc.
- Gives an opportunity to observe the things which are not under study.

Instrument for Interview

a. *Interview schedule:* A questionnaire is read to the respondent and formed about facts and situations involved.
b. *Interview guide:* It provides ideas but allows the interviewer freedom to pursue relevant topics in depth. To use interview guide or not depends upon the policy and attitudes of the interviewer.

Preparatory Process on Technique of Interview

- Based on scientific knowledge
- Understands the problem which are under study
- Preparing interview schedule and interview guide
- Training of field workers
- Selection of informants, appointment with respondents
- Seeking and providing information about respondents.

Process of Interview

- Get cooperation from the leader and the community
- Select proper time and place
- Introduction with respondents
- Put systematic, clear and unambiguous questions
- Precautions to be taken regarding emotional point of view.

Technique of Interview

- Establish contacts and rapport with the informants
- Start the interview in a scientific and attractive manner
- Help the respondents to recall things correctly and encourage to come out with proper information

- Ask probing questions
- Encourage and guide the informants in proper line.

Qualities of Good Interviewer

- Attractive personality
- Pleasing manners
- Tactful
- Initiative
- Should win the confident of the informant
- Objective observer
- Avoid too much inquisitiveness.

Types

On the basis of objectives and qualities.

i. Clinical interview: To know the cause of certain abnormality thereby remedy can be sorted out. It studies individual's life experiences.
ii. Selection interview: To select a person on the basis of certain traits and qualities, e.g: Job interview
iii. Diagnostic interview: To find out certain serious causes of some social events or problems.
iv. Research interview: To find out the cause of problem, a comprehensive study of social problems in detail.
v. Directive interview: Predetermined questions, which the interviewer will ask the respondent.

On the basis of functions and methodology

1. Non-directed interview: Uncontrolled interview asked through conversation. The informant is encouraged to exhibit and express his knowledge and views. The interviewer collects the information.
2. Focused interview (Controlled interview): To test a particular or specific experience hypothesis. The questions are predetermined and preplanned, which are formed on the basis of behaviour of respondent.

3. Repeated interview: To study the dynamic functions and attitudes that influence, guide and determine the behaviour of certain individuals. These interviews are carried out after certain interviews in repeated manner.
4. Respondent interview: To study the specific development of a social or psychological process.
5. Depth interview: The respondent will be fully encouraged to respond. The interviewer must be perfectly trained.

On the basis of number of informants or respondents

1. Individual interview: Information will be gathered from an individual.
2. Group interview: Collecting information from the group of respondents.
3. Structured/Formal/Standardised interview: Interviewer cannot adopt questions for a specific situation, the interview is not permitted to change the specific wording of the questions.
4. Unstructured/Informal/Non-standardised interview: The interviewer will have freedom to develop each questions in the most appropriate manner for the situation.
5. Semi-standardised interview: The interviewer may be required to ask a number of specific major questions, beyond which any number of further questions may be asked.

Advantages

- Possible to study the events that are not open to observation (hidden factors), e.g: Feelings, attitudes, fear, emotions, reactions
- Complete answers are possible
- Clarification can be made if respondents had done so, that misunderstanding can be minimised
- Questions can be pursued in depth
- A higher response is possible and the reliable information can be obtained

- Inflow and outflow of ideas can be possible between interviewer and respondent.

Disadvantages

- The data collected are of a doubtful character
- Costly method
- Validity measurement problem due to difference in social characteristics, e.g: Race, ethnicity, perceived status differences
- Too much dependency of the memory of the respondent
- Possibility of change in meaning
- Lot of subjectivity, individual feelings, inferiority complex.

Social Medicine

Knowledge of human behaviour with an interdisciplinary approach to understand human needs in the context of societal problems. It is a social system approach to understand human behaviour. The interpersonal orientation, group influence and socio-cultural factors helps to find solutions to problems which are arising due to mass complex nature.

In the recent time the fields of sociology is extended towards medical science known as 'Medical Sociology' which describes medicine as a social science as 'health' is a complex whole, state of physical, mental, social, spiritual well-being of an individual and not merely an absence of disease or infirmity. There is a dire need to integrate the behavioural sciences with medicine in educating health care professionals. Social medicine is having components such as education, medicine, health care and socio-behavioural sciences. The health care professionals should adequately trained up to practice the science of medicine and the art of professional with health care systems, to keep on-line in the path of social progress by keeping scientific pace with an understanding of the structural realities in contemporary societies.

It also studies the relationships between health phenomena and social factors in medical context. It develops integrate knowledge as it relates the life processes to the existing social phenomena and health in a meaningful manner. It provides information concerning the process, scope and organisation of the elements of the medicine which will affect the individuals. It enables the practitioners to have sound knowledge about medical institutions, the study of diseases, socio-cultural perspectives, attitudes and values, treatment facilities and its patterns.

It is the study of various broad socio-cultural, economic, political forces, health problems and health practices that shapes health services system of a country at the macro-level, and health behaviour of the people and health institutions at micro-level.

The field of 'Medical Anthropology' has direct relevance to help management programmes consists of three sub-fields, i.e., Ethinomedicine, Medical Anthropology and Cultural Ecology. It analyses the medical-clinical-curative systems in different societies. It is the branch of science of man, which studies biological, cultural aspects of man in understanding the medico-social and public health problems of individuals. It is the holistic study of health, illness, cultural aspects, social roles, status and institutional networks, which will help in the health enhancement process and identifies cross cultural similarities and variations in the pattern of social behaviour.

Social Telesis

It is a planned progress and purposeful use of natural and social forces. It is a total process of cultural transformation, e.g: Adult education, satellite programmes, free education. Powerful indicator for quality of life, social change, and social development; positive social control, *Bogardus* describes social telesis is an economic development, regional development and rural development.

Previous Years University Questions

1. Define sociology and discuss the importance of sociology in nursing profession. (15 m, MP State, RGUHS, 2004)
2. Define anthropology and sociology and discuss its relationship with each other. (15 m, MP, 2004)
3. Define sociology. Discuss the relationship between sociology and anthropology. (15 m, MP, 2003)
4. Define sociology and discuss the importance of its study in India. (15 m, MP, 2000)
5. Define sociology and discuss its importance. (15 m, MP, 1998)
6. Define sociology and discuss its scope.(15 m, MP, 1997)
7. Discuss how sociology is related to other social sciences. (15 m, MP, 1997)
8. Explain the need of studying sociology in nursing. (15 m, RGUHS, 2000)
9. Explain how a nurse can make use of knowledge of sociology in patient care. (10 m RGUHS, 2001)
10. Define sociology and explain the scope and importance of sociology. (8 m, RGUHS, 1997)
11. Describe the nature and scope of sociology. How does sociology help in the nursing profession. (10 m, RGUHS, 2002)
12. Define sociology. (2 m, RGUHS, 2002)
13. Social medicine. (2 m, RGUHS, 2001, 04)
14. Explain the need for studying sociology or nurses. (10 m, RGUHS, 2001, 03, 5 m, RGUHS, 2002)
15. Write 2 definitions of sociology. (5 m, RGUHS, 2002)
16. What is social telesis. (2 m, RGUHS, 1999)
17. Explain how social factors influence health and illness. (10 m, RGUHS, 2000)
18. What is sociology? Explain the importance of study of sociology. (10 m, RGUHS, 2000, 02)

19. Write the meanings of the root words from which the term sociology is derived. (2 m, RGUHS, 2000)
20. Describe the origin and development of social medicine. What is its application in nursing. (5 m, RGUHS, 2002)
21. Describe the sociological research methods used in nursing profession. (5 m, RGUHS, 2002)
22. Describe the relevance of sociological principles in nursing. (10 m, RGUHS, 1999, 2000)
23. Uses of sociology in nursing care. (5 m, RGUHS, 2001)
24. Social factors and health. (5 m, RGUHS, 2001)
25. Describe the role of family in health and disease of individual. (10 m, RGUHS, 2000)
26. Social disease. (5 m, RGUHS, 2000)
27. Describe the importance of sociology for nurses. (19 m, NTRUHS, 2002)
28. The learning of 'sociology' in the nursing facilitate 'social interactions among nurses'. Explain. (15 m, NTRUHS, 2002)
29. What is sociology? Explain about the importance of study of sociology for nurses. (15 m, NTRUHS, 1999)
30. Discuss the importance of sociology to nursing. (15 m, NTRUHS, 1998)
31. What is the relationship of anthropology to sociology? Discuss in detail. (15 m, NTRUHS, 1998)
32. Define anthropology and how study of anthropology is useful to nurses in their profession. (NTRUHS, 1996)
33. Define sociology and explain its scope and importance in nursing profession. (NTRUHS, 1989)
34. Why it is important for nurses to study sociology, how will improve social status of nurses in India. (NTRUHS, 1998)
35. Definition of sociology and discuss it. (NTRUHS, 1984)
36. Is sociology a science and discuss. (NTRUHS, 1986)
37. Explain the need and utility of sociological knowledge to the student of nurse. (NTRUHS, 1987)

38. Explain with examples how the knowledge of sociology is useful in nursing care of patients. (10 m, SVIMS, Tirupati, 2003)

MGR University Question Papers

1. Bring out the importance of the study of sociology in health and nursing with particular reference to attitude towards illness and treatment in Indian context. (15 m, MGRU)
2. Social anthropology applied to nursing. (MGRU, 5 m)
3. Define sociology and describe its importance in the field of nursing. (15 m, MGRU)
4. Bring out clearly the importance of the study of sociology in health and nursing with special reference to attitude towards illness and treatment in Indian context. (15 m, MGRU)
5. Discuss how far the sociological knowledge is helpful for a nurse in her career. (15 m, MGRU)
6. Explain the meaning and importance of sociology in nursing. (15 m, MGRU, Nov-98)
7. Sociology. (2 m, MGRU, Nov-01)
8. Public opinion. (2 m, MGRU, Nov-01)
9. Importance of sociology. (5 m, MGRU)
10. Social anthropology. (2 m, MGRU)
11. Prove sociology as science of society and discuss its scope, subject matter and importance. (10 m, MGRU)
12. How far the sociological knowledge is helpful to the nurses in their clinical and social settings and rehabilitation measures. Discuss. (10 m, MGRU)
13. Explain the concept of 'Sociology'. (5 m, MGRU)
14. Describe the importance of sociological knowledge in nursing profession. (15 m, MGRU)
15. Describe the scope and importance of sociology in India. (15 m, MGRU)

16. Define social anthropology and discuss its applicability to nursing. (15 m, MGRU)
17. Importance of sociology. (5 m, MGRU)
18. Write an essay on the relationship between society and nursing. (15 m, MGRU)
19. Social anthropology. (2 m, MGRU)
20. Justify the scientific nature of sociology and explain the importance of it. (15 m, MGRU)
21. Social anthropology applied to nursing. (5 m, MGRU)
22. Write an essay on the concept and uses of the study of sociology. (15 m, MGRU)
23. Social anthropology and health. (5 m, MGRU)
24. Define sociology. Discuss the nature, scope and importance of sociology. (20 m, MGRU)
25. Anthropology in nursing. (5 m, MGRU)
26. Sociology as a science. (5 m, MGRU, Nov-03)

CHAPTER TWO

Individual and Society

INDIVIDUALISATION

Definition

'Individualisation is the process by which, an individual is made independent of his group'.

'It is the process of attaining to one's own self. It makes him independent and self-determining'. It is carried out by individual himself and it is mainly a mental process, which is spread through the prevailing ideas. Socialisation brings man in relation with others.

Aspects of Individualisation

- The process of becoming different from other people
- Democratisation
- Free competition
- Social mobility
- Aware of one's own specific character
- A new kind of evaluation
- The individual will consider himself superior to others and evaluates himself in high terms
- A feeling of self-glorification

- It is the wishes through objects
- Social mobility may also bind the individual to specific wishes
- Family conditions
- The feeling of loneliness may lead the individual to introspection
- In big cities, the community does not have much influence on the individual and so he develops a feeling of privacy and partial isolation. It leads to individualisation.

Society

The term 'society' is derived from Latin word, 'Societus' means 'companionship or friendship'. Man is a social being, gregarious in nature. Mans needs society, enjoys group life, human life individual and society always go together.

Definition

- 'A number of like-minded individuals who know and enjoy their like-mindedness and are therefore able to work together for common ends'.
- 'The sum of formal relations in which individuals are associating together or bounded together'—*Giddings*
- 'Society is a system of usages and procedures, authority and mutual aid, of many groupings and divisions of controls of human behaviour and of liberties'— *Maciver and Page*
- 'A group of people, the complex pattern of norms of interaction, that arise among and between them'— *Lapierre*
- 'Collection of individuals united by certain relations or modes of behaviour which mark them off from others who do not enter into these relations or who differ from them in behaviour'—*M Ginsberg*

Meaning

A complex of groups in reciprocal relationships interacting upon one another enabling human organisms to carry on their life activities and helping each person to fulfill his wishes and accomplish his interest in association with his fellows. – From functional point of view.

The total social heritage of folkways, mores and institutions, of habits, sentiments and ideals. —From structural point of view.

Elements of Society

- Mutual interactions of individuals
- Mutual interrelationship between individuals
- A pattern of system
- Reciprocal awareness is an essential ingredient of social relationship
- We feeling/common propensity
- Like-mindedness
- Society also implies difference/diverse/variations
- Interdependence
- Cooperation.

Man lives in the society for his mental and intellectual development. Society safeguards our culture and transmits to future generations. The mind of man without society remains the mind of an infant at the age of adulthood. The cultural heritage directs our personality.

Though the individual is a product of society, sometimes there may be a conflict between societal members. Sometimes the individual may develop a personality, which is incompatible with the environment, in which he is placed.

Deterioration of the societal system may also cause opposition between the individual and society. So individual and society are interdependent. The relationship between them is one sided. Individual and society interact with each other and depend on one another. They are complementary and supplementary to each other.

Characteristics of Society

- It is composed of people

- People in the society have mutual awareness, continuous reciprocal interaction and interrelationship among societal members
- Society has likeness and differences too, e.g: Similarities like needs, activities, occupation, aims, ideals and values, etc.
- Differences among the people will exhibit vivid interests, wants to enjoy enthusiastic life. People differ in their looks, personality, ability, talents, attitudes, tastes, intelligence and faith, etc.
- People have cooperation and common interests, holds responsibilities by means of division of labour and delegation of authority. Division of labour is based on speciality. Individuals satisfies their desires and fulfill their interests with joined or continued efforts and it promotes social solidarity and social cohesion
- Interdependence is observed among the groups, communities, societies and also nations and it is essential to meet the societal needs.
- Society is dynamic; changes may take place abruptly or slowly or gradually or suddenly
- Society has its own ways and means of social control. In society we will observe existence of all types of social processes, i.e. cooperation, conflict, accommodation and assimilation. The behaviour and activities of the people will be controlled through formal and informal means of social control, e.g: Customs, traditions, folkways, mores, manner etiquettes (informal means) and laws, rules, regulations, standards, constitution, legislation, police (Formal means)
- Each society has its own distinct culture; it is the expression of human behaviour, e.g: Attitudes, judgments, morals, values both society and culture go together.
- Man gregarious in nature (tendency to live in group)
- Society controls individual's talents, and capacities

- Society shapes the personality of the individual, and meets the basic needs and provides material comforts.

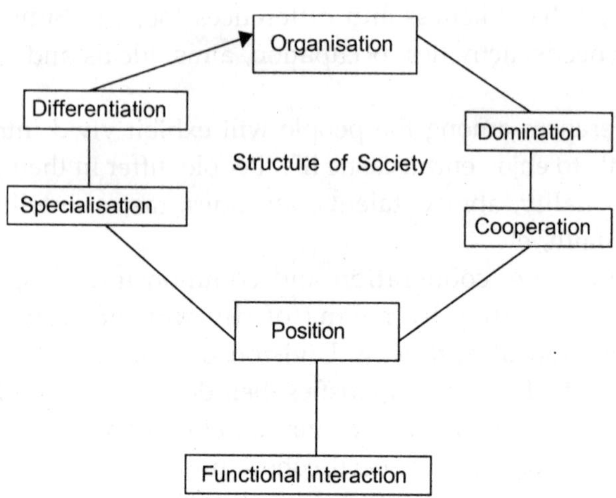

Relationship between Individual and Society

Individual is a core of society. Lot of individuals is present in galaxy of society.

Historical Evidences

Earlier sociologists have made an attempt to understand the relationship of individual and society. Basing on their intusions, theories have been formulated, however these theories, some criticism is lying. They attempted to understand the social phenomenon existed in the society.

By means of human touch, the living organism is made into social beings. He undergoes the process of socialisation to survive in the society.

Individual has certain biological, anatomical, physiological features with that, he cannot satisfy the needs of society; he should form social relationship through social interaction.

The earlier thoughts of former sociologists were :

Divine Origin Theory

Human beings are born to enjoy the relationship between male and female. God has created them and also created the society, e.g: Conjugal union of *Adam and Eve.*

God has created the rights for individuals, but no script was available. This theory is not fully explaining the various social phenomenon, societal relationship that exists in the society, e.g: Polyandry, sex ratio.

Social Contract Theory

T. Hobhouse, Locke explained how the individual is preceding the society.

All the individuals are born free and equal to fulfill the needs, which he cannot fulfill by alone. Through socialisation process he is performing his functions in the society. The individuals formed several groups, they have created the norms and laws.

Organic Theory

Plato in ancient period and *Herbert Spencer* were explained, according to this theory, the individual is a living organism, the various systems has to coordinate to maintain his living functions. Individual is a part of social system, various social systems has to coordinate to meet the societal needs. Cell cannot survive or existence of its own; but the individual can survive apart from the society.

The cell cannot think on its own, whereas the individual can stay alone, forms new groups, new communities, can adopt themselves, to stay in different social structures.

In the society if one system fails, the individual can survive in another area.

In physiological systems, the cells will join together to form as an organ and fulfill its function just like that, even in the society, each individual has to function cooperatively for effective functioning as a member in that society. In society, if an individual fails to perform their function other individual may come and occupy and fulfill those functions, but it is not so with the cells, each system has its own function, one cannot replace the other. In the social system, several specialised systems, structured organisations are present.

Group Mind Theory

Maciver and Page described this theory. Collective thinking, cohesiveness among the group members and cooperativeness are main features of this theory. Individuals in the society develop rules, regulations, and norms in the social system. Group mind facilitates collective thinking, collective acting, each group exhibits their own goals, needs which have emerged out of interaction of group, within the society, vested interests, different needs of individuals formed into different outlook. To some extent, collective thinking does not exist in our India, e.g: Different castes, cultures, identity, affinity was developed. Universality among diversity is observed. Individual and society are not separate entities. Individual neither precedes society nor society precedes the individual. They are interdependent, leading symbiotic life, mutually dependent on each other; they are interrelated. People will cohesively interact with each other to solve their problems.

Evolution Theory

From single cell to homosapions, the individual is evolved, e.g: Ferral cases in anthropological studies. We cannot conduct tests in labs. Individual and society are mutually interdependent. Individual needs society for socialisation.

For example: Ferral cases

Children were brought out in different environment; one was placed in jungle in the midst of animals. No single social factor was observed in this individual. Child behaves like an animal. After the child's death, postmortem studies revealed that the brain was not developed. This case proves that the individual needs society.

For example 2: Kamala and her sister was placed in jungle were brought out by wolfs. After some time, these two children were brought into the society, one dies and the other was crawling like the wolf. It indicates that individual needs society to be socialised.

For example 3: Hema, 6 months old child is placed in a room after her mother's death. The child was found like a creature without any sign of social being.

These ferral cases have amply throw light that society is a must to precede the individual. Man is social by nature, they like to live in company of others, and they are gregarious in nature, crave for other's company and interact with others and establish relationship. They do not like to live alone. Man likes to share the values, feelings with others. Socialisation is unending. Individual precedes the society, the necessity compels us to be within the society. We acquire many traits from the society.

Society determines the personality of the individual. Individual is the product of society in which individual is socialised and cannot survive independently without society. Society teaches where and how to behave. It makes the individuals to be as a member of society and compliment each other.

Role of a Nurse in Indian Society

The health care services (preventive, promotive, curative, rehabilitative and restorative) bringing closure to the doorstep of the community, who require the services at most, more particularly to the weaker, deprived sections of the interior corners of society. The public health nurse should shoulder the responsibilities specially for the provision of first level care in the community, thus acting as a changing agent in bringing good quality of life to the people at large.

Direct Health Care Provider to the Community

The nursing professional who are working in the community should conduct domiciliary visits, observe the pattern of living, practices of the families. Thereby they can be able to identify family health problems and meet the health and well-being needs of the members in the family by adopting principles of community health nursing process and by implementing nursing models. Nurses should orient the community the importance of health maintenance and qualitative living. Nurse should be sensitive to the individual health needs in the context of broader social changes. Nurse will act as a direct health care provider in meeting the health needs of the community by implementing appropriate, suitable nursing interventions.

As a Health Educator

To achieve 'Health For All' and to attain social development, nurses should carry out health educational activities and conduct health awareness campaigns to make the community to understand the importance of health by practicing good health life styles and develops healthy behaviour. Nurse should focus the social consequences of illness and its effects and they should motivate the community to actively participate and involve in planning and implementing health care programmes for the attainment of qualitative life. Nurse has to educate the public to identify and fulfill their health needs.

Manager and Supervisor

The nurse will act as a community organiser and leader in planning, organising and implementing health services through community participation.

Planner

- Identifies beliefs, practices, customs which are affecting the health and illness of the community

- Formulate the community diagnosis by identifying the socio-cultural barriers and promotes activities related to treatment, prevention of diseases and promotion of health
- Identifies the various community resources who are interested in community developmental activities
- Selects suitable health education methods
- Develops plan of operation by involving local people and others who are engaged in community development by keeping the social realities in mind
- Plan for supportive supervisory activities.

Researcher

Nurse conducts research projects in the community by identifying the social problems and needs of societal members, for the solvation of the existing social problems.

HEREDITY AND ENVIRONMENT

Heredity and environment both play an important role in developing the personality of the child.

Heredity

Definition

- 'A biological mechanism as a result of which the child gets something from his ancestral stock through his parents'— *DR. SK Mangal*
- 'The sum total of inborn individual traits'— *BN Jha*
- 'It consists of all the structures, physical characteristics, functions or capacities derived from parents, other ancestry or species'—*Douglas and Holland*

Nature of Heredity

Physical Heredity

The entire physique of the individual, e.g: Size, structure, appearance form, colour of skin and eyes, muscles, etc.

Psychological Heredity

For example: Intelligence, mental traits such as memory, reasoning, imagination, thought processes, etc. instincts, and tendency to commit crime.

Determinants

Hereditary factors are determined by the pairing of the male germ cells and female germ cells. The childs' life begins from the conception of the child within the mother's womb. The fertilized nucleus in the mothers' womb consists 23 pairs of chromosomes of the father and 23 chromosomes of the mother. Each chromosome consists of gene, these are physical substances passed from parents to off springs and they are real carriers and determinants of heredity. There are about 2 million different types of pairing of genes.

Principles

According to *Weisman (the Germ Plasma theory)*

- Heredity of the child is ancestral
- Child does not inherit the acquired personality traits of his parents
- Mental traits earned are subjected to transmission (according to *McDougall and Pavlov)*
- Heredity of the child may transmit from remote ancestors—according to *Sir Francis Galton* (25% from father, 25% from mother, 25% from grand parents, remaining 25% from great grand parents). The hybrids produce pure parental type with dominant character– according to—*G. Mendel and Dr. BN Jha*
- *Sir Charles Darwin's theory*—The universe and life in all its aspect are a product of development.
- Struggle for existence and survival of the fittest: New generation tries to adjust in the new surroundings of the universe. They also develop new and useful traits. This

development of new traits is due to the changes in the genes. These new genes produce new characteristics in the off springs. Such changes are called mutations.

Laws

Like begets like: A child receives characteristics from the parents such as size, colour, intelligence levels. This is due to the continuity of the germ plasma.

Law of variation: The variations among the off springs can arise because of:

- Pairing of chromosomes.
- Physical and mental condition of the parents at the time of each conception.
- When 2 dissimilar chromosomes combine there are chances of variation.

Law of Regression: In successive generations variations tend to move towards the average of species of which they form a part.

Transmission of acquired traits:

- Parents are only the trustee of the germ plasma. (*Weismann's* theory)
- Favourable variations are passed on to the next generations (*Darwin and Camarck*)
- Acquired habits are in some degree transmissible (*McDougall*)
- Instincts also transmitted.

Importance of Heredity in Education

1. Heredity determines the physique of the child. (The teacher should keep in view the health of children while assigning any social duty). For example: Weak children should be assigned easily performed activities.

2. Special hereditary traits like aptitude, reflexes, drives, temperament, interest, instincts, emotions, capacities (endowments). The teacher should provide suitable environment for their expression and development.
3. Determining the intelligence limit.
4. Correlation between intelligence and character.
5. Traits gained through heredity:

Physical traits—Structure of the body, eye movement, hair texture, colour, complexion

Certain diseases—Colour blindness, emotional imbalance, cancer.

Family character traits—Interests in music, art, dance.

Mental traits—Intelligence levels, attitudes, attention span, emotional make-up.

ENVIRONMENT

The surroundings of the child from birth to death.

Definition

- 'Environment covers 'all the outside factors that have acted on the individual since the child begins the life'— *Woodworth*
- 'Environment is everything that affects the individual, except the genes'—*Boring, Congfield and Weld*

Types of Environment

Physical Environment

All the physical features that have an effect on the individual. For example: Land, food, climate, shelter, temperature, clothing.

Emotional Environment

Intellectual atmosphere at home, school and community. The child learns new experiences unconsciously, which become a part of his mental make-up.

Social Environment

Family, school, society, community, peer group, playmates, the place where he is working and living and nation.

Cultural Environment

Social values, traditions, customs, cultural traits, e.g. symbols, belief, knowledge, sentiments, etc.

Function of Environment

Child is born with some hereditary traits. They are raw and imperfect at this stage. A healthy environment that has fuller development and in right direction. It provides good opportunities for development.

Role of Environment

- The adaptation of individual to environment. (*Lamarck*)
- Struggle for existence and survival of the fittest. (*Darwin*)
- Improving the environmental tasks IQ of children (*Woodworth*)

Importance of Heredity and Environment

Both are important for moulding the life and personality of the child.

One competes the other. Heredity – inborn traits, instincts, IQ, reflex action, etc. Environment – for the growth and development of all physical, mental traits and social traits are complementary to each other, like seed and soil, ship and sea. Both are required for individual development.

Heredity – Raw material out of which the child is to be developed.

Environment – The technique and other material for the proper manufacture of the child into a good citizen.

Thus individual is a product of the two. The individual has an opportunity to unfold the traits and fulfill them to make necessary improvements if possible.

'Improvement through a better environment. Both heredity and environment are essential to achievement and co-acting influence'—*Garrett*

Man's capacity for adaptation—*Darwin's* theory of evolution. Man has a wonderful capacity for adaptation. He can adapt the environment for himself through the wonders of science.

Heredity and environment cannot be separated, both are equal, which cannot be eliminated or isolated with each other.

The Role of Parents

Parents should provide a conducive and healthy environment at home. They should have all sympathy for the child and their aspirations like:

- Meet the needs of the child
- Identify the talents of children and encourage them to develop it
- Avoid pampering the child
- Give responsibility and freedom for the child to do things themselves
- Keep a conflict free atmosphere at home and surroundings
- Keep a vigilant eye on child, if they commit any mistake try to correct in a peaceful atmosphere.

Role of Teacher

The child spends most of the time in school apart from family. Teacher will act as a 'role-mode'. The child tries to follow teacher in all means.

Physical Development

School should be an attractive place for the child with well-ventilated environment and adequate playground for free movement to learn physical exercises.

Mental Development

School environment should encourage broad social interest of the child and the child should know about the society and their role in it. Encourage the child to participate in debates and other cultural activities.

Social Development

The social environment of the school is 'social heredity' for the children.

For example: Playmates, encourage the child to contribute the best for the societal development with adequate exposure to cultural life.

Previous Years University Questions

1. Write an essay on 'individual and society.' (15 m, MP, 2002)
2. Discuss how individual and society are inter related. (15 m, MP, 1998)
3. Evolutionary theory of origin of society. (5 m, RGUHS, 2003)
4. 'Man is a social animal'. Comment. (5 m, RGUHS, 2004)
5. Characteristics of human society. (2 m, RGUHS, 2001, 02)
6. Role of nurses in society. (5 m, RGUHS,1999)
7. Individualisation. (2 m, RGUHS, 2002)
8. Write the meaning of the word 'Society'. Why it is important for people in the society to have interaction with each other. (19 m, NTRUHS, 2003)
9. Describe heredity and environment. (19 m, NTRUHS, 2002)

MGR University Question Papers

1. Social factors influencing health status. (5 m, MGRU, Nov-03)

2. Anthropology and health. (5 m, MGRU)
3. How are society and health related? (15 m, MGRU,Dec-03)
4. Environment and health. (5 m, MGRU, Dec-03)
5. Geological, biological and socio-psychological environment and health and illness. (5 m, MGRU)
6. Society and health. (5 m, MGRU)
7. Society. (5 m, MGRU)
8. Discuss the relationship between man and environment with suitable examples. (15 m, MGRU)
9. Interdependence between man and society. (5 m, MGRU)

CHAPTER THREE

Culture

Culture is dereived from the English word 'kulthra' and Sanskrit word 'samskar', which denotes social channel and intellectual excellence. Culture is a way of life.

Definition

- 'Culture is a complex whole, which includes knowledge, belief, art, morals, customs and any other capabilities and habits acquired by the man as a member of society'— *EB Taylor*.
- 'Culture is a symbolic, continuous, cumulative and progressive process'— *Leglic AY White*
- 'The cumulative creation of man; the handwork of man and the medium through which he achieves is ends'— *Malinowski B*
- 'An accumulation of thoughts, values and objects; it is the social heritage acquired by us from preceding generations through learning, as distinguished from the biological heritage which is passed on to us automatically through the genes'— *Graham Wallas*
- 'The instruments constituted by man to assist him in satisfying his wants'—*CC North*

- 'The body of thoughts and knowledge, both theoretical and practical, which only man can possess'—*EV DeRoberty*

Meaning

Culture is an organisation of phenomenon of acts (patterns of behaviour) objects (tools) ideas (belief, knowledge, sentiments) attitudes values the use of symbols. Culture is an organised body of conventional understanding manifested in art and artifact (indication) which persisting through tradition, characterises the human group—Redfield.

Characteristics

1. Culture is an acquired quality or learned way of behaviour. It is learned through experience, imitation, communication, concept, thinking and socialisation process.
2. Culture is transmitted by vertically or horizontally and thus it is communicative. Vertical transmission is from generation to generation, horizontal transmission is from one group to another group within the same period. Knowledge is accumulative. Language is the chief vehicle of culture. The expression, body movements, gestures, feelings, attitudes, thinking also exhibit the culture.
3. Culture is social but not individual. The patterns of thinking, feeling, acting are characteristics of culture. Culture can be shared by members of group and kept relatively uniform through group pressures.
4. Culture is idealistic. The learned ways of behaviour which make up the culture are regarded as ideal patterns to which members are supported to conform disparities often occur between ideals and practice but members will understand and be aware of ideal means of culture.
5. Culture fulfills some needs and desires of individual to fulfill group functions.

6. Culture is adoptive. It may institute changes in the environment as a means of adopting, instead of altering themselves to the changing environment.
7. Culture is integrative. The parts of culture display a tendency to be moulded in an integrated consistent pattern.
8. Culture evolves into more complex forms through division of labour, which develops special skills, the interdependence of members within the society.
9. Culture is continuous and cumulative. Culture is a growing whole which includes in itself, the achievements of the past and the present and makes provision for the future achievements of the mankind. Culture is the social heritage of man.
10. Culture is dynamic. Culture is subjected to slow but constant changes. Change and growth are latent on culture and is responsive to the changing conditions of the world. It is the process of adjustment.
11. Culture is gratifying. Culture provides opportunities and provides means for the satisfaction of our needs (biological and social) and desires.
12. Culture varies from society to society. Every culture has a culture of its own/unique. Cultural elements are not uniform everywhere, e.g: Customs, traditions, morals, ideals, values, ideologies, beliefs, practices, institutions etc., and culture varies from time to time.
13. Culture is super organic. Culture is independent of physical and physiological properties and characteristics. People are proud of their cultural heritage. e.g: The 'flag' represents the nation.

Types of Culture

Culture is unique, every culture has its own varied and diverse; culture is based on society. Certain cultural similarities and variations will be observed, e.g: People worship different Gods but the basic concept is religion. People will hold different occupations but ultimate aim is 'living and earning'. Some 'rituals' 'ceremonies' 'customs' may have similar or of little variation. The content culture is of two types:

1. Material culture: Man made objects, which may be experienced with senses, e.g: Pen, table, pad, etc. It is concerned with external, mechanical and utilitarian objects. The devices and instruments by which nature is controlled. It includes technical and material equipments like: Housing, press, locomotive, media. Material culture represents 'the whole apparatus of life' or 'civilisation'. It can be easily communicated and makes our life more comfortable, meaningful and luxurious. It has thus extrinsic value, e.g: Housing – when people are constructing the houses they will take the opinions of elders, customs, traditions and 'vaastu' apart from suggestions of engineers.
2. Non-material culture: It includes the concepts, values, and ideas, e.g: Monogamy, democracy.

Functions of Culture

1. Culture makes man as a social being.
2. To regulate the conduct and prepares the human being for group life through the process of socialisation.
3. It defines the meaning of situation.
4. Provides solutions to complicated situations as it provides traditional interpretation to certain situations.
5. Defines values, attitudes and goals.
6. Broaden the vision of individuals.
7. Provides behaviour pattern and relationship with others.
8. Keeps the individual behaviour intact.
9. Creates new needs and interests.
10. Moulds national character.
11. Defines myths, legends, supernatural believes.

Organisation of Culture

Cultural Trait

The smallest unit of culture is 'cultural trait'. It may be material or non-material. These traits develop concurrently and collect together to gain the importance in terms of degrees of significance they have for the behaviour of human being. This collective group behaviour is called 'Cultural complex', e.g: Joint family system, caste system.

Cultural Pattern

The combination of material and non-material traits into a functional whole, which reflect the dominant characteristics of culture in standardised manner among the members of group, e.g: Child rearing practices, childs' behaviour in school.

Cultural Area

Refers to a geographic locality, which shares common cultural climates, e.g: Tribal areas, industrial belts.

Folk Ways

The word 'folkways' literally means 'the ways of the people'. Conformity to folkways is expected but is not absolutely insisted upon. These are accepted ways of behaviour. Folkways make man in unique means of adapting himself to the environment.

The customary traits and ways of behaviour of people that are binding. A group through trail and error influences or may arrive some possibilities of behaviour. It is passing through generation to generation.

Definition

- 'Behaviour patterns of everyday life, which unconsciously arises within a group'—*Gillin and Gillin*

- 'The ways of acting that are common to a society or a group, that are handed down from one generation to the next'—*AW Green*
- 'Typical or habitual beliefs, attitudes, styles of conduct observed within a group or community'—*Lundberg*
- 'Social habits or group expectations that have arised in the daily life of the group'—*Merill*

For example: Eating pattern, habits, communication, dressing, walking, working, greeting.

Nature of Folkways

- *Social in nature:* Products of man's group life. For sustaining, maintaining, to get social recognition individuals has to conform the folkways.
- *Repetitive in character:* If majority of people observe constantly and regularly, it becomes folkways. Practices become standardised by constant repetition.
- *Unplanned origin:* Spontaneous, automatic, unconscious in origin. No advance planning is required, e.g: Hairstyle, dressing style, conversation style, etc.
- *Informal enforcement:* Folkways are informal means of social control. If the individual is not following the folkways, it becomes 'ridicule' or 'gossip'.
- *Varied in nature:* It differs from group to group; society to society, e.g: Table manners, eating pattern.
- *Numerous and diverse:* Depending upon society and group varied folkways are observed.
- *Subjected to change:* Based on social conditions, situations, environment the folkways will be varied. Based on cultural traits, people will adopt certain cultural practices.

Characteristics of Folkways

- Spontaneous in origin, automatic
- Approved behaviour

- Distinctiveness (recognised ways of behaviour)
- Hereditary
- To meet the needs/problems of the society, e.g: Greeting, lunch in the noon, dress pattern.

Importance of Folkways

Folkways, if so internalised (fully assimilated) they become personal habits. They save our energy and time, solve the social problems and strive towards achieving the targets or goals. It meets felt needs of the individuals, thereby tension, stress, and strain over the society is reduced. It helps us to handle the situations, to maintain social relations and makes the individual to live in a comfortable manner. Folkways constitute social structure. It provides predictability to both of our behaviour and that of them. It informally controls the behaviour of the individuals.

MORES

The standards of behaviour which influences the moral conduct of people conformity to mass is called as, 'mores'. It is more vital (security) of society than folk ways, e.g: Eating with right hand.

Prescribed accepted behaviour patterns. The word 'mores' was a Latin word and ancient Romans means 'more' as a respected and sacred customs. The term 'mores' was introduced in sociological context by *Summer.* The folkways, which are considered by the group to be essential for its welfare and existence are called as mores; certified mores are called 'laws'.

Definition

- 'When the folkways have added to group welfare and high standards, that are converted into mores'—*RN Maciver and CH Page*

- 'Customs and group routines, which are thought by the societal members to be necessary to the group's continued existence'—*Gillin and Gillin*
- 'Customs, which can note fairly strong feeling of the rightness or wrongness of mode of behaviour'—*Edward Sapir*

Types of Mores

Positive Mores

It prescribes behaviour patterns. They provide instruction and guidance for the people to behave in a particular manner, e.g: Giving respect to elders, protecting children; care of diseased and aged, doing correct things, speaking truth.

Negative Mores/Taboos

It prescribes, which they should not exhibit through behaviour taboos prohibits certain behaviour patterns, e.g: Instructions like not to have anti-social behaviour.

Characteristics of Mores

- *They regulate the social behaviour:* It dictates the right attitudes and shapes the personality of the individual. They are compulsive and everybody should follow it and if anybody violates, they will be punished.
- *Relatively persistent:* Mores are long lasting, conservative in nature.
- *Varied from group to group:* Some group prohibit one kind of more, others may accept or practice it, e.g: Some follows monogamy, others accept polygamy.
- *Mores are backed by values and religion:* Religious sanction, values are shared by mores.

Social Importance of Mores

- Determines individual behaviour

- Moulds personality of individual and character formation
- Restrains our tendencies
- Powerful means of social control
- Identifies the individual with the group and maintains social relationship; essential for satisfactory living
- Preserves social solidarity
- Helpful for framing the social laws which will govern our social relations.

Differences between folkways and mores

Folkways	Mores
Simple in nature	Wider and general in character
Maintains good relationship and comfortable means in solving social problems	Value judgment about the folkways
May have chances to disobey; rewards will be given if people adapt folkways but isolation may not be punished	Profound conviction violation of the mores brings the individuals for wider chances of disapproval and punishment
Folkways are subject to change, varied from society to society	Compulsive, persistent, regulative, rigid and effective influencing factors over the individuals behaviour
Maintains social relationship, bondage developed when it is followed	Moulds the personality, restricts the tendencies of individuals
All folkways may not be equally important, if the folkways are added to the group welfare, transferred to mores	Promotes right living, group welfare
Less deeply rooted in society and change more rapidly	Deeply rooted, less frequently subject for change
Less dominant over individual's life	More stable, dominant

NORMS

Groups tends to develop the characteristics ways of doing things normally. The norms of larger social groups are usually embodied in laws, customs, traditions. In small groups, norms may appear in formal rules and regulations or they may be unwritten laws learned by all members through participation in the group. In one way or other, the group communicates its norms to its members, so that the individual is usually well aware of what the group norms are—whether formal or informal, whether to accept or not; the group norms will serve as criteria of conduct for the group members, specify the range of tolerable behaviour for members in good standing. It focuses on the social rules for individual behaviour; group ideology focuses more on group purposes, group assumptions about reality; possibility and value. Group develops frame of reference, assumptions (goals, characteristics way of coping with problems and evaluating themselves and others) about themselves and their environment.

'Social norms' constitute foundation of the social structure. No society exists without norms, they serve the individual as guides to conduct. Norms are based on social values; is a pattern setting limits on individual behaviour. Norms determine, guide, control and also predict human behaviour.

Definition

- 'Group shared expectations'—*Young and Mack*
- 'An abstract pattern held in the mind, that sets certain limits for behaviour'—*HM Johnson*
- 'The rules that guide behaviour in everyday situations and are derived from the values'—*Donald Light Jr. S. Keller*

A cultural norm is a 'set of behavioural expectation and cultural procedures, how people are supposed to do'.

'A standardised expected ways of feeling and acting which the members of society follow more or less perfectly'.

Norms are, 'standards of group behaviour', it is a 'behavioural expectation shared by group members against which the validity of perception is judged and the appropriation of feeling and behaviour is predictable'.

Norms gives order to the social relations to have smooth cohesive society. It determines and guides institutions judgment of individual and of others.

Characteristics

- *Universal:* To maintain social order norms will be formulated. They are essential for smooth functioning of the society.
- *Related to the functional order:* These are based on actual behaviour of the people. Society regulates the behaviour of its members and exercises influence on the normative system.
- *Incorporates value judgments:* The concepts of norms are evaluated by the group and incorporate value judgments. Discrete or classifies or judges the situations into good or bad; needed or not needed' right or wrong, etc. norms denotes expected behaviour/ideal behaviour of man.
- *Relative to situations and groups:* Norms vary from society to society; they differ from group to group. e.g: Some norms are applicable for men alone and some for women alone. Culture exhibits high degree of integration.
- *Norms are not always obeyed by all:* Some norms are obeyed at time; some are disobeyed or ignored at some other time; according to the interest or intension of the people.
- *Norms vary with sanctions:* Norms are the group's rules of proper behaviour. Sanctions are the group's punishments for violations of the norms. Thus sanctions are the rewards or punishments used to enforce the norms in a society. Proper observation of behaviour by the individuals has to be rewarded, e.g: Smile, approval, praise, appreciation.
- *Norms are normally internalised by the people:* Norms become part and parcel of personality of the individual through the process of socialisation. The individual internalises the group norms.

LAWS

It serves as 'reinforcement to the mores'. If the individual is not following the rules and regulations laid by the legal authority are punished. Laws are the most powerful means of social control. Government forms various laws.

Definition

- 'Form of social rule emanating from political agencies'—*JS Roucek*
- 'An authoritative canon of value laid down by the force of politically organised society'— *Roscue Pound*
- 'Rule formally enacted by a political authority and is backed by the power of the state'—*Ian Robertson*

Characteristics

- Not universal, e.g: Laws were not observed in tribal societies
- The human activities prescribed by the state for its members
- It is the product of conscious thought careful planning deliberate attempt made by the political authority
- Law is clear, precise and definite
- Applicable for all without any exception
- Violation of the law is followed by penalties, punishments determined by the state
- Written ones
- Maintenance of legal order depends upon the moral climate of a society
- It preserves societal behaviour
- Laws are enforced with the help of court, police, armed forces.

Functions of Laws

- Eliminates the homicidal activities of individuals
- Persuades individuals to pay attention for the rights of others as well as to act in cooperation with others
- Protects the individuals and society
- Promotes social welfare.

CUSTOMS

Informal means of social control, which are universal and pervasive. Socially accepted ways in which people do things together in personal contacts.

Definition

- 'Group accepted, socially approved techniques of control which are well established, taken for granted, passing to generation to generation by tradition'—*Bogardus*
- 'The uniform socially approved ways of acting, which are passing from one generation to other'—*Anderson*
- 'Rule or norm of action supported on the emotional side of forces, sentiments'—*Ginsberg*
- 'Socially accredited ways of acting'—*Maciver and page*
- 'Practices that have been repeated by a multitude of generations, practices that tend to be followed simply as they followed in the past'—*Kinsley Davis*
- 'Established modes of thought and action'—*Duncan Mitchell*
- 'Folkways that persists over a big period of time, attain formal recognition to be passed from one generation to other'—*Lundberg*

Nature

- Customs is a social phenomenon, which is socially recognised got social significance and normative in nature. Custom represents routine acts of daily life of the people, they enjoy social sanction
- Normative, maintains social order, inherited, external social sanction
- It has great social significance, inherited
- Custom are considered to be conducive to the welfare of the society
- Unconsciously customs are maintained as they are strongly imbedded in group life

- Customs are varied in nature, e.g: For the performance of marriage; varied religions performs in different manner
- Origin of custom is obscure—it is very difficult to ascertain the exact way in which customs are emerged
- Customs are relatively durable, spontaneous in nature
- All customs are not traditional.

Social importance of customs

- Regulates social behaviour, it makes the people to bind them together, assimilate their actions to be accepted standards and control their egoistic impulses
- Constitutes the treasury of our social heritage. Preserves the culture and transmits to succeed generations, develops social relationships, maintain security
- Supports laws. Customs provides solid grounds for the formulation and establishment of laws. If the state enforces them as rules to bind the citizens, it becomes law
- Moulds personality of the individual
- Customs are universal
- It is democratic and totalitarian of self-expression.

Differences between Culture and Civilisation

Civilisation	*Culture*
It is a more complex and evolved form of culture. Culture becomes civilisation only when it possesses written language, science, philosophy a specialised division of labour and a complex technology. It is a later phase of super organic culture.	Culture is a complex whole which includes knowledge, belief and morals, customs and any other capabilities and habits acquired by the members of society.
It includes useful material objects and the methods of producing and using them.	It consists of ideals, values, mental, emotional aspects of group.
The authority of man over natural phenomenon as well as special technology or mores which control man's behaviour.	It includes the basic elements, which will bring satisfaction and pleasure to man.

Contd...

Contd...

Precise standard of measurement based on utility value.	Has no quantitative or qualitative standard of measurement because culture is an end itself. The elements, needs, values and thoughts, etc. changes in accordance with time and place.
Is an organised advancement as mechanisation, communication, transport system, etc. are advanced.	It is not organised advancement.
Transmitted without effort, based on utility and connected with external life of human beings.	Efforts are needed for transmission. The adoption of culture depends upon personality and nature.
It is easily adopted, we may enjoy the products without sharing the capacity which creates them.	
Borrowed without change or loss.	Cannot be acquired without any modification.
Is an external process.	Internal traditional pattern.

Cultural Variations/Cultural Growth

Culture is acquired behaviour of group. It is a distinctive character of nation/group/a period of history. The development of culture is a continuous process.

Factors of Cultural Variations

- Historical accidents, e.g: Monogamy, polygamy
- Geographical environment
- Mobility of human beings
- Inventions, discoveries which influence technology, customs, traditions, believes and faith
- Individual peculiarities
- Change on modes of production
- Dominant cultural themes.

Process of Cultural Variation

Cultural Diffusion

Is the process by which the cultural traits invented or discovered in one society will spread directly or indirectly to other societies. In the course of transmission of this, it may be difficult to trace the origin of cultural trait. The culture of one society be borrowed by other society, but the physical isolation may influence the cultural contact of various culture, e.g: Buddhist thought—spread from India to China, Japan, Burma (Myanmar).

The factors influencing cultural diffusion:

- Relation
- Communication
- Needs
- Desire (New Traits)
- Competition of old traits and objections to them
- Respect and recognition of new traits.

Accommodation

The new ideas, which have been acquired through diffusion, have to be accommodated with the features of other culture. It becomes as part of its life and has added to its progress.

Cross Fertilisation

The conjunction of two cultures is beneficial to both. These processes of mutual give and take is known as, 'cross fertilisation'. Due to this it retains vitality and life to culture.

Acculturisation

When conjunction of two cultures occurs causing cultural growth and they are intimately related to each other rather than identified by its own process is called as, 'acculturisation'. When we are exposed to different cultures, naturally the cultivation of the culture of the dominant group will result, e.g: Learning to speak their language, cooking new dishes and way of dressing, etc.

Assimilation

When one culture becomes so intimate with other culture as it looses its individuality.

Accumulation

The experience gained is accumulated and passed on one generation to its successive generations through social heritage.

Enculturisation

'When a growing child learns to conform to his own cultural traditions' is known as, 'enculturisation'.

Ethnocentrism

It is the belief that one's own culture is superior to all others and using it as preference to one's own self or group or relatives. It is tendency for each group to take it granted the superiority of the group. It promotes group cohesion, loyalty and morale. This reinforces nationalism and patriotism. Without ethnocentrism, a vigorous, national consciousness is impossible as it protects against change.

Cultural Lag

The term cultural lag was coined by, 'Ogburn'. The other synonyms are: Cultural clash, technological lag, cultural ambivalence. The word lag means, 'crippled movement'. Hence cultural lag means 'the faltering of one aspect of culture behind another'. The material culture progresses far better comparison with non-material culture.

For example: The sphere of fashion, dressing, art—constitutes rapid change.

Religion, nations—constitutes slow change.

The main course for cultural lag is the various elements of culture it passes varying degrees of changeability. It is responsible for creating international tensions due to individual psychological means or dogmatism.

According to some sociologists, cultural lag is artificial and imaginative. It creates disequlibrium occurring in the process of social change. One thing progresses forward another lag (restricts) the behaviour. It is faltering of one aspect of culture to another. The time interval between the arrival of change and completion of adaptation is called as 'cultural lag'. It is related to differing rates of changes in society and it describes the disharmony between the related parts of a single culture produced through unequal rates of change.

Ogburn writes, 'the strain that exists between two correlated parts of culture that change at unequal rates of speed may be interpreted as a lag in the part that is changing at the slower rate for the one lags behind the other, if the society is to maintain its equilibrium it has to seek ways and means of bridging this gap'.

Cultural Beliefs Related to Health

- Getting up early in the morning and taking bath
- Drinking *Tulsi* water every day will give good health
- Drinking water stored in the copper vessel
- By keeping Jasmine flower, over the breast of the post natal women will suppress the secretion of milk and consumption of garlic will produce more milk in lactating mother
- Early to bed, and early to raise (in the morning)
- Circumcision of male child is a cultural trait commonly observed in Muslim families, is one way to prevent urinary tract infection
- Occurrence of chicken pox, measles, mumps are due to the curse of the Goddess and the affected child is bathed with neem leaves and taken to the place of worship and isolation will be followed

- In a chicken pox affected children's family keeping the neem leaves at the entrance, prevents the spreading of the disease to the neighbourhood
- Eating *papaya* fruit during the first trimester and last trimester will induce abortion and premature delivery
- After burn injury (due to fire), applying honey will induce better healing process
- Pardah system by Muslim women still followed which causes vitamin-D deficiency
- Giving iron object during convulsion period will reduce the intensity of fits
- Wearing gold ornaments below waist level is prohibited
- Following *vaastu sastram* will benefit the family
- Cleaning of the house, taking hygienic care and putting *rangoli* in front of the house, offering *pooja* will give blessing for the entire family
- Quarrelsome environment has to be avoided
- Women should not lie in supine position while in the group
- Doing meditation will increase concentration and attention
- Mental illness can be treated by placing the client in the *Masjid, and specialised temples*
- Out-reach families are not following contraceptive devices stating that, children are God's gift
- Polygyny is accepted social phenomena in certain religion
- Untouchability by the forward caste people, is a social stigma
- Male child is preferred by the Hindu parents as they believe that the son will perform their last rights
- Respecting and following instruction of the elders will bless the younger generation
- During the time of stress, the individual appeals to the God to get moral support and protection
- Following *devadasi system*
- Wearing of foot wear inside the house is prohibited by some castes.

Cultural Belief Related to Food

- Periodic fasting will help in cleansing the G.I.T. (weekly fasting by the Hindus, during the month of Ramzan by Muslims, following 1enti days by Christian)
- *Brahmins, and Vysyas* will not consume garlic, onions and non-vegetarian foods
- Drum-stick will not be consumed some sects.
- Avoiding cold food (butter-milk, curds, cucumber, guava fruit) items during common cold
- In post-operative period, consumption of *channa dhal* and fatty foods to be avoided
- Excess eating of mangoes will cause heat boils in the face and body
- Pregnant women will eat mud/ash/chalk powder/lime powder as it enhances the normal development of the foetus (*pica*)
- Beet-root consumption enhances blood production in the body
- Rich people consume more often, saturated food, which causes obesity
- Alcoholism, drug abuse are indications of rich class and complex society's culture
- Brinjal, egg, fish will produce allergies
- Eating raw vegetables like cucumber, carrot in the night will reduce obesity; keeping the cut cucumber over the closed eyes will bring coolness to the eyes.

Previous Years University Questions

1. Define culture and give its characteristics. (15 m, MP, 2004)
2. Cultural lag. (4 m, MP, 2003, 04)
3. Culture is the man-made part of environment–discuss. (15 m, MP, 2003)
4. Write an essay on diversity and uniformity of culture. (15 m, MP, 2003)

5. Explain the concept of culture and discuss its various characteristics. (15 m, MP, 2002)
6. Discuss 'cultural lag; in the process of change. (15 m, MP, 2002)
7. Discuss critically the theory of cultural lag given by *Ogburn*. (15 m, MP, 2000)
8. Man's cultural past. (5 m, MP, 1998, 2000)
9. Cultural change. (5 m, MP, 1998)
10. Unity in diversity is the characteristics of Indian culture – discuss. (15 m, MP, 1997)
11. Critically examine the theory of cultural lag. (15 m, MP, 1997)
12. Explain the concept of culture-lag. (5 m, RGUHS, 2000)
13. Effects of culture-lag. (5 m, RGUHS, 2001)
14. Folkways and mores. (5 m, RGUHS, 1997)
15. How folkways differ from mores. (5 m, RGUHS, 2002)
16. Point out the functions of culture. (5 m, RGUHS, 2002)
17. Difference between culture and civilisation. (5 m, RGUHS, 2003)
18. Define culture. (2 m, RGUHS, 2003)
19. What is custom? Describe the role of customs and laws. (5 m, RGUHS, 2004)
20. Culture. (2 m, RGUHS, 2002, 04)
21. Ethnocentrism and mental health. (2m RGUHS, 2001)
22. Ethnocentrism. (5 m, RGUHS, 1999, 2000, 01)
23. Food beliefs and health. (5 m, RGUHS, 2001)
24. Elements of culture. (5 m, RGUHS, 2002)
25. Write the meaning of social mores.(2 m, RGUHS, 2002)
26. Explain cultural diffusion. (2 m, RGUHS, 2002)
27. Social mores. (5 m, RGUHS, 2000, 01)
28. Define culture-lag. (2 m, RGUHS, 2000)
29. Acculturation. (2 m, RGUHS, 2000, 03)
30. Write any *two* specific beliefs in Indian culture which has adverse health effects. (2 m, RGUHS, 1999)
31. Write any *two* specific beliefs in Indian culture which has beneficial health effects. (2 m, RGUHS, 1999)

32. Health beliefs relating to food. (5 m, RGUHS, 2000)
33. Explain the process of enculturation. (2 m, RGUHS, 2003)
34. Culture-lag. (5 m, RGUHS, 1999)
35. Define 'culture'. Describe the factors influencing cultural change in urban India. (19 m, NTRUHS, 2003)
36. Discuss the influence of culture on personality. (19 m, NTRUHS, 2002)
37. Describe the factors influencing cultural change in rural India. (19 m, NTRUHS, 2001)
38. What are the factors influencing cultural change and cultural lag. (19 m, NTRUHS, 1999)
39. How does culture influence an individual? Why should a nurse know about the culture of her patient. (19 m, NTRUHS, 1998)
40. What are the cultural difference between rural and urban communities and mention some cultural practices which influence the health of people. (NTRUHS, 1996)
41. Write the meaning of culture and discuss the diversity and uniformity of culture. (NTRUHS, 1996)
42. Culture is socially acquired discuss. (NTRUHS, 1989)
43. What is culture and mention its characteristics and function. (NTRUHS, 1985, 87)
44. Can you distinguish between society and culture. (NTRUHS, 1986)
45. Describe any three negative beliefs and three positive beliefs-related to pregnancy and child birth with examples. (9 m, SVIMS, Tirupati, 2003)
46. Consequences of cultural lag. (5 m, SVIMS, Tirupati, 2003)
47. Explain with examples how the socio-cultural beliefs influence health and illness. (13 m, SVIMS, Tirupati, 2002)

MGR University Question Papers

1. Cultural heritage. (5 m, MGRU)
2. Culture and civilisation. (5 m, MGRU)

3. Describe the role of culture in defining health and illness. (15 m, MGRU, Nov-98)
4. Customs and law. (5 m, MGRU, Nov-98)
5. Culture. (5 m, MGRU, Nov-01)
6. Cultural lag. (5 m, MGRU)
7. Acclturation. (5 m, MGRU)
8. Define culture and discuss the sociocultural constraints and barriers in promoting health status of the people in the society. (15 m, MGRU)
9. Mores. (2 m, MGRU)
10. What is the role of culture in understanding health and illness of an individual? (15 m, MGRU)
11. Folkways. (5 m, MGRU)
12. Culture and civilisation. (5 m, MGRU)
13. Culture, health and illness. (5 m, MGRU)
14. Norms, values, folkways and mores. (5 m, MGRU, Dec-2003)
15. Folkways and mores. (5 m, MGRU)
16. Impact of culture on human behaviour. (5 m, MGRU)

CHAPTER FOUR

Social Groups

Social group is a basic social unit when two or more persons interacting with each other, interrelationships are directed towards fulfillment of certain common goals or purposes. Inter-stimulation and response are the key factors in the process of social interaction.

Definition

- 'A social group grows out of a situation which permits meaningful inter-stimulation and response between the individuals, focusing of attention on common situation or interest, the development of certain common drives, motivation or emotions'—*Gillin and Gillin*
- 'It is system of social interaction'—*HM Johnson*
- 'Any collection of human beings who are establishing human relationships with one to another'—*Maciver RM and Page*
- 'Two or more individuals come together and influence one another'—*Ogburn and Nimkoff*
- 'Two or more individuals who have common objects of attention, stimulating to each other, who have common loyalty and participate in similar activities'—*ES Bogardus*

Characteristics of Group Life

- The members of the group are related to each other and possess a sense of 'we' feeling
- Group involves a sense of unity
- The interests, ideals, values of the group members are common
- Similarity of behaviour among the group members is observed
- There are certain norms, customs and procedures which are acceptable and everyone in the group to obey the norms, rules and regulations of their own group
- The members of the group are affected by its characteristics.
- Homogeneous
- Good interpersonal and interactional relationship
- Collective perception of their identity and unity
- Shares certain goals, values and beliefs
- Emerges social control over the behaviour
- Cooperation
- Power relations
- Members behave in a natural and relaxed manner
- Membership is by voluntary, automatic in informal groups, with some purpose in formal groups
- Joining in a group may be motivated by a variety of personal needs
- Individuals who has similar values and beliefs will join together.

Classification of Groups

Charles Cooley: Primary group, e.g: Family, friends. Secondary group, e.g: Social institutions, or social organisation.

WB Sumner and Kellerr: In group and Out group.

Miller and PA Sorokin: S: Vertical and Horizontal.

Gidden's: Public and Private.

Elwood: Sanctioned and Unsanctioned.

Gillin and Gillin: Based on blood relationship, physical traits, situation proximity, cultural interests.

Charles Elwoods: Voluntary and Involuntary.

WB Sumner and Keller Classification

In Group

- The members in the group will have 'we' feeling a common attitude and treats the group members as one, e.g: Family, group of friends.
- Based on ethnocentrism.
- People exhibit good behaviour with one to another.

Out Group

- People will develop a sort of hatred feeling on a particular group and treat the group completely away from them.

Cooley's Classification

Charles Cooley has classified social groups on the basis of importance and the form of relationships among the group members.

Primary Group

- People will have intimate face-to-face, close, cooperative relationship
- Play fundamental role in forming the social nature and ideals of an individual
- Participation in primary group leads to a fusion of individualities in a common whole
- Wholeness involves the sympathy and natural identification for which 'we' is the proper expression
- People will have close intimacy and nearness in relationship

- It is very important to form satisfaction of the child and also the development of childs' personality.

Characteristics

- Physical proximity: The relationship among the group members is close and they will have intimate contact with each other. Exchange of their ideas and opinions will take place
- Small in size (to develop intimate and personal relationship, the group should be small)
- Stability in nature (to promote closeness)
- Continuity in relationship (by meeting frequently and by exchanging thoughts, the intimacy increases. When this chain is broken, the relationship does not remain the same.
- Common aims among the members (every member will share pleasure, pain, worthy for common interests. Relations are ends in themselves. The relationship between members will have mutual pleasure and contentment)
- Spontaneous, personal and inclusive relationship (every member of the group feels intimacy for others in a natural way, there is nothing like compulsion or pressure between them)
- Maximum control over group members in the family affairs.

Importance of Primary Group

- To develop personality
- The efficiency of the members will be increased and persons of the group get help, inspiration and cooperation from one to another
- Satisfaction of total needs (physical, emotional, psychological, social and spiritual) of the individual
- Group members will provide love, security, belongingness to the persons and satisfy their desires of loving and be loved, a person gets the benefits of companionship,

sympathy, exchange of thoughts and satisfies most of their psychological needs
- Socialisation process will take its origin within the family and maintain the control. Family teaches the person to work in the society according to their roles. The primary groups are the foundation of the whole society, the individual acquire the basic attitudes towards people, social institutions and the world around them
- The individual acquires the attitudes of kindness, tolerance, love, generosity, mutual concern and affection.

Secondary Group

- Groups are constituted for some specific aims, after achieving the goal the members will not maintain required relations within the group. The relationships are indirect, short and formal
- Individual do not have any interest in the pleasure and pain
- Relations among them are competitive, casual and impersonal
- Demands of person receive segments of their time and attention.

Characteristics of Secondary Group

- Position of a member depends upon their role and status
- Individuality develops in the persons because their relations are based on self-interest
- Self-dependence among members
- Large size
- No physical closeness
- Formed for some purpose after attaining it they are no more required
- Group cannot exercise control to that extent due to large size

- Lacks stability and personal relationships. The group covers wide area, but not formed on the basis of identical, common ends. Status is determined by the function
- Has the limited acquaintance and responsibility
- Group form with definite objective, its function is not spontaneous
- Members play active and passive role
- Possibility of development in individualism.

Importance of Secondary Group

- The needs are satisfied in the group with the advance of technology and associated with social change. This group will satisfy the changing needs of society and individual. The growth of social group has created some problems and many benefits
- Rules formed by the group, will increase the efficiency of the work
- Delegation of authority, coordination and planning of the activities will be implemented
- Channels of opportunity is wide, individuals can develop themselves by using their talents
- Wider outlook: It has to accommodate large number of members/localities which widens the outlook of its group
- It breaks the barriers of class, caste and province
- Must articulate with primary group.

Differences Between Primary and Secondary Group

Primary group	*Secondary group*
Size—small	Large
Relations—direct, personal, face-to-face, intimate, inclusive, spontaneous.	Indirect, impersonal, formal, exclusive.
Natural situation	Artificial situation
Aims, purpose, interest, values are same for the members	Individual interest is dominant

Contd...

Contd...

Foundations of relations are important	Relations are not important
Found mostly in traditional societies	More commonly seen in urban society
Concern with total personality	Concern with only one aspect of personality
Warm relation	Cold relation
Qualities of love, affection, sympathy will flourish	Self interest will flourish
Control by elderly person	Control is exercised by designated persons, laws, norms
Good social control exist	Less social control
Permanent relationship	Temporary relationship
Groups are complete, good deal of cooperation among its members	Partial cooperation exist
socialisation based on culture or blood relationship	Are born after socialisation and they don't have any common bond of culture or blood

Group Morale

Every individual in the group will possess certain attitudes that range over the entire spectrum of human behaviour. The group leader has concerned for their group morale, which they lead, job satisfaction is an individual phenomena whereas morale is a group phenomena. Group morale increases the work satisfaction of the individual in job area. When individual needs are satisfied and the degree to which the individual desires satisfaction from his total job situation. Group morale emphasises social reaction and concentrate on attitudes towards group values, e.g: Cohesiveness, interest, optimistic views, etc. it describes the attitude levels (favourable or unfavourable) collectively to all aspects of their work, i.e. tasks, activities; working environment towards colleagues, superiors. It is also describes the thinking capacity and feeling of the personnel about their functions. It denotes the strong emotional elements associated with values. Higher the group morale, higher will be the productivity, if leadership is effective along with proper production facilities and individual's ability that organisation will be benefited.

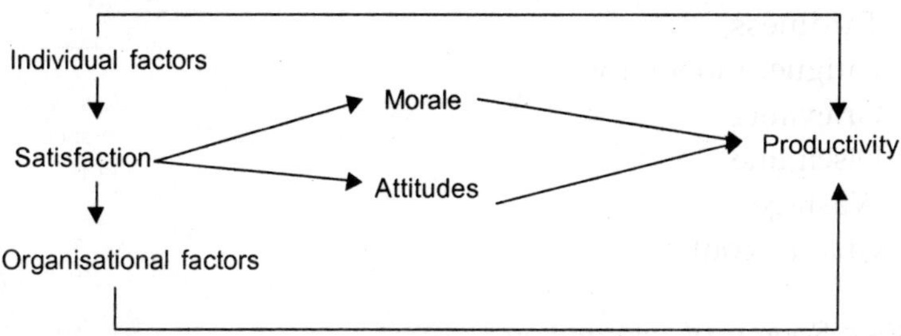

Productivity and satisfaction of individual's results with the interaction of several factors like individual factors, organisational factors. The successful leader recognises that behavioural management requires a positive integration of goals so that people working together will achieve the desirable high morale with high productivity. If the members in the group show their resistance, dissatisfaction and limited interaction leads to low productivity.

Morale Measurement

Information will be gathered by conducting public opinion, attitude, survey and observation of set of values.

Surveys

Objective, projective and descriptive types of questionnaires will be used to collect the information related to morale.

For example: Objective questionnaire viz multiple choice, yes/no, fill up the blanks, rating scale, check-list.

Descriptive questionnaire: Open-ended questions

Projective questionnaire: The respondent is given situation and he is asked to comment on these.

By observation of comments morale can be measured indirectly, e.g: Thematic Apperception Test.

Indices of Morale

- Turnover, absenteeism, withdrawal
- Productivity

- Tardiness
- Fatigue, monotony
- Grievance
- Discipline
- Wastage
- Quality control.

Other Source of Information

- Counseling reports
- Exit interviews
- Accident reports
- Training records
- Medical records
- Suggestion system
- Complaint box system.

Uses of Morale

- To take decisions related to group
- Morale is one of the basic ingredients of the conducive organisational climate which will influence the people to behave in a particular manner
- To introduce or modify group practices, which are conducive to the people in organisation
- To control the difficult situations
- Ensures group communication in upward direction. Through group morale people can convey their actual feelings, the leader can make special action to ensure the free flow of communication
- Provides opportunity to the group members to interact with higher authority. Individuals will feel their importance and motivated, both the parties shows real interest and expresses their feeling outwardly to relieve their tensions
- To assess the needs of people as a whole, i.e. social functioning of the individuals in group activities

- Identifies gaps; wherever assistance is required, provides training to fill up the gaps
- Creates an awareness on morale consciousness.

Morale Building

Is a continuous process and responsibility of group leader. He should possess sound management skills, periodic information on the status of individual's morale in the particular direction should be collected.

Sound Manpower Management

Leader in the group has to influence the group behaviour, inspire, motivate and activate the group members' interests in effective implementation of activities to fulfill their group responsibilities. Every group leader has to function as an efficient personnel manager. The group leader has to deal specifically the group grievances, handle safety measures, discipline rules and welfare activities. He should identify the abilities, limitations, intellectual skills of every individual in the group, based on their efficiencies leader has to involve them in implementation of group tasks. It will help them in improving individual morale, prevent absenteeism, turnover and withdrawal nature and provides satisfaction

Human Relations Approach

Humanitarian approach, trustworthy, authentic, interpersonal relationship has to be adopted, interact with the members frequently, recognises the individual felt needs and tries to meet and assist group members needs are some of the functions of group leader. Develop interpersonal competence, inter-group cooperation, flexibility, provide opportunity for each member to develop fullest potentiality, provide exciting, challenging environment which will give more satisfaction to them to work efficiently, cooperatively. Develop team spirit, recognise and appreciate the contributions of the team members.

Management of Attitudes

Cultivation of favourable attitudes with morale building objective is necessary for the group process. Develop positive attitude to others, and provide group activities among members which will have effect over the individual's behaviour. Involve the people in acquiring varied interests, abilities, capacities and behaviour patterns in which they feel that, their contribution to their group is more appropriate. Effective use of persuasion, communication, showing genuine interest to perform adequate activities, will raises the level of group morale.

Group Formation, Membership and Development

Persons who are bound together by specific relationships, which set them apart from others and work together to achieve common goals or aims. Groups vary in size from two persons to millions—related to their degree or organisation and the degree to which the members function together in a coordinated way, e.g.: Organised groups like family, school or any social institution; unorganised group will have greatest influence on our lives and behaviour.

Needs of the individuals are the basis for the formation of groups. Group formation provides security for their members to carry specific responsibility and perform defined, scheduled activities. It provides social experiences where an individual enjoys cohesiveness and feels protected.

Groups form more or less spontaneously by the mutual agreement of people, who share common interest or are facing with a common threat. For continuation and to meet changing needs, it may expand in size and organisation, sometimes, it may be formed largely through the activities and persuasive powers of a particular articulate person. New groups may also be formed by elections or appointment by larger groups already in existence. The way the group is formed will strongly influence the role expectations and activities.

For example, members in appointed group would have their goals and functions laid out by the organisation.

- Leader formed group, the main initiative of activities may be held on group leader.
- Members of group formed by mutual agreement will feel more personal responsibility in determining the goals and activities of the group.

Individuals attain group membership by birth (ascribed status); by choice, by invitation and by mutual consent (achieved status), e.g.: Political parties, marriages. The groups formed by achieved status, the extent to which the member perceives the group as related to the meeting of his needs is likely to be a key consideration in membership decisions.

In determining the performance and effectiveness of the group, the composition of the group is essential (e.g.: In terms of age, sex, interests, capabilities and values).

Group Attractiveness to the Individual

- Commonality of interests, values, goals: The individual tends to join and participate in groups whose purposes and values are congruent with his own success and status of the group.
- Individuals tends to be attracted to groups which have a demonstrated record of competence and success, which have high status among their peer group.
- Difficulty of gaining entrance in the group: Individuals often place a high value on membership in a group to which it is difficult to gain entry.
- Measures of security or anxiety reduction: To avoid loneliness, confusion, alienation, the individual joins the group as it provides him with ready-made purposes, values and norms.

Group Structure

Is based on stability, group norms, standards, positions/ authority, and responsibilities. Group structure is developed to regulate the actions of its group members. The group power (expert power, legitimate power, assumed power) is the ability to control some aspect of the behaviour of others by giving some rewards or punishments. Group structure may be based on communication, as communication is essential in transforming information and coordinating the activities of individuals in groups. Stabilisation of particular line of communication is essential, e.g.: Two-way communication in family, students and teacher relationship.

The sociometric structure is the pattern of personal attractions (interaction, social relationship) within the group among members.

It tends to lengthen the channels of vertical communication, increases the difficulty of upward communication in large organisation. Group structure has an impact over the quality of employees' relations; flat structure increases the group morale by decreasing the length of vertical communication. Self-actualisation, self-realisation, independent activities and effective thinking raise the morale of an individual.

Participation

Improves members morale; when the leader recognises individual's efficiencies whatever the leader decides the activities for effective functioning of the group, members has to give respect and actively participate in implementation of group welfare activities at the same time the leader has to give respect, exhibit concern, identify their efficiencies and utilise their services. Participation is a natural way of management by means of integration and self-control. Managerial actions, suitable degree of participation in situations like the nature of problems involved, individual responsibilities and their nature also has to be cited.

Job Enrichment

Provides opportunity to overcome monotony, fatigue, disinterest and create the environment to satisfy high order needs resulting in high morale enriched job satisfaction.

Handling of Conflicting Situations

- Carefully the leader has to handle the clashes of opposing demands
- Healthy, conducive and peaceful environment has to be created
- Show concern for the group interest and their welfare
- Measures to increase potentials of individuals
- Resolution of group conflicts, maintaining adequate interpersonal relationship results in positive team spirit and cooperation
- Conflict resolution is one of the important responsibility of a group leader
- Control of absenteeism and tardiness
- Collect factual information, analyse and take necessary actions to over come the problems
- Identify fatigue and monotonous jobs, provide varied activities.

Group Dynamics

Kurt Lewin is a social psychologist of the university of Iowa, USA was the founder of group dynamics.

Aspects of Group Discipline

- Formation and structure of group
- Group activities
- Composition of group
- Interaction among the group members
- Working pattern

- Growth, decline and resolution of the group
- Dissolution of group
- Pattern of achieving unity and handling of conflict situation
- Change and adapt themselves to meet the needs of group
- Task performance
- Measures adopted for group members satisfaction

Thus, 'group dynamics' is the study of the forces or processes that are responsible for various group phenomena. Group influences individual behaviour in many ways, individual/followers also will have influencing tendency over the group; thus mutually dependent groups appear to satisfy many needs, but they often lead to performance or decision-making. Group dynamics is the study of group behaviour. Many groups are part of our organisation or large social system, e.g: Corporation.

Group Interpersonal Relationships

Interaction among group members leads to the formation of social bonds or relationships. It may be warm, intimate or impersonal, harmonious or conflicting, which may be supportive or destructive in nature. Interpersonal patterns are extremely complex and keep on changing and can be a source of greater satisfaction or frustration of personal growth and self-fulfillment.

Communication and interaction in groups are corner stones of cooperative group activities, which facilitates group processes and behaviour, e.g: Goal-setting, group problem solving, decision-making, socialisation of members, task performance, group cohesiveness, introduction of change and so on. Interpersonal relationship promotes better understanding, a sense of well-being.

Goals

- To maintain group cohesion
- Organisations of goals and objectives

- To promote better understanding
- To resolve group conflicts.

Facets of good interpersonal relationship

- Interpersonal goals
- Perceptions and attraction
- Accommodation to each other.

GROUP NORMS

Definition

'Standards of behaviour and performance expected of members'.

'Represents group's shared beliefs and ideas about proper conduct and behaviour of its members in important areas of group activity'.

'Norms are blue prints for behaviour setting limits within which individuals may seek alternative ways to achieve their goals'—*Broom and Seiznick*

Meaning and Nature

- Norms relate to both interpersonal behaviour, task performance, conduct and behaviour
- In primary group—norms are unwritten and informal, secondary group—written and formal
- Based on social values which are justified by moral standards and aesthetic judgment
- Members will conform to group norms to retain their group membership and to strengthen their associations with the group and to avoid penalties
- There are also social pressures in the group which force the members to conform to norms
- It incorporates value judgments
- Norms are related to factual world.

Purposes of Norms

- Established norms on members' behaviour and performance are needed for group survival, credibility and effectiveness
- To ensure that the members will behave in a consistent, predictable and proper manner, maintains good interpersonal relationship
- To serve as rules of conduct, e.g: Do's and don't which members are expected to observe in their action behaviour within and outside of the group
- Conformity to norms by members is an important aspect of group functioning, group cohesiveness
- Provides structure, balance and discipline to the activities of group members
- Man needs a normative order to live in society
- Determines and guides intuitive judgments of others.

Conformity of Norms

- Norms are formed in matters of consequence to a particular groups goals or objectives
- Social norm operative in one social system may not be operative in another. Conformity to norms is always qualified in view of the socially defined situations in which they apply
- Violators of norms suffer with loss of prestige, ridicule, fines and imprisonment
- Higher the status of man the more likely he is to conform to the norms
- A norm need not to be carried out to the later in order to influence the behaviour.

CROWD

Definition

- 'Crowd is a collection of individuals' united temporarily and close proximity in each other, whose objective may be diverse kinds'—*Kimball Young*

- 'Crowd is a gathering of a considerable number of people around a centre and a common point of attraction'—*Maciver*
- 'A physically compact, aggregation of human being brought into direct temporary and unorganised contact with one another whose curiosities, values and emotions are temporarily identical and which arises because of common interest or common stimuli'.

Characteristics

- Physical presence
- Temporary social group
- Organised
- Large in group
- Direct contact
- Irresponsible
- Anonymity
- Narrow attention
- High suggestibility because of high emotion
- Low mental level.

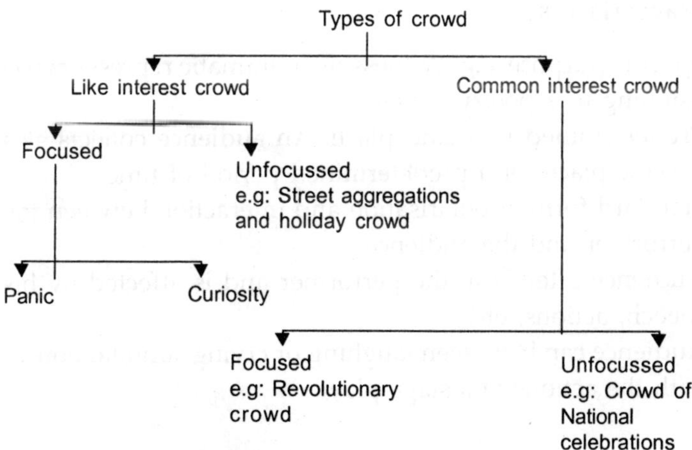

PUBLIC

Public is non-contagious and transitory mass of individuals with the common or general interest.

Characteristics

- Transitory mass
- Its related to problem of common interest
- Public ends in the problem, but no longer remains
- Any individual can be member of many public simultaneously
- Difficult to oppose the opinion of public.

AUDIENCE

Audience is a form of institutionalized crowd.

- 'A crowd formed for a specific period of time based on some specific laws'—*Kimball Young*
- 'An accepted pattern of conduct, a formal beginning of a formal end'—*Sprott*

Characteristics

- Specific purpose, e.g: Witnessing a dramatic representation listening to a poetry recital
- Predetermined time and place: An audience collects at a specific place for a predetermined period of time
- Standard form of polarisation and interaction between the performer and the audience
- Audience attends to the performer and is affected by his speech, actions, etc.
- Audience can been seen laughing or crying simultaneously with the actions in a stage play.

Difference between Crowd and Audience

Crowd	*Audience*
No predetermined aims	Predetermined aims
Gather by itself	Is invited
No definite time or place	Time and place are determined
Uncertain behaviour	Behaviour by definite modes
Stands shoulder to shoulder and stimulate one another	Behaviour is not stimulated by the members
Members react to the influence of an internal stimulus of the crowd	People are reflective and keep in mind the propriety or otherwise of any conduct
Intellect of almost all the members become inactive	Members do not loose their discrimination
Uncontrolled, unorganised and disordered	Controlled, organised and orderly
No definite pattern of polarisation and interaction	Definite pattern of polarisation and interaction
Attraction point in some incidence	Focal point can be any such thing as an idea, incident, etc.
Power increases with number	Numerical strength does not have much influence

Similarities Between Crowd and Audience

- Many people gather near one another at one place
- Both have some common focus of attention or interest
- Some emotions in both
- Polarisation should be in only one direction.

Audience is composed of all kinds of individuals, some of them visit such occasions to express the intension of creating disturbance and do so at the slightest excuse. This creates disorder even in an organised audience and it takes the form off a crowd.

SPATIAL GROUP

The spatial groups are those which are constituted because of spatial contiguity of their members, e.g: Clan or sib, tribe, band.

CLAN OR SIB

It is an important part of the tribal organisation. It is only an extensive form of lineage constituted blood relations.

A clan is constituted by including all the relatives of either the mothers' or the fathers' lineage and the off spring of one ancestor constitute a lineage.

All the lineal descendants of the family are introduced by combining the lineages of both the mother and the father. It is invariably unilateral. Its descendants are of either matrilineal or patrilineal lineage.

Definition

'Collection of unilateral families whole members believe themselves to be the common descendants of a real or mythical ancestor'. It is that exogamous combination of unilateral families, whose members are related by some common ties.

Characteristics

1. Exogamous group: They believe themselves to be descended from a common ancestor. Consequently they do not marry any member of their clan. Marriage is contracted only out of the circle of one's own clan.
2. The members of a clan believe in one common ancestor – real or mythical.
3. It is a unilateral group. It consists of all the families either on the mother's side or the father's side.

Types of Clan

Matrilineal Clan

All the off spring of one woman is held to be members of one clan. At the same time the sisters and brothers of the woman are also members of this clan, e.g: It includes a woman, her off spring, her sisters and their children.

Patrilineal Clan

It includes a man, his children, his brothers and sisters, the children of the brothers, but not of the sisters.

Clans have different names based on various grounds

After the name of:

- Seers, e.g: Shandilya, Bharadwaj
- Totem, e.g: Kunjam, Naagsari
- Substitute, e.g: Kamar, Jagat
- Topography, e.g: Mahanadiya, Jaunpriya.

Function of Clan

Mutual Assistance and Protection

- Members of clan possess 'we feeling' because of their belief in descent from a common ancestor.
- They are prepared not merely to assist one another but even to lay down their lives for each other.
- When one member of the clan is injured, all the members share the pain.
- Two prevalent sayings are:
  a. Strike my clan brother and you strike me.
  b. The blood of the clan is my blood.

Control Over Members

The clan exercises great control over its members, thereby saves its members from doing unsocial acts. Individuals indulging in unsocial acts are extradition from the class proves more effective and disastrous than even a death sentence for the member. In this way, the conduct of clan member is controlled.

Legal Function

Punishes miscreants and maintain peace in an orderly manner.

Exogamy

It arranges marriages from outside the group.

Cordiality

Increases cordial relationship with the members of the other clan.

Governmental (administrative) Function

Heads of the various clan meet and takes political decision in time of war and peace. It avoids conflicts between men for a woman within the clan.

Religious Function

Caters to the religious needs of its members. Usually, the head of the clan is also a priest. He consummates the religious undertaking of all the members.

Property

On the village where agriculture is carried out, it is the clan, which arranges for agriculture land. The head of the clan distributes the land. When a person is deprived of the membership of the clan, he is also deprived of this land. Members can only rent the land.

Difference between Clan and Caste

Clan	*Caste*
Well organised group based on a mythical ancestor.	It is a real, actual, organised group.
Exogamous, members can marry outside the clan.	Endogamous, they cannot marry outside the caste.
Individuals possess the same status.	Individuals possess higher and lower social status.

TRIBE

Introduction

The second largest group of the backward class of the unprivileged section consist of 7.5% of total population is scheduled tribes. Gandhiji called them as 'Girijans', the constitution of India has referred them as scheduled tribes.

Definition

- 'Group of families bearing a common name, speaking a common dialect, occupying or professing to occupy a common territory and is not usually endogamous though originally it might have been so'—*Imperial Gazette of India.*
- 'A social group in which there are many class, nomadic bands, villages or other sub-groups, which usually have a definite geographical area, separate language, singular and distinct culture and either a common political organisation or at least a feeling of common determination against strangers'—*George Peter Murdock (Sociology dictionary)*
- 'A collection of families or groups of families bearing a common name, members of which occupy the same territory, speak the same language and observe certain taboos regarding marriage, profession or occupation and have developed a well assessed system of reciprocity and mutuality of obligations'—*DN Majumdar*
- 'A group of total communities which live in a common area, speak a common dialect and follows a common culture'—*Gillin and Gillin*

Characteristics of Tribe

Definite Common Topography

The tribe inhabits and remains within a definite topography. Common habitat is essential for a tribe. In the absence of a common topography, the tribe would also loose its other features like community sentiments, common language, etc.

Consciousness of Unity

Members of a tribe are possessed with a sense of unity.

Common Language

Members of a tribe speak a common language. They also help to generate and evolve a sense of communal unity among them.

Endogamous

Members of the tribe marry within their group.

Ties of Blood Relationship

The main basis for communal unit is the tie of blood relationship between its members. The members of the tribe have faith in their real or mythical ancestor.

Experience of Need for Protection

A political organisation of the tribe is established and all authority for administration is vested in one person. This leader employs his mental power and skill in protecting the entire group.

A tribal committee is formed to render assistance in the form of advice to the tribal chief. The chief solve the problems of their own groups and act according to the direction of the tribe.

Political Organisation

It has its own political organisations, which maintains harmony and avoids notes of discord among its members and protect them.

Importance of Religion

The tribal organisation is based on religion because social and political laws become invisible once they are granted religious sanctity and recognition. Religion rendered service in developing the habits of obedience. The authority of a common religion is an important characteristic of the tribe.

Common Culture

Resulting from a feeling of unity, common language, common religion, common political organisation.

Organisation of Clans

A tribe is constituted of many clans. There exist laws of mutual reciprocity among its members.

Distinct Between Tribe and Clan

Tribe	Clan
Lies on a definite common territory	No definite territory
Common language	No common language
Endogamous group	Exogamous group

Distinct Between Tribe and Caste

Tribe	*Caste*
Endogamous group*	Endogamous group*
Local group	Social group
Common inhabitation	Originated on the basis of division of labour
Have their own political organisation	No political organisation
Occupy any profession as they like	Ancient period—definite occupation, now transforming
Opposes Hindu rituals even though indulge in worshipping of God	Own religious pattern
Rank and status is low	Rank and status is vivid
Names are based on totem	Based on family names, saints or God

* *with the advancement in transportation, communication both the groups promoting exogamy.*

The tribes are gradually being converted into castes. Four processes in this transformation:

- By changing one's lineage.
- By accepting the principles of any school of Hindu religion.
- 'By entering into relations with Hindus without changing name'—*Risley*

- 'A tribe can enter Hindu society by adopting class and name of caste'—*DN Majumdar*

As a result of these changes, the differences between tribe and caste are being continually reduced.

Indian Tribes

Indian tribes constitute roughly 8% of the nation's total population, concentration lives in a belt along the Himalayas stretching through Jammu and Kashmir, Himachal Pradesh and Uttar Pradesh in the west, to Assam, Meghalaya, Tripura, Arunachal Pradesh, Mizoram, Manipur and Nagaland in the northeast. Another concentration lives in the hilly areas of central India (Madhya Pradesh, Orissa and to a lesser extent, Andhra Pradesh); in this belt, which is bounded by the Narmada river to the north and the Godavari river to the southeast, tribal people occupy the slopes of the region's mountains. Other tribals, the Santals, live in Bihar and West Bengal. There are smaller numbers of tribal people in Karnataka, Tamil Nadu and Kerala, in western India Gujarat and Rajasthan and in the union territories of Lakshadweep and the Andaman and Nicobar islands.

The extent to which a state's population is tribal varies considerably. In northeastern states 90 % of population is tribal. The largest tribes are found in central India, although the tribal population there accounts for only around 10 % of region's total population. In south, about 1 % of the population are tribal.

There are 573 communities recognised by the Government as scheduled tribes and therefore eligible to receive special benefits and to compete for reserved seats in legislatures and schools. On occasion, an entire tribe or part of a tribe joined a Hindu sect and thus entered the caste system en masse.

Tribal society tends to be egalitarian, its leadership being based on ties of kinship and personality rather than on hereditary status. Tribes typically consists of segmentary lineages whose extended families provide the basis for social organisation and control. Unlike caste, religion, which recognises the hegemony of Brahman priests, tribal religion recognises no authority outside the tribe.

Language is not always an accurate indicator of tribal or caste status. Especially in regions of mixed population, many tribal groups have lost their mother tongues and simply speak local or regional languages. Linguistic assimilation is an ongoing process of considerable complexity. In the highlands of Orissa, for example, the Bondos- a Munda-language-speaking tribe–use their own tongue among themselves. Oriya, however, has also supplanted the native tongue as the language of ritual.

Economic and Political Conditions

Most Indian tribes are concentrated in heavily forested areas that combine inaccessibility with limited political or economic significance. Historically, the economy of most tribes was subsistence agriculture or hunting and gathering. Improved transportation and communications have brought ever-deeper intrusions into tribal lands; merchants and a variety of Government policies have involved tribal peoples more thoroughly in the cash economy. In 1970s, the gains tribal peoples had made in earlier decades were eroded in many regions, especially in central India. Migration into tribal lands increased dramatically, and the deadly combination of constabulary and revenue officers uninterested in tribal welfare and sophisticated non-tribals willing and able to bribe local official was sufficient to deprive many tribals of their landholdings.

Government policies on forest reserves have affected tribal peoples profoundly. Wherever the state has chosen to exploit forests, it has seriously undermined the tribes' way of life. Government efforts to reserve forests have precipitated armed resistance in the part of the tribal peoples involved. Intensive exploitation of forests has often meant allowing outsiders to cut large areas of trees (while original tribes inhabitants were restricted from cutting), ultimately replacing mixed forests capable of sustaining tribal life with single-product plantations. Where forests are reserved, non-tribals have proved far more sophisticated than their forest counterparts at bribing the necessary local officials to secure effective use of forest lands.

Efforts to improve a tribe's educational status have had mixed results. Recruitment of qualified teachers and determination of the appropriate language of instruction also remain troublesome. Commission after commission on the 'language question' has called for instruction, at least at the primary level, in the students' native tongue. In some regions, tribal children entering school must begin by learning the official regional language, often one completely unrelated to their tribal tongue. The commitment of tribes to acquiring a formal education for their children varies considerably. Tribes differ in the extent to which they view education positively. Schooling has helped tribal people to secure political and economic benefits. The education system there has provided crops of highly trained members in the professionals and high-ranking administrative posts.

Tribal Problems

1. *Problem of geographic separation:* Some tribes are living in unapproachable areas, e.g: Deep valleys, dense forest, hills, and mountains. They are far away from civilised society.
2. *Economic problem:* Majority of the tribal people live below the poverty line, tribal economy depends majority on agriculture, many of them live as bonded labourers, young women often sold to brothel houses.
3. *Cultural problem:* The customs, practices, beliefs, traditions are of their own, cultural gap exist between civilised and the tribal people.

4. *Social problem:* Tribals are traditional and custom bound, they become the victims of superstitions, beliefs, meaningless practices with harmful habits. The prevalence of problems includes child marriages, infanticides, homicides, animal sacrifices, black magic and exchange of wives. They believe in ghosts and spirits.
5. *Educational problem:* One-third of tribals are illiterates, even though the Government formulated reservations, relaxations in rules, for entry in the school, still they are below in educational standards. Establishing schools in the tribal areas is also problematic, they won't believe in formal education.
6. *Health problem:* Mainly they believe in customs, traditions, spirits, ghosts, black magic for curing the diseases, results in more incidence of communicable diseases, which takes a heavy toll of tribal life. Their skepticism and disbelieves in modern medicine leads to multiple problems.
7. *Lack of transportation and communication facilities:* As they live in hilly, mountains, deep valleys, the Government is unable to provide transport facilities.

Tribal Welfare Activities

Central and state Government have undertaken tribal welfare measures along with the help voluntary agencies, to elevate the tribal from ignorance, illiteracy and poverty.

- Constitutional safeguard—article 15 provides equal rights and opportunities to all the citizens of nation including tribal without any discrimination, article 16 shows reservation in employments for Girijans. 320 and 335 articles, seats were reserved for legislations, 330, 332 and 334, describes the tribals can make property and enjoy it in any part of the country, article 275, funds related to tribal welfare activities, 338 empowers the President of India to appoint commissioner and other official agencies for implementation of tribal welfare activities.

- Economic facilities—tribal sub-plans, integrated tribal development projects for economic improvement of the tribals, loans will be given for the purchase of necessity things in life.
- Education facilities—schools are established in some tribal areas, for tribal students concessions like free tuition, stipend, scholarship, supply of stationary equipment, midday meal, relaxation for entry into various courses, and for job opportunities.
- Medical facilities—establishment of hospitals, mobile units in tribal areas, conducting free medical camps, awareness campaigns to inspire the tribal people for effective utilisation of medical services.
- Carrying out research activities—permission to conduct intensive studies related to culture, customs, and identification the problems of tribal people, sanctioning of funds for tribal welfare activities.

REFERENCE GROUP

The concept of reference group behaviour was developed by *Hayman, Later, Turner, Merton and Sheriff.* It is the desired behaviour learned by an individual through the process of imitation. The desire to imitate other individuals or groups is instinctive in them. If one is progressing by adopting certain strategies, it is the natural tendency for the second to imitate and compare themselves with the first and begins to behave like first in order to reach the status and position of the first person. This is called as reference behaviour.

Definition

- 'Particular individual in a society, whose standards or values become the ideals for other people and are imitated by others'—*Hayman*
- 'An individual in a group situation accepts the group norms or imitate the behaviour of the distinguished people. He relates himself psychologically'—*Sheriff*

- 'It aims to systematise the determinants and consequence of those processes of evaluation and sub-appraisal in which the individual takes the values or standards of other individual groups, as a comparative frame of reference'—*Merton*

Reason for reference group behaviour:
- Social and economic situation.
- Psychological level of the individual.

Kinds of members in reference group behaviour:
- Aspiring members: Individuals who aspire to enter a reference group, but lacks the capacity to enter. Position is non-member.
- Potential members: No desire the others group, but forced to enter.
- Actual members: The members who possess the imitative behaviour.

Characteristics of Reference Group Behaviour

- Individuals or groups considers the behaviour of others as ideal behaviour and imitates it.
- Compares with other group members behaviour.
- Desire to rise higher in the social scale.
- The feeling of relative weaknesses or defects leads to the deprivation feelings and he takes the values or standards of other individual whereby he changes his behaviour.
- Assimilates the values, goods and standard of the others.
- Feels stress and strain by imitating others, which leads to grouplessness or de-grouped situation.

ISOLATION

Social interaction involves contact. Contact need not mean the infringement of one directly upon the other. The stimulus carries a meaning and unless the sensory contact carries a meaning, it is not social.

The social behaviour of human beings consists of acquired responses to the meaningful responses of others. So social interaction is communicative interaction.

Definition

'The absence of communicative interaction or social contact' is called as isolation.

TYPES

Absolute Isolation

The individual has no contact with other individuals at any time.

Spatial Isolation

It is external and enforced deprivation of contacts, e.g: Criminals, putting to solitary imprisonment.

When somebody is punished from the community, the individual in such cases is deprived of protection of his group and becomes aggressive and show a greater propensity for anti-social behaviour. It leads to melancholy and other mental disorders, sexual abnormalities and anti-social attitudes.

Organic Isolation

Caused by certain organic defects of the individual, e.g: Deafness or blindness. It is not imposed by an external authority. They may become suspicious, distrustful, irritable in nature. He may give up the hope of obtaining a normal position in life and may even become a broken personality.

Partial Isolation

Shyness

It is an inability to make adequate responses in certain spheres of life. It occurs due to psychic shock suffered during childhood and disturbed personality which hinders the normal decisiveness of the individual.

Privacy

An individual withdraws his inner-self and the external circumstance creates a set of attitudes and feelings. Excessive privacy may lead to split-mind personality.

Physical Isolation

Certain geographical factors like mountains. Broad river and jungles creates physical isolation.

Linguistic Isolation

The constitution of India recognised only 14 languages, but hundreds of languages are spoken. The people who lives closer are unable to communicate with each other as they speak different dialects. Linguistic differences causes barrier to social contact among people, which limits inter-group communication subjected to stress and strain among individuals. It also affects traditions and leads to cultural cross-fertilisation.

Societal Isolation

Ethnocentric attitude where integrity is enforced, which promotes the stability of the group, which leads societal isolation.

RACE

Anatomical variations, which occur among groups is called 'Race'. Sometimes it is used as synonymous with nationality. Race is a recurrent ingredient in the ethnosemantics of group identity and inter group relations. 'Social races' are composed of socially defined and significant groups. The study of social race thus is a fundamental aspect of the study of social structure, especially in stratified state societies. In 1950 UNESCO replaced the word race with ethnic group.

Definition

'A race is a group of people having certain genetically transmitted characteristics, which vary within certain range and differentiate them from other groups of people'.

Meaning

The race is a group of inter-marrying people who are born of common ancestors, possess similar physical traits and 'we' feeling. Inbreeding renders physical characteristics of the race permanent and due to them one race may be distinguished from another. A race originates due to mutation, migration, selection and adaptation.

Social races are composed of subjectively significant groups, unrestricted by age and sex criteria, in which membership is sociocentric (i.e. appears the same to all egos), is established at birth, endures for life, and confers special behavioural obligations or privileges.

Classification of Human beings on the Basis of

- Skin colour, e.g: Black race, white race, yellow race.
- Physiological recognition of an individual, e.g: Negroes, European.
- Nation wise, e.g: Irish, Japanese, Germans.
- Linguistic minorities, e.g: Aryans, Dravidians, Jews.

Determinants of Race

Indefinite Physical Traits

Colour of the skin: The colour of skin alters with the effect of the climate and subtle variations will observed.

Leucoderm: Caucasian.

Xanthoderm: Mangolian.

Melanoderm: Negro.

Blood-red white skin: Kashmiri people.

Pale transparent wheatish skin: Superior castes of Northern India.

Texture and colour of hair: On the basis of texture.

Leiotrrichy (soft, straight hair): Mongols and Chinese.

Cymotrichy (smooth curly hair): Indians, Western Australian, Europe.

Ulotrichy (thick curly hair): Negroes.

Structure and colour of the eyes: White, grey and yellow.

Orifice of the eye is usually horizontal.

Diagonal eyes are found—Southern Europe, North Africa.

Definite Physical Traits

1. Stature

   Tall stature: 170 cms (5 ′ 7″) or above.
   Average stature: 165 cms (5′ 5″)
   Short stature: 160 cms (below 5′ 3″)
2. Structure of head

   $$\frac{\text{(The width of head} \times 100)}{\text{Length}}$$

   Dolicoephalic: Cephalic index: 65%
   Mesocephalic: -do- : 75 – 80%
   Brachycephalic: -do— : 80%
3. Structure of the nose: The length of nose as 100, the % of its width is calculated. The sesultant figure is called as the 'Nasal Index'.

   Leptorrhine (thin)
   Mesorrhine (medium)
   Platyrrhine (thick)
4. Blood group: The blood group is unaffected by changes in the environment, e.g: A, B, AB, O. The proportion of their blood group members differs from race to race.

5. Length of the hands and feet: Among different races the length of the hands and feet do not coincide.
6. Perimeter of chest: Differences in the chest measurements between people of different races are found.

Races are undoubtedly determined by the above mentioned traits, but it is almost impossible to find all the traits of one race in the people of any country. Now all the races of the world have been inter-mixed. Hence there is no pure race anywhere. Some members of the race may possess some of the racial characteristics associated with the race and deviate from the racial norm in others.

According to *Sir Herbert Risley:*

- Pre-Dravidian race—Primitive tribes of the hills and jungles
- Dravidian type—Southern peninsula upto the gangetic valley
- Indo-Aryan type—Kashmir, Punjab, Rajputana
- Aryo-Dravidian type—Gangetic valley
- Cytho-Dravidian type—East of Indus
- Mongoloid type—Assam and foot hills of the eastern Himalayas
- Mongo—Dravidian type.

Race and Social Consciousness

The racial background indicates the differences are cultural experiences rather than biologically determined. Race is being a biological term, it is also indicative of a sociological fact. It has a hand in social consciousness, e.g: People may marry their own group members, it increases social consciousness.

The concept of race continues from generation to generation, e.g: Inter race marriage in India is forbidden because of race distinction. The idea of race has a direct and strong influence on the behaviour of the individual.

One finds serious and important differences in the living standards, facilities, privileges, etc. on the basis of race, e.g: Due to racial discrimination, though unconstitutional that

Negroes are deprived of their fundamental rights like entering the hotels, restaurants.

Race influence the personalities and social institutions, e.g: White, blacks. The social consciousness confirms to this notion of basic differences. In this way, even though the concept of race lacks any scientific basis, it plays an important role in developing social consciousness.

Fallacies of Racism

Imagination of a Pure Race

There is no nation in the world, which can boast of a pure race.

Some race stand lower on the scale of evolution than do others

Some racists assume that the Negro more closely resembles the gorilla and chimpanzee than does the white. Thus, the Negro is given a low place on the scale of evolution.

All races stand at about equal distance from their common ancestor.

Racial Intermixture Leads to Degeneration

It is a superstition as

- Hybrid vigour often results from the crossing of racial stocks, which are radically different in physical appearance.
- Crossing of diverse racial strains serves to prevent the manifestation of recessive defects in grouping.

Confusing Race with Culture

- Emancipation or downfall of culture is dependent exclusively upon the race.
- Culture is a social phenomenon while race is a psychological or biological factor. The elements of culture are poetry, art, philosophy.

- Culture spreads through cultural contact, but race cannot spread in a different area without actual crossing.

Interpreting Language as a Characteristic of Race

- Language and race have no relation. Language is a part of culture and it can be learnt by any individual of any race. It cannot be associated with race.

Identifying Race with Nationality

- Race and nation are two different and distinct concepts. Many different racial elements can be admixed in the organisation of a nation. Race can be physical and material element of the nation. Nation is a social concept, while race is a genetic concept. Nation has a geographical unit while race has no specific limits.

Nation is created with a view to attain some definite purpose. The creation of the race is the outcome of natural processes.

Nation is subjective.

Race is objective—based on common psychological characteristics.

Race Prejudice

It splits mankind into warring camps. There is much injustice to one race caused by another, e.g: Race slavery.

Man's inhumanity to man is often based on race. Race prejudice is threatening the world peace.

Prejudice – is an attitude that predisposes a person to think, perceive, feel and act in favourable or unfavourable ways toward a group or its individual members. Prejudice means to prejudge. We prejudge readily when emotion forces us to a conclusion without much thought. Strong emotion blocks thought and blinds us. Once prejudice takes place even facts will not be able to eradicate it.

Source of Race Prejudice

1. Economic advantages
   Negroes: Inferior, given lower jobs, without any of improvement.
   White people: Employers, economic interests are benefited, dominant group.
2. Political advantages
   South Africa: Negroes – denied the right to vote and hold public office.
   Whites: Continue to enjoy the political power high status quo.
3. Ethnocentrism
   It is a feeling whereby the natives come to despise foreigners and feel superior to them.
4. Compensation for frustration
   Individual frustration due to dishonesty, hostility one's failures are not due to one's inaptitude but due to the intrigues and machinations of individuals. Of a certain group whom he characterises as inferior, mean and unscrupulous.
5. Lack of proper education.

Eradication of Race Prejudice

Racism acts as a strong barrier to cooperative social action. Educate properly the youth on the right lines and teach the indisputable fact that colour of skin, class, religion belief, geographical or national origin are no tests of social adaptability.

A citizen is to be judged not by the colour of the skin, but solely by the readiness with which he fits himself into the social structure and by the value of his contributions to the development of the country.

The expansion of communication with its corresponding multiplications of contacts will also help in breaking down the race barriers whenever they exist. Accurate knowledge of the subject of race, information as to how cultures grow and why they are different and recognition of the fact has to be imparted in educational institution.

Minority Groups

The achieved status of an individual or a group is by income, education or occupation. Ascribed status is by birth in a family, particular religion or caste.

Definition

'A group having an inferior, subordinate position in the society. Traditionally, 'racial, ethnic and religious groups'.

Features

- Subordinates social status
- Lack of effective powers to combat, unfavourable treatment by dominant groups
- Susceptible to prejudice and discrimination
- Exclusion from full participation in the life of society
- Subordinated of complex society
- Inferior status
- Low self esteem, physical and cultural traits
- Self conscious units bound together by the special characteristics where the group members share the disabilities which these bring together
- Descent is capable of affiliating succeeding generations even in the absence of apparent special cultural or physical traits
- Pattern of relationships, distribution of power and employment opportunities provided to them
- They become object of contempt, violence and ridicule
- In power relationships, conflicts exists in degrees of intensity and explicitness between dominant and minority group
- Minority groups attempt either to gain autocracy or to achieve equal status and opportunity

- The relationship between major and minor vary by the degree of difference in culture, language and race.

Religious Minority in India

Muslims

11.21% of total population consists of Muslims, which is largest minority group in India. Earlier, they felt insecure, to overcome Muslims minority issue, Government has made provision to include their festivals in the gazetted holidays.

Christians

Twenty six percent of the total India's population constitutes Christians and 22% of Kerala's populations are Christians. Christians are regarded as aliens by Hindus and Muslims, the problems related to Christianity are: Right to propagate religion and missionary activities. They are dedicated for service and are made as one group of backward caste and their festivals are published in the Indian gazette.

Sikhs

1.89% of India's populations are Sikhs. After bifurcation of Punjab state 78.62 % are Sikhs, the community fairly treated.

Anglo-Indians

Microscopic minority where it possess all the characteristics of minority, i.e. racial, religious, linguistically combined the community.

Parsis

Constitutes 0.1% of country's population, nearly 70% of them are concentrated near Mumbai alone. Now a day their number is decreasing and less of religious identity. They represented the core of political struggle in India and also led the economic revolution in India. The members are economically well off and they are predominantly urban.

LINGUISTIC MINORITIES

Definition

'Who are residing in the territory of India, any part there of, having a distinct language or script of their own'.

'Any group of people whose mother tongue is different from the principal language'.

According to linguistic survey of India, there are 17 languages and 544 dialects, 4 district groups, Indo-Aryan, Dravidian, Austro-Asiatic and Tibeto-chinese.

If one state people start educational institutions in another state, they are considered as linguistic minority educational institutions.

India is divided by language horizontally, vertically by religion, whatever may be division, each will overlap with other.

In Indian constitution, article 350 states, 'each state of local authority should endeavour to provide adequate facilities for instruction in the mother tongue atleast in the primary stages of education to the children belonging to linguistic minority groups.

In secondary schools, medium of instruction will be in the regional language. Government recruitment can be made without any bar related to the medium; regarding efficiency can be tested in the scheduled language before the end of 'probation'.

Government has taken action to promote Urdu language at university level and produce literature in the same language.

Previous Years University Questions

1. 'India is a museum of races' explain. (15 m, MP, 2004)
2. What is crowd? Explain its characteristics. (15 m, MP, 2000, 03)

3. Define religion and discuss its sociological importance in society. (15 m, MP, 2002)
4. Public. (5 m, MP, 2000)
5. What do you mean by social group. Describe the characteristics of primary group. (15 m, MP, 1998)
6. Social significance of religion. (5 m, MP, 1998)
7. Describe the characteristics of primary and secondary groups. (10 m, RGUHS, 2000)
8. Effects of social isolation. (5 m, RGUHS, 2000)
9. What are social mores. (2 m, RGUHS, 2000)
10. Explain the difference between primary and secondary groups. (10 m, RGUHS, 2001)
11. In-groups and out-groups. (5 m, RGUHS, 2001)
12. How does crowd differ from audience. (2 m, RGUHS, 2001)
13. Examine the various sources of prejudice. (5 m, RGUHS, 1997)
14. Types of crowd. (2 m, RGUHS, 1997)
15. Meaning of secondary group. (2 m, RGUHS, 1997)
16. Bring out the feature of crowd. (5 m, RGUHS, 2002)
17. Define tribe. (2 m, RGUHS, 2001, 02)
18. Importance of primary group. (5 m, RGUHS, 2003)
19. What are in-group. (2 m, RGUHS, 203)
20. Crowd, public and audience. (5 m, RGUHS, 2003)
21. Define social group. Describe briefly the classification of social groups. (10 m, RGUHS, 2004)
22. Crowd behaviour. (5 m, RGUHS, 2001)
23. Social benefits of isolation. (5 m, RGUHS, 2001)
24. Functions of social control. (2 m, RGUHS, 2001)
25. Characteristics of in-groups. (5 m, RGUHS, 1999,2002)
26. Uses of social isolation in patient care. (5 m, RGUHS, 2002)
27. Classification of social groups. (5 m, RGUHS, 2003)
28. Negative effects of social isolation.(5 m, RGUHS, 2003)
29. Health benefits of social isolation. (5 m, RGUHS, 2000)

30. Adverse effects of in-groups. (5 m, RGUHS, 2000)
31. Influence of religious practices on health. (5 m, RGUHS, 1999)
32. Health problems of tribals. (5 m, RGUHS, 1999)
33. Health effects of social isolation. (2 m, RGUHS, 1999)
34. Define race. Give a brief account of the different races and their features. (5 m, RGUHS, 2001)
35. Describe the functions of primary and secondary groups. (10 m, RGUHS, 2000)
36. Achieved status and ascribed status. (5 m, RGUHS, 2003)
37. What is the meaning of 'social group'? describe any two types of social groups in brief. (19 m, NTRUHS, 2003)
38. Discuss the effects of social maladjustments on effective functioning of social groups. (19 m, NTRUHS, 2003)
39. Describe the factors of group integration. (9 m, NTRUHS, 2002)
40. Define social group and distinguish it from nation and crowd. (NTRUHS,1992)
41. What is social group and describe its characteristics and functions. (NTRUHS, 1989)
42. Define social group and examine the need of group life to the individual. (NTRUHS, 1987)
43. Short notes on primary group. (NTRUHS, 1987)
44. Characteristics of primary and secondary groups. (NTRUHS, 1985)

MGR University Question Papers

1. Define role of primary and secondary groups. (5 m, MGRU)
2. Formal and informal groups. (5 m, MGRU)
3. Functions of primary and secondary groups. (5 m, MGRU)
4. Collective behaviour. (5 m, MGRU)
5. Characteristics of primary group. (5 m, MGRU)
6. Secondary groups. (5 m, MGRU)
7. Crowd. (2 m, MGRU)

CHAPTER FIVE

Social System

Definition

'Plurality of individuals interacting with each other according to shared cultural norms and meaning'.

'An orderly and systematic arrangement of social interaction'.

Meaning

It is an organisation where orderly and systematic arrangement of social interactions and consists of a network of interactive relationships. The people will interact with each other according to shared cultural norms and meanings. The individual has a role to play. He influences the behaviour of other individuals and he himself influenced by their behaviour. The behaviour of individuals and groups in society is controlled by social institutions. The various groups do not act in an independent and isolated manner. They are the coherent parts of an integrated whole. They act in accordance with social norms. On the basis of their interactions and interrelationships creates a pattern called 'social system'.

Elements

- *Belief and knowledge:* Any proposition about any aspect of the universe that is accepted as true. It may be true or false, verifiable or not, but the people considers it as true. It furnishes the cognitive basis for social action
- *Sentiment:* Represents what we feel about a particular stimulus. It is articulated in the internal pattern of the social system, results from interaction. These are acquired as a product of experience and cultural conditions
- *Goal and objective:* Members in the social system will expect to accomplish particular goal through appropriate interaction
- *Norms:* Standards to determine right or wrong, appropriate or inappropriate, good or bad in social relationships
- *Status:* It is a position, which an individual has in society. The place in a particular system in which an individual occupies at a particular time in his status with reference to that system
- *Role:* Expected behaviour of the individual with in that society observed by his performance
- *Rank:* The importance of the individual has for the system in which the rank is accorded
- *Power:* It is the capacity to control others and exhibits authority
- *Sanction:* The society will reward or punish the individual depending on the efficiency of their work performance
- *Facility:* It is a mean used to attain ends within the system to enable the individuals to perform functions and their roles efficiently.

Type-I	*Type-II (Durkheim)*	*Type-III (Sorokin)*
Political	Mechanical	Sensate
Educational	Organic	Ideational
Religious		Idealistic
Economic		

Characteristics

1. Social system is based on social interactions.
   When a number of individuals act and interact their interactions produce a system, which is called as 'social system'. An individual alone cannot produce it, he has to interact with number of individuals then only social system is formed.
2. The interaction should be meaningful.
   It is an orderly arrangement of the various expressions of social relationships. They find expression in tradition, customs, mores, laws and in institutions. Aimless and meaningless interactions do not produce social system.
3. Social system is a unity.
   Where the various parts/subsystems are arranged in an integrated manner and constitute a social style. It implies order among the interacting units of the system.
4. The parts of social system are related on the basis of functional relationship.
   Each system has its assigned role and performs it in accordance with united to the each other. It is an arrangement of interdependent interactive parts based on functional relationship.
5. Social system has environmental aspect.
   Social system changes with the change in time. This change does not disturb the social equilibrium, but may be disturbed for some time. In spite of social changes social system continues to exist.
6. Social system has the quality of self-adjustment.
7. It is the system of interdependent action consists of mechanisms of socialisation and social control.

Pre-requisites

1. Biological, e.g: Family size.
2. Functional, e.g: Obedience to social norms, social control, interest towards positive action

3. Cultural, e.g: Language, symbols.
4. Communication, e.g: Social interaction can take place through language, symbols, scripts, gestures, telephone.

Social Values

'Cultural standards' which are desirable for organised social life. These are assumptions, which are important for society, they provide the ultimate meaning and legitimacy for social arrangements and social behaviour; these are ideals or the abstract sentiments. Social values are concern for group's welfare, these are organised within the personality of the individuals, regulates individual's thinking and behaviour, moulds personality. The desirable behaviour based on actions or ideas that fulfill the needs of communal life. Values are absorbed into the culture. If the social values are achieved, the social progress also noticed.

The value of a thing in its desirability or worth, value clusters around:

- Activities and attitudes which serves the needs of the group
- Customary or habitual ways of life requires little conscious adjustments
- 'Disturbance of one part of the complex, threatens others'—*Gillin and Gillin*

'Value' has different meanings related to varied dimensions, e.g: In economics—'value' denotes price; philosophical treatment—value is a part of ethics; social value—constituent part of social structure.

Definition

- 'Group conceptions of the relative desirability of things'—*GR Leslie and others*
- 'General standards regarded as higher order norms'—*HM Johnson*
- 'Assumption, unconscious of what is right and important'—*Young and Mack*

- 'A belief that something is good and 'worthwhile'—*Michael H*
- 'General conceptions of 'the good', ideas about the kinds of ends that people should pursue throughout their lives and many different activities in which they engage'—*Peter Worsley*

Meaning

Social values are measures of goodness or desirability. These provide general guidelines for the behaviour of the people. It is a part of culture, it explains the way, the social processes operate in a given society. These are the social sources of patterned interaction, maintain stability social order, serves as a guideline for conduct, facilitates social control. People will use values as a criteria where people can use in assessing their lives, arranging priorities, measuring their pleasure and pains, hosting alternative course of action.

Function

Provides goals or ends for the members to aim for:
- Maintains stabilities and uniformities in group interaction, social solidarity
- Brings legitimacy to the rules that govern specific activities and adjustment between different sets of rules.

Aspects of Values

General Values

More significant abstract and pervades in many aspects of life, e.g: Democracy, freedom, respect for fundamental rights, dignity of labour, patriotism, religious, social equality.

Specific Values

Range form highly abstract to specific level, e.g: Value for physical health.

Hierarchical arrangement of values:

a. Means values—'Instrumental values' efforts to achieve specific values.
b. Ends values—valuing the work, groups view, e.g: Enjoying the health as a fundamental right (end value) and mean value are adequate nutrition, hygiene, etc.
c. Dominant values—it influences the condition of the behaviour of the people to a great extent, e.g: Extensiveness, duration, intensity, prestige.
d. Ultimate value—it gives meaning, substance and direction to the lives of people, e.g: Attainment of physical health ultimate value is provision of longevity of life span.
e. Explicit value—clearly stated, deliberate thoughts, e.g: Enjoyment of democracy, freedom, fundamental rights, social quality.
f. Implicit value—leaders may not stress upon it, but implicitly related, e.g: Respect for elders, taking care of elder parents.

Conflicts Between Values

In a complex society, multiple values which are over-lapping and sometimes even opposing, e.g: Right to dissent, conformity, respect for authority and elders.

Social Security

The idea of social security springs from the deep desire of men to free them from the fear of want. The causes of insecurity must be removed, wherever possible, the individual must be assured of that protection against the common risks of life, which his own efforts do not avail to provide.

The social security has arisen out of the deep and eternal need of man for some measure of security for his immediate future. A man or a woman has to face a number of contingencies or risks right from birth. The contingencies includes unemployment, injury, accidents, occupational diseases, invalidity, disableness, childbirth, old age, burial, widowhood, orphanhood.

Definition

'Social security is the security that society furnishes, through appropriate organisation against certain risks to which its members are exposed'.

Social security is a programme of protection provided by society against those contingencies of modern life—sickness, unemployment, old age, dependency, industrial accidents and invalidism against which the individual cannot be expected to protect himself and his family by his own ability or foresight.

Main forms: Social insurance, public assistance, public service—all the social risks like incapacity to work, inability to find job, need for medical care can be covered. The benefits are paid as matter of right on the fulfillment of certain prescribed conditions according to a fixed scale.

Early history

The family unit of social organisation is the original cell of security. The reciprocal obligations of the parent to support the child in infancy and of the child to support the parent in old age are represented in social insurance by the solidarity of generations.

The family is the first line of defense, which can cope only with limited misfortune. The sense of responsibility of the larger group needs to be evoked and sustained by religious sanction.

Social Security in India

The care of the needy and the helpless has always been regarded as a pious duty. In the past, the institutions like joint family, the caste system, the village Panchayat and individual charity and philanthropy were instruments in affording protection to persons without means and without capacity to work. But the impact of western civilisation and the industrialisation of the country, these institutions have fallen into decay and are no longer able to meet the situation adequately. Some institutions to help orphans, widows, blind, deafness and other handicapped persons were started by voluntary organisations, but they are incapable of meeting of the challenge. It is now regarded as the duty of the state itself to promote social security.

A beginning in the social security programme was made in 1923, when the *Workmen's Compensation Act* was passed with benefits such as pension, provident fund, gratuity and some other welfare amenities for many years *like Maternity Benefit Act* also in force from 1929 onwards. *Employees State Insurance Act* is passed in 1948 onwards.

- Coal mines provident fund—1948.
- Sickness Insurance Act—1948 (old age pension)
- Bonus Scheme Act—1948
- Employees provident fund scheme—1952
- Industrial dispute (Amendment Act)—1953

Social Assistance

- Old age and invalid pensions—1957
- Mother's pension
- Unemployment assistance
- Medical benefit
- Rehabilitation of disabled persons
- Disability pension scheme—1962
- Handicapped pension scheme—1963
- Widow's pension scheme—1963

Services for Physically Handicapped

Physical handicapped includes all persons who have either completely lost the use of or can make only a restricted use of one or more of their physical organs. They are capable of performing all the functions of a normal person except in so far as they are limited by their handicap.

Categories

1. Persons lacking one or more physical sense, e.g: Blind, deafness or dumb
2. Orthopedically handicapped and crippled, e.g: Short limb, amputation
3. The defects of the internal organ of the body, e.g: Heart defects, TB, diabetes.

Suggestions to solve the problems of handicap

- Proper treatment
- Special grants and other aids
- Employment facilities
- Special training
- Asylum establishment
- Rehabilitation centre.

Services

- Old age pension scheme
- Homes for the aged
- Family foster care
- Medical assistance.

Mentally Handicap Services

- Help people to overcome inner conflict and to regain mental health
- Medical and psychiatric treatment
- Special orientation in education to develop mental outlook
- Education on mental hygiene
- Child guidance, counselling services has to be provided.

Social Mobility

It is the movement of individuals, families, and groups from one social position (social status) to another. The study of social mobility relates, present to a past social position. It thus forms part of the more general study of social selection, i.e. of low people get distributed into different social positions. It is hardly possible to study effectively the influence of past social position except in the context of other influences that determine the individual's present social status.

Types

Intergenerational Mobility

It compares the social position of parent and offspring.

Open society: Adult status of offspring is independent.

Closed society: Adult status of offspring is dependent on parent's social status.

Career Mobility

Compare the social positions of the same individual at different times.

Group Mobility

It is concerned with the changes in social position of groups possessing a relatively homogeneous status, e.g: Castes, intellectuals.

Changes in Social Position

Primary variations in:

- Occupation (Professional, entrepreneurial, clerical and skilled)
- Prestige
- Political and moral values
- Income
- Wealth
- Parental status
- Power
- Social class (Upper, middle, lower)
- Education
- Life span of individual

Societies are also sometimes viewed as being more or less open according to thee frequency with which social mobility occurs, e.g: High status parents' children fall to low social status. All children of low status parents achieve high status.

Social Mobility Table

The social positions between which movement may occur remain a series of discrete, qualitatively different categories. The study of social mobility is, however, closely related to questions concerning social achievement, and more particularly, concerning the role of the parental social position in determining final status, then to the amount of upward, downward mobility or the amount of non-movement.

Determinants

Father's Occupation

- Education and intelligence: That affect the son's occupational locus
- Race
- Occupational locus
- Knowledge
- Experience
- Incentives
- Opportunities for access to it.

Educational Level

The relation of education to status achievement is free from an intermediate dependence on parental status, and the effect of these variations on status certainly cannot be ascribed to parental status. There will be correlation between status achievement and education.

Intelligence

Part of the effect of education on status achievement is due to the correlation of education with intelligence. In the process of status selection, variations in intelligence operate to influence the achieved level of social status, both by leading to variations in educational level and by facilitating the advancement of those of greater intelligence.

Certain educational attainments have, however, become such decisive prerequisites for entry into many occupational positions that intelligence without the added attainment of a corresponding education is unable to produce its full potential effect. Dependence of achievement on motivational and other personality characteristics like intelligence has a major genetic component, parental intelligence has a major social component. Parental status, education and intelligence play a significant role in determining filial status.

Discrimination

The various modes of discrimination increase the dependence on parental status.

Other Social Handicap

The social handicaps are high-grade mental deficiency, physical disabilities, chronic disease, mental disorder, and alcoholism act as powerful handicap to occupational achievement.

Neglected Source of Downward Mobility

For example: Parent-son status relationship and unmarried and married subjects with or without children. Since marriage and sometimes fertility are associated with greater occupational stability, mental and physical health, general achievement. A neglect of those sources of influence in the parental occupational situation that exercise a direct influence on the son's occupational destiny by giving him special knowledge, incentives and opportunities with respect to particular occupations, the child will attain a given status position. The motivations and aspirations of young people in different sectors of society obviously play an important role in determining the manner in which various individual and family assets and handicaps exercise their influence.

Social Mobility and Social Structure

The relation of social selection and social mobility to the principal institutional structures of society. The occupational distribution process is a dual process, in which two sets of preferences and decisions, those of the employee and employer or manager, confront each other and that the distributive outcome is affected by the supply and demand of various qualities.

Even the most suitable political, juridical and economic institutions of a society are of capital importance for the mobility process. Thus, the occupational selection process in western society is decisively influenced by the nature of the labour contract, by laws relating to freedom of movement and ultimately by the distribution of political power, together with the political and social sentiments associated with this distribution.

Rights of Women

History and background of creating special rights in favour of women:

Women have been oppresses class around the globe in all societies at all times. In 1948 UNO (United Nations Organisation) made declaration of women rights, as per that 'Every individual born in this world is born with dignity, equality and equal rights'.

The early part of 19th century is a remarkable period as for as women movement is concerned. Social thinkers like *Raja Ram Mohan Roy, Keshav Chandra, Eswar Chandra Vidhya Sagar* and so on struggled hard to eradicate many social evils like *Sati*, child marriage, etc. At their instance in 1937 women secured right in the property left behind by her husband. In 1935 women were given political right to vote.

Post Independence Period

- After independence Indian constitution was drafted and which came into force from January 26th 1950. It made elaborate provisions for providing equal and special provisions for women.

- Article 14 guarantees to all citizens' equality before law and equal protection of laws.
- Under article 15 (3) for the advancement of women and children state is empowered to make special provisions, e.g: Reservations of seats in education, employment, etc.
- Article 21 guarantees right to life, that means to live with human dignity.
- Under 73rd amendment women have been given 1/3 rd reservation in Gram Panchayat and local bodies.

Criminal Procedure Code 1973

Under this a legitimate wife can claim maintenance, if her husband is living with another women and he has neglected to maintain her.

Hindu Law

Under Hindu law women have been given right of marriage, divorce, maintenance, adoption rights—which were denied to her earlier and right in the ancestral property and father's self acquired property.

Dowry Prohibition Act 1961

Under this Act, women have been given special rights. If any unnatural death takes place of bride within 7 years of her marriage, it is presumed to be dowry death unless proved otherwise. The punishment is imprisonment of not less than 7 years and it can get extended to the remaining period of life.

Factories Act 1948

To protect women labourers, it is the protection given to women labourers that they should not be employed near hazardous machines.

Maternity Benefit Act 1961

As per this Act, before the delivery women should be given 6 weeks holiday and after the delivery 6 weeks.

In case of abortion she should be given 6 weeks holiday with pay.

After delivery for the protection of child's health and until the baby is 15 months old she should be allowed to feed baby twice a day during working hours.

Minimum Wages Act 1948

Women have been given right to claim minimum wages fixed by the Government. Even though women agrees to work for less than the minimum wages she should not be allowed to do it.

To protect dignity of women in work places, in the case of *Vishakha and others vs State of Rajasthan* the Hon'ble Supreme Court has cast duty upon employer to see to it that women work in free and peaceful environment.

In cases where women are arrested on the allegation of having committed an offence they should be examined by women police only and arrested women should be kept in separate room.

Apart from passing from various laws the Government has also extended certain facilities. They are:

In district levels legal services authority has been set-up to extend free legal facilities for needy women.

National Commission for Women

Has been set-up, which makes various recommendations to Government for maintaining security of women at all places and bringing necessary constitutional amendments. It also deals with women adults, and family counselling centres.

In Karnataka under companies Act of 1956 women's development corporation has been set-up to identify women entrepreneurs and making facilities for bank loan and giving advice as to market the products of women entrepreneurs.

Conclusion

Though Government at all levels is trying its best to provide equal opportunities for women, it is for the society to make best use of it.

RIGHTS OF AN INDIVIDUAL IN DEMOCRATIC SOCIETY WITH SPECIAL REFERENCE TO INDIAN CONSTITUTION

Introduction

In a social system, individuals have to perform certain roles and fulfill the responsibilities by utilising their fundamental rights. Democracy is based on equality, liberty and fraternity. It is the duty of Government to conduct awareness campaigns to enhance the awareness of the public about their fundamental rights and duties so that they will function accordingly. Article III of the Indian Constitution has stated the 'Fundamental rights' of its citizens. These are regarded as the soul of the constitution.

Fundamental rights are essential to provide security and equality of citizenship and there by helping the process of nation building. To provide certain standards of conduct, citizenship, justice and fairplay. Rights are fruits of duties.

Definition

'Those conditions of social life without which no man can seek to be himself at his best'—*Laski*

'A legally enforceable right governing the relations between the state and the individual'—*PB Gajendra Gadkar*

Need of Fundamental Rights

It is a right of liberty permissible under the law, which enables an individual to develop his personality and his faculties to lead his life in his own interest and in the interest of the community as a whole. It is the responsibility of the Government to make all the citizens to appreciate that equality between one section and another in the matter of all those rights, which are essential for the material and moral perfection of man. It safeguards the individual from the encroachments of the legislature.

Fundamental Rights

Right to Equality

Article 15 prohibits any discrimination on grounds of religion, race, caste, sex, income, place of birth between citizens. It abolishes untouchability and ensures quality of opportunity in the matter of public employment. No citizen shall be unreasonably prevented from using wells, tanks, bathing ghats, roads and public resorts maintained wholly or partly out of state funds. Every citizen should be treated equally and alike, equal protection of laws will be ensured by this right implementation. Special provision may be made in favour of women and children, socially and economically backward classes of citizens.

Right of Freedom

Article 19 (1) of the constitution grants freedom to every citizen the right.

- Freedom of speech and expression
- Assemble peacefully and without arms
- Form association or unions
- Move freely across the length and breath of the country
- To reside or settle down in any part of India
- To own or dispose of property
- To practice any profession, trade or business
- Free to have friendly relations with foreign countries, public order any decency and good conduct
- The states are authorised to restrict the freedom of the press in order to check slanderous articles and promotion of disaffection towards or contempt of court.

Freedom of Religion

Article 25 indicates the freedom of religion that:

- All persons shall be entitled to freedom of conscience and the right to practise and propagate their religion freely
- Any religious institutions can be opened and function for the welfare of nation
- Article 28 warns against imparting religious instructions in any educational institution wholly maintained out of state funds; but it does not apply to institutions established under any endowment or trust
- Article 26 says that subject to public order, morality and health every religion shall have the right to establish and run institutions for religious and charitable purposes and to own, acquire and administer such property
- Article 27 prohibits raising funds through taxes to promote religion
- It gives secular character to our state.

Cultural and Educational Rights

Article 29 of the constitution allows all the minorities in India to preserve and promote their language, script and culture.

- It permits all the minorities whether based on language or religion to start and run their educational institutions and get financial aid without any discrimination from the state
- No citizen can be refused admission in any educational institution maintained or aided by the state.

Rights Against Exploitation

- Our constitution recognises the dignity of the individual and protects him against any form of exploitation either by the state or by the privileged classes in the society
- Article 23 prohibits forced labour and declares that slavery or use of women for immoral or other purposes is a punishable offense

- It prohibits the employment of children below 14 years in any factory or mine
- The state reserved to itself the right to secure compulsory service from the people for public purposes, e.g: Compulsory military training
- It has protected the people particularly women and children against maltreatment.

Right of Property

Article 31, 31A and 31B guarantee the right of the individual and trust to own and administer their property.

- No person shall be deprived of his property except by a lawful authority
- Without compensation, the state alone can compulsorily acquire any property for a public purpose.

Right to Constitutional Remedies

Article 32 provides for the enforcement of fundamental rights by the Supreme Court. It confers on the people the right to move the supreme court in case of encroachment on the fundamental rights by the state.

Right to Work

An individual can opt all the types of work according to his capacities, skills and talents, place of work also not restricted.

Right to Leisure

Individual can spend leisure time freely according to his interest in a constructive and conducive manner.

Right to Free Education and Material Security

Free education will be given by the Government up to university of education is implemented.

Every individual irrespective of sex, who is aged above 30 years and citizen of the nation, can be a candidate for the election irrespective of education or societal status.

Reservation for women and weaker societal sections in the Parliament legislation is available.

Minorities also suitably represented.

Any one who has the majority support in the legislation can become higher cadre like chief minister or prime minister irrespective of social status.

Unitary Elements of the Indian Constitution

Single Citizenship

All citizens are equal, the law guarantees equality of opportunity to every citizen irrespective of his place of birth, race, caste, sex or religion. They can move from one place to another without any problem of citizenship. Single citizenship curbs provincialism and promotes the feeling of oneness in the country.

Distribution of Powers Favours the Centre

It strengthens state and centre.

Proclamation of Emergency

The president can issue directives to the state Government, constitution of India empowers the president to declare emergency in the event of threat to the security of India whether by war, aggression or a major internal disturbance. When proclamation of emergency in an operation, the president can issue directives to the state government and thus empower the union parliament to make laws for the whole or any part of India with respect to any matter mentioned in the state list.

Extension of Union Parliament Authority

In normal times, it can be extended to the state list in terms of national interest, parliament becomes authorised to exact laws for one year period.

No Right of the States to Secede

Indian constitution does not give the states the right to frame separate constitutions or break away with the union.

Right of the parliament to temper with the territorial integrity of the states

The parliament is empowered to alter the boundaries and name of any state.

Unequal state representation in the council of states

The states are represented not uniformity but in proportion to their size and population.

Appointment and Removal of Governors by the President

The Governor holds office during his term, he has to report to the president about the state affairs and to execute the directions issued by the president in emergency times.

Centre's right to give directions to the states and supersede them in cases of non-compliance

If any state has failed to comply with or to give effect to, any directions given in the exercise of the executive power of the union under any of the provisions of the constitution.

Governor's powers to withhold the bills passed by the state legislature reserve them for the asset of the President

Governor can delay the implementation of the bills, which they do not like.

Right of parliament to enforce any treaty, agreement or convention

Parliament has power to make any law for the whole or any part of territory of India.

Power of parliament to legislate for 2 or more states by consent and adoption of such legislation by any other state

The same Government can rule both the centre and state or different Government for the centre and the state.

Constitution ensures uniformity in basic matters

Indian constitution provides for all administrative services uniform, civil and criminal codes, a controller and auditor general to guarantee for fair elections in the country.

Fundamental Duties of Citizen in Indian Society

- To abide by the constitution and respect its ideals and institutions, the National Flag and the National Anthem
- To cherish and follow the noble ideals which inspired our national struggle for freedom
- To uphold and protect the sovereignty, unity and integrity of India
- To defend the country and render national service when called upon to do so
- To promote harmony and the spirit of common brotherhood amongst all the people of India transcending religious, linguistic and regional or sectional diversities; to renounce practices derogatory to the dignity of women
- To value and preserve the rich heritage of our composite culture
- To protect and improve the natural environment including forests, lakes, rivers and wild life and to have compassion for living creatures

- To safeguard public property and to adjure violence
- To strive towards excellence in all spheres of individual and collective activity so that the nation constantly rises to higher levels of endeavour and achievement.

'We the people of India, having solemnly resolved to constitute India into a sovereign socialist secular democratic republic and to secure to all its citizens, justice, social, economic, political, liberty of thought, expression, belief, faith and worship, equality of status and of opportunity, to promote fraternity assuring the dignity of the individual, the unity and integrity of the nation, do hereby adopt, enact and give to ourselves this constitution'.

Responsibilities of an Individual in a Democratic Society

- Every individual should participate in the elections either as a voter or as a candidate, every individual aged 18 years or above has a right to vote
- Women should take part in the democratic process so that they have due representation in all public bodies, they can represent their grievances and their needs
- Minorities should feel themselves secure under the democratic rule
- An individual, who becomes a member of any legislation, parliament or any public institution should consider himself as a public servant and discharge his duties without fear or favour
- Religious freedom has to be given to everybody, that, they should not hate any other religion
- The abled individuals should join the defence forces and contribute their services in maintaining peace and tranquility.

The duties and responsibilities are mentioned in part IV-A "Fundamental duties of the Indian Constitution'.

WOMEN'S EMPOWERMENT

Introduction

The year, 2001 has been declared as a year of "Empowerment of women' by Government of India. It is a base for human liberation and empowerment for all. Achievement of equity and equal mindedness in society. Women are needed to be empower in all walks of life as it is multidimensional, e.g: Economic, social, political, education, health care, nutrition, and legal. Women's empowerment is a global issue, women empowerment is the control over material assets, intellectual resources and ideology. Empowerment of any society is possible only when women are empowered, strengthens family as a basic unit of any civic society. Family is a conducive instrument to empower women. It nurtures the potentials of women in different walks of life.

Definition

- 'It is the process of challenging existing power relations and of gaining greater control over the sources of power'.
- 'The manifestation of redistribution of power that challenges patriarchal ideology and male dominance'—*Chandra 1997*
- 'Process aimed at changing the nature and direction of systematic forces which marginalize women and other disadvantaged sections in a given context'—*Sharma 1992*
- 'It is a process of awareness and capacity building leading to greater participation to greater decision-making power and control and transformation action'
- 'It is a social process that neutralises women's oppression, women's decision to be empowered'.

Reasons for Choice of Women for Empowerment

- Willingness to be empowered by the women
- Intention to develop one's potential

- Interested to lead a meaningful life with productivity
- It has to be forced in all stages of life cycle
- Need of stronger positions to support others and to make substantial contributions to society
- It requires women to face the facts of their lives at all levels of social organisation.

Prerequisites of Empowerment

- Active participation in social economic and political spheres
- Process of decision making empowerment
- Desired self-respect
- Social dignity
- Involvement of women in decision-making process.

Levels of Empowerment

Welfare

The basic needs of women without attempting to solve the structural causes, provision of welfare services.

Access

To make meaningful progress, equality of access to resources, e.g: Educational opportunities, land and credit. The path of empowerment is initiated when women realise their lack of access to resources as a barrier to their growth and development and take action.

Conscientisation

Women has to take appropriate action to close gender gaps of gender inequalities, they have to recognise the role they can play in reinforcing the system that restricts their growth.

Participation

Women should take decisions along with men equally. Mobilisation of women is necessary by organising themselves and working collectively. Women will be empowered and gain increased representation which will lead to increased empowerment and ultimately greater control.

Control

The balance of power between men and women should be equal, they should not dominant with other. Women are able to make decisions over their lives and childrens'lives and play an active role in the development process.

Phases and Aspects of Women Empowerment for Collective Empowerment

- Women can be independent and they will be empowered in diverse social settings
- They can develop their own religious beliefs and practices. It will be helpful for women to search for survival and fulfillment
- Mutual support in work setting and outside home is vital to women empowerment through work
- Women connect their biographies with history, seeing the influence of broad social structure on their lives, they will be empowered
- Mutual support of women is necessary.

Categories

Empowerment or
- Marginal groups
- Process-oriented
- Holistic nature
- Strategic
- Cognitive, psychological and economic components
- Democratisation
- To understand the character of literacy that empowers
- Context
- Sustainability

Qualitative Indicators

- Increase in self-esteem, knowledge on women's health, nutrition, reproductive rights, legal rights, literacy, etc.
- Changes in role and responsibilities in the family and in the community
- Changes in social customs, e.g: Child marriages, dowry, discrimination
- Visible increase or decrease in levels of domestic and other forms of violence
- Increase participation in public meetings and training programs
- Formation of women groups, self-help groups, DWACRA groups
- Positive change in social attitude among the community members
- Women's economic contribution in sharing family responsibilities
- Increased decision-making power related to work, income and expenditure in her control.

Quantitative Indicators

- Demographic trends
- Number of women participating in different development programs, political processes at local level
- Access and control over community resources and Government schemes
- Visible changes in health, nutritional status, changes in literacy.

STATUS

Every individual in the society or social organisation occupies a particular status. It may be high or low. Social change also is based on change of status and role. Social status is the position of an individual within social relationships. It is recognised by a pattern of symbols, actions, prestige and respect.

Advantages of Women Empowerment

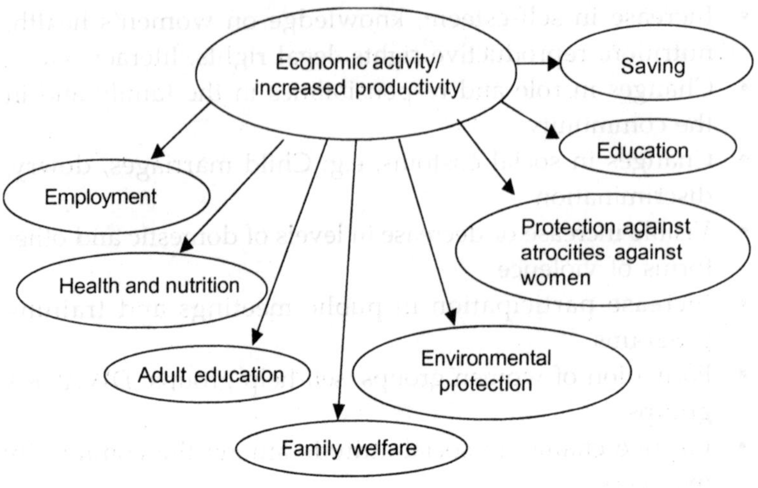

Definitions

- 'It is the position, which the individual occupies in the group by virtue of his sex, age, family, class, occupation, marriage and achievement'—*Elliott and Merrill*
- 'It represents the position of the individual in the group'—*Ogburn and Nimkoff*
- 'A defined position in the social structure linked to a social role, i.e. a pattern of expected behaviour'.
- 'A position in the social system'.
- 'A ranked position in a social hierarchy or stratification system, an individual's social standing in society'.
- 'The place in a particular system, which an individual occupies at a particular time will be referred to his status with respect to that system'—*Linton*
- 'To designate the comparative amounts of prestige, difference or respect accorded to persons who have been assigned different roles in group or community'.
- 'The worth of a person as estimated by a group or a class of persons'—*Secord and Bukman*

- 'Position in the general institution system, recognised and supported by the entire society spontaneously evolved rather than deliberately created, rooted in the folkways and mores'—*Davis*
- 'Location of an individual within the group, his place to the social network of reciprocal obligations, privileges, duties and responsibilities'—*HT Mazumdar*

Types

1. *Ascribed status:* By virtue of birth, without any individual effort, e.g: Nationality, religion, caste.
2. *Achieved status:* By his own efforts or capabilities; social position is secured through individual choice, e.g: Placement of an individual in an organisation.

Determinants of Ascribed Status

Sex differences—In Indian society, men are accorded with high and dominant status in the family and in the community; lower status have been given to the women.

Age—In traditional societies elders are respected and youngsters are under the control of older generation.

Family and kinship—Members are ascribed to status according to the family to which they belong. Each family will have a name. The status of a person is judged according to the name of his family, e.g: Based on the family name, fixation of marriage occurs.

Physical attributes—Beauty of a female; well built physique in male will increase person's esteem in the society.

Race—In America, white race always have superior status when compared to black and Mongoloid.

Caste—In Indian society Brahmins, Vysyas will be given a high status.

Determinants of Achieved Status

Wealth—It gives power to an individual, controls other individuals by the power of wealth.

Rewards—Persons are awarded high status if their attributes are rewarding to each member of the group.

Occupation—Certain occupations like doctors, teachers, engineers are more reputed in the society than others.

Political authority—Ministers, MLA, MPs, Government officials will hold high status.

Marriage—Automatically it gives a status of husband, wife, son-in-law, brother-in-law, sister-in-law, mother-in-laws.

Individual achievements—In the field of education, occupation, sports, literature, art and science will give high status. According to their efforts, talents and abilities individual will achieve the status.

Nature of Social Status

To designate the comparative amounts of prestige, respect, accorded to persons, who have been assigned different roles in a group or community; if the person's role is important in the organisation, he will achieve high status. Thus status indicates/place/the location of the individuals within the social network.

Elements

- Status is a part of the whole society
- Society is divided into different groups based on status
- Status is determined by the cultural situation and relevance of other members in the society.

Importance

An individual wins respect in society by virtue of social status. Symbols of respect change along with social status. Different roles are conjoined with different social status. Differentiation in status within the society facilitates division of work among the people, based on their ability. It indicates a particular back ground, a person is known by his society to which he belongs. It influences the individual life, the society to which he belongs and the personality; certain cultural activities will be performed based on social status, e.g: Marriages, it entitles to enjoy several roles and specialisation of functions, promotes sense of responsibility and cooperative living.

Differences between ascribed status and achieved status

Ascribed Status	*Achieved Status*
By birth (Nationality, family)	By the result of individual efforts, abilities and potentialities
No pre-condition for the status (Elder in the family is bound to be respected)	Pre-conditions are necessary (Ability, efficiency, status)
Based on age, sex, race, caste and kinship	Based on capacities, abilities and characteristics
Stable and rigid	Unstable and flexible
In traditional societies it occupies respect	In modern societies based on achievements and personal qualities respect can attained

SOCIAL ROLES

Introduction

'A set of behaviours expected a member who occupies a particular position in the group'. The expected role of each member in a specific group will be specified, e.g: Father in the family is holding responsible role to feed the members of the family; an employee in an organisation will perform the activities specified by the employer. Individual members of a group may develop perceptions of their own roles; it differs in the degree of their clarity and compatibility. The higher the clarity, the greater is member's and group performance and satisfaction. The role of a person is determined by his social status. Social roles are part and parcel of an individual's behaviour when interacting with other people in various situations.

Members will play several roles:

- Task-related
- Relation-oriented
- Self-oriented

The same individual may have to perform different roles at the same time in a group, e.g: A girl is a daughter to her parents, sister to brother, wife to husband, teacher (based on occupation) to the students. If the social organisation has to function in a proper manner when social status and roles function effectively. Status and role has to be defined clearly; Roles are continuously changing and multiplying. Role represents dynamic aspect of status.

Definition

- 'A set of expectations and behaviours associated with a specific position in a social system or a certain group situation'.
- 'The part a person plays as a result of each status'—*Elliott and Merrill*
- 'A set of socially expected and approved behaviour pattern consisting of both duties, privileges associated with a particular position in a group'—*Ogburn and Nimkoff*
- 'Pattern of behaviour applying to persons occupying specific positions or fulfilling definable functions in the society'.
- 'An obligation which an individual has towards his group'.

Attributes Related to Role

- *Peripheral attributes:* Optional which will admit alternatives, peripheral characteristics which may not alter the role status.
- *Sufficiently relevant:* Certain attributes if they are absent, the relevancy of the role will be lost.
- *Basic or pivotal attributes:* Absence or variation of certain attributes changes the whole identity of the role and the interaction which will normally provoke.

Types

- *Occupational role/Service role:* For fulfilling definable functions, allotting to the individuals certain position/role, rendering services to others which involve in contractual relationship.
- *Recruitment role:* 'The authority which will have function of recruiting employees in an organisation'.
- *Achievement role:* 'Individuals are free to choose as a goal or objective'.
- *Asymmetrical role:* 'No precise hierarchy, no definite focus or pivot I the series, e.g: Friend, enemy, lover, patriot'.
- *Interactive role:* 'Role are designed to meet/interplay having a given efficiency'.
- *Distributive role:* 'Indirectly interactive representing the basic fact about all roles, e.g: Belief, origin, age, residence, personality'.
- *Authority/supervisory/leadership role:* 'Influences the group members behaviour and functions'.
- *Expressive role:* 'They communicate the ideas, emotional experiences through manipulating, applying odds expressive symbols current in the society'.
- *Dependent role:* e.g: Wife role in the family, employee's role in an establishment.
- *Independent role:* e.g: Conducting a research project by the investigator.

Relationship Between Role and Status

Status	*Role*
Determined by socio-cultural values and related to other members of the group which is justifiable	Based on position and expected performance in a specified group, it is also influenced by societal situations and other members of the group
Almost all the societies have similar status	Roles are expressed in different forms
Properly understood in the background of social aspirations and ambitions	Properly understood the roles in the requirements of society

Contd...

Contd...

Represents only a part of social set-up	Different individuals performs different roles
According to the status the society is divided into different groups of various categories, ranks	Society is not divided but based on roles
Provides prestige and respect	Role discharges in relation to the prestige of status and value attached

Terminology

- *Social role*: The pattern of expected behaviour of a person occupying a particular position in the group
- *Role expectation:* The behaviour prescribed for an individual occupying a given position in the group
- *Role conception*: The way the individual perceives his role, which may be different from the way it is perceived by others
- *Role acceptance:* The degree to which the individual finds his role compatible with his values, needs and self-concept
- *Role performance (role behaviour):* The way in which the individual actually plays or performs his role in group
- *Role conflict:* The contradictory role demands resulting from multiple group memberships, e.g: Wife role in the family, conflicts with her administrative role in a social institution.

Previous Years University Questions

1. Explain social mobility. (5 m, RGUHS, 2000)
2. What are social norms. (2 m, RGUHS, 2001)
3. Social mobility. (5 m, RGUHS, 1997, 2000,01, 03)
4. What is meant by social system. (3 m, RGUHS, 2002)
5. What are norms. (2 m, RGUHS, 2002)
6. Define social system. (2 m, RGUHS, 2000, 03)
7. Role and status. (2 m, RGUHS, 2003,04)
8. Principle types of social system. (2 m, RGUHS, 2001)
9. Rights of women. (5 m, RGUHS, 2002)
10. Education and social mobility. (5 m, RGUHS, 2002)

11. Define social role. (2 m, RGUHS, 2002)
12. Explain 'life style' . (2 m, RGUHS, 1999)
13. Types of social system. (5 m, RGUHS, 1999)
14. Examine the different social systems of society. (5 m, RGUHS, 2001)
15. Social distance and social mobility.(2 m, RGUHS, 2002)
16. Critically examine where's concept of stain a power. (NTRUHS, 1991, 5M)
17. Norms of behaviour. (2 m, RGUHS, 1999)
18. Describe the social legislations related to Indian women. (13 m, SVIMS, 2002)

MGR University Question Papers

1. Social structure. (5 m, MGRU)

CHAPTER SIX

Socialisation

INTRODUCTION

At birth the human being comes to the world, as a biological organism with animal needs subsequently in a gradual manner moulds into a social being. Individual acquires the ways in dealing with social activities. Man is not only social, but also cultural. Culture provides and moulds personality. This process of social training is called, 'Socialisation'. It affects personality development of its members. Socialisation and culture conditions the personality. Thus socialisation is a process of learning that enables the learner to perform social roles and ability to participate in social system.

Definition

- 'The process of working together, developing group responsibility or being guided by the welfare needs of others'—*Bogardus*
- 'The process by which the individual learns to conform to the group norms'—*Ogburn*
- 'The process of transmission of culture, whereby individuals learn the rules and practices of social groups'—*Peter Worsley*

- 'It enables the learner to perform social roles and transmits culture'—*Harry M Johnson*
- 'Complex process of interaction through which the individual learns the habits, beliefs, skills and standards of judgment that are necessary for his effective participation in social groups and communities'—*Lundberg*
- 'The process by which the human beings establishes wider and profound relationship, dependent, sense of obligation and responsibility for one to another, in which individuals develops personality of themselves and other to form a complex social situation'—*Maciver*
- 'The process of educating the individual into the social and cultural world, making him a particular member in society and its various groups by inducting him to accept the norms and values of the society'—*Kimball Young*
- 'The development of we feeling in associate and their growing capacity and will act together'—*Ross*
- 'The individual develops into a functioning member of the group according to its standards, conforming to its modes, observing its traditions and adjusting himself to the social situations'—*Gillin and Gillin*
- 'The child acquires a cultural content along with selfhood and personality'—*Green*
- 'One internalises the norms of his groups so that a distinct 'self' emerges, unique to that particular individual'—*Horton and Hunt*
- 'Original nature is transformed into human nature and the individual into person'—*Mazumdar*

Concept of Socialisation

Human behaviour is acquired. The existence of society and social processes is possible with socialisation. Individual exposed himself to the varied experiences in the society, follows the procedures and practices of social groups and develops his distinct personality. The individual shares the culture of the group and acquires the ways of behaviour through methods of learning, e.g: Imitation, conditioning, and specific training.

Meaning

The newborn is moulded into a social being through the process of socialisation. It shapes the total personality of the individual; he follows the norms, regulations and performs social roles, develops social assets. The individual acquires the conventional patterns of human behaviour. Every man tries to adjust himself to the condition and environment predominantly determined by the society of which he is a member. It designates all the social processes and pressures by which the norms and standards of the group or community are inculcated in the beliefs and behaviour of individual members. He acquires a set of attitudes, habits, skills, standards, values, likes, dislikes, goals, and purposes, judgments and a pattern of behaviour that are necessary for individual's effective participation in social groups and communities. The child acquires through socialisation cultural content along with social bond. The individual tries to adjust to the condition and environment in the society. The process of adjustment is called as 'socialisation'. He establishes good interpersonal social relationships.

In a nutshell, it can be said that, socialisation is a learning process initiated at birth continues through the life processes and ends at death.

Aims

- To become social and cultural being
- To maintain social order by following social norms, standards
- To develop hidden or latent talents in order to have contended life

- To lead qualitative, meaningful life
- To learn and fulfill social roles
- For existence of specified pattern of behaviour
- To mould and shape total personality of the individual.

Characteristics

- Continuous process
- Tool for transmission of culture
- Learning process
- Establishes limits on the individual through social interaction.

Importance

The individual becomes as a person and expresses himself more effectively the hidden and latent talents through the process of socialisation. Through constant training, the newborn child transforms into social being by moulding his personality. It prepares the child to lead approved way of social life, at the same time the individuality also develops. Through socialisation, the individual learns the values, ideals, aims, objectives of life and the means of attaining them. Socialisation makes the individual to become socially disciplined and helps him to live according to the social expectations.

Each individual has to maintain various social roles in his life and every role is having their own expected specified set of attitudes and norms. The socialisation assists him to learn the norms associated with roles imparting skills, which are essential for effective social life (economic, professional, educational, religious and political roles, etc.) are transmitted to younger generations. Socialisation helps the individual to develop right aspirations, which are complementary to the interests of society. It directs or channelises the whole energy for the realisation of total aspirations and desires fulfillment.

According to the cultural goals, ideals, traditions the individual leads social life. It contributes to the stability of social order. Socialisation reduces the social distance between different caste, class, religion and disorganisation. It brings people together, guides them the ways to solve social problems. It changes the destiny of the individual for a bright future. Transmits culture from one generation to other. Thus socialisation is a social learning.

Process

Socialisation process starts before the birth of the child and continues until death associates with various life processes. Prenatal care forms an integral part in family welfare activities. The activities such as parents' marital selection, marital life, customs related to pregnancy and birth and the whole family cultural practices, etc. are important for the child's growth. Thus the social circumstances precedes the childbirth affects a large extent on the child's life, which indirectly influences his growth in society. Socialisation is a process, where the individual is entering into social life through the process of social learning. Direct socialisation will take place after birth only. Man's behaviour is influenced by reflexes, instincts, surges, capacities, comprehension and educability. Each individual tries to adjust himself through socialisation to the conditions of his social environment. The gradual development of 'self' or ego where the personality shapes and mind starts functioning.

Factors in Socialisation Process

Imitation

The child learns the social behaviour patterns through imitation. It may be spontaneous, deliberate, conscious, perceptual, ideational or unconscious. Child performs social activities exactly, which he observes (imitates others' activities). He learns language, pronunciation through imitation. They imitate indiscriminately the same personalities like family members, teachers, close friends.

Suggestion

It can be given through languages, pictures or certain/specified media, communication transformed from one to another, rational persuasion can be given by means of influencing the behaviour with others. In the field of education, occupation, trades industry, politics, etc. people will be acquainted. Propaganda, advertisement are based on principles of suggestion. Suggestibility of an individual decreases as the age advances, here the mental maturity is heightened. Intellectual ability, temperament, educational levels, emotional excitement influences the pattern of suggestibility.

Identification

Identification increases as the age advances. It is sociable. In the childhood, the activities are random and cannot be able to distinguish between organism and environment. As the child grows, he will identify the things, which will satisfy his needs. Such things become the objectives of identification.

Language

Language is the powerful medium of social interaction. It is a means of cultural transmission. Language is a key factor, which moulds the personality of the individual.

Role of Socialisation

Socialisation is important factor in total personality development. The human behaviour and mentality will be developed through the process of socialisation, e.g: A child who is kept all alone in a isolated room and brought out after few years, the child cannot talk, walk or do anything. He was expressionless and indifferent to everything and cannot move on his own. The child is unaware of social relationship. The absence of socialisation will affect the communication and contact. Later efforts were made to teach the child, first the response was less; later responded, ultimately reached to the normal level of development. Isolation, deprivation of communication affected the child's behaviour.

Theories of Socialisation/Development of the Self

The core/essence of socialisation is the development of the self. According to *Cooley,* self is 'I' 'me' or 'myself'. According to *Murphy,* 'A person what he is consciously or unconsciously conceives himself to be the self-concept, total perception about himself especially, attitude towards himself'.

The child at birth is not conscious of any of the self and other relationships. The fulfillment of his development will be possible through socialisation. Biological organism will transform into self by possessing sense of identity endowed with values, ideals and ambitions. For individualisation, socialisation is a must. 'Self' is a social product.

Cooley's Theory (Looking-glass self)

American social psychologist, *Charles Horton Cooley* made sustained attempt to explain the concept of self. He placed two primary propositions.

1. Mind is social.
2. Society is mental.

Self and society are twinborn, two sides of a coin. He concluded that the idea of 'self or ego or I' can arise only in relationship with other people. Our ideas, loyalties, attitudes, view points are derived from others. Self-ideas, self-attitudes developed by imagining process elements.

- Our imagination or perceptions of how we look to others
- Our perception of their judgment of how we look

- Self feelings like pride or mortification about these judgments.

The self-knowledge is gained from primary group, i.e family, later by secondary groups. Man will not form opinion by himself, when others' perception, feelings, opinions about him observed or witnessed, he develops the process of self. The perception and reaction of others gives an idea of their social self. The individual perception may differ from the images others have or actually formed. Significant variation between individual's perception and others' perception may be noticed. This theory assures the child and their assumed roles, i.e. praise, blame, acceptability, unacceptability in terms of others. Thus, it is clear that we are prone to look at ourselves through others' eyes. Depending upon others views, man develops his attitudes according to this theory. Thus Cooley concluded that the self is social and self-conscious would not exist in the absence of society, where as the individuals normally have their own attitudes towards social roles and adopts the same, the self thus arises when the person becomes an object to himself.

George Herbert Mead's Theory

According to *Mead,* American social psychologist, through social interaction man becomes aware of himself, the individual comes to know about himself by 'role playing'. The individual in order to get picture of himself, plays the role of others, but putting himself in the place of others; the others includes family members, teachers, friends, associates, colleagues, community. Thus the child is enabled to see himself objectively from the eyes of others. Self is the product of social interaction arises in social experience constantly changing and adjusting to new situations. Thus self grows in a social context, i.e. communicative contact with others.

Sigmund Freud's Theory

According to *Freud*, Austrian psychiatrist (father of modern psychology), self and society are not identical. Human mind consists of three components: Id—works on pleasure principle and represents instinctive desires, Ego is working on reality principle and acts with ideals, norms, Super Ego works on morality principle.

W I Thomas Theory

The situation in which the child finds himself has already been defined for him. Group, where the child is born determines the norms, rules and regulations, which the child has to follow. The child cannot behave according to his own wishes, he must compromise his wishes with societies' expectations or wishes. Society frames order, discipline for the child to follow. Any deliberate action calls for an appraisal of the situation within which the person finds himself. Once the situation is defined for him, he can act appropriately in it in the normal life. First, the primary caregivers, i.e. parents frames the social situation for the child.

Durkheim's Theory

The individual becomes socialised by adopting the group behaviours, i.e. 'collective representations'. The individual unconsciously depends upon his society for his ideas, attitudes and behaviour. The group frames standards, rules what the child has to follow.

Stages of Socialisation

Socialisation is a gradual continuous process of social learning, where the newborn child throughout life processes acquiring the social values, standards, norms to lead productive social life. It proceeds from simplicity to complexity. Socialisation will be carried out through social groups and social institutions, where the child adjusts and learns to adapt and confirms him within the broader social network, performs the social roles effectively. The internalisation of social roles performed by him and with other persons is spectatory. The child must internalise the roles that he is expected to perform by him and the roles of others with whom he interacts. At each stage of socialisation the child internalises a system of roles.

The Oral Stage (First Stage)

By crying, the child establishes dependency and over hunger drive. It starts from birth and continues up to one year. In womb the child enjoys comfortable environment, as he comes out, he has to face first crisis, i.e. must breath, exert himself to feed, must be protected from physical discomforts, child learns to give signals for his felt needs. The child is involved in him and his mother. Internalisation of two roles is difficult for the child. It is the stage of 'primary identification' as the child merges his identity with that of the mother.

The Anal Stage (Second Stage)

During the toddler period the child exhibits anal stage. It varies based on society, social class and family. The child completely not dependent on mother, he starts to take some degree of care for himself like toilet training, wearing clothes, etc. the child internalises two separate roles, i.e. himself and his mother. The child learns to receive love and care and return by smiling. He is able to distinguish between right and wrong correct action is rewarded and incorrect action is punished. Mother, the primary caregiver plays a dual role, she participates in the interaction of child and family, mediates between sub-system and larger system, flexible in nature, yielding to the child's demands and some other times resisting its tendencies.

The child has to express his aggression withholds faeces or releasing at wrong time. The positive sanction for correct performance is mother's love. The child contributes by means of expressive, helps to integrate the system by cooperating and giving love. However, the child is, too young and dependent, to contribute very much for task accomplishment.

Oedipal Stage (Third Stage)

It starts from pre-school period extends up to puberty. The child becomes as a member of the family as a whole. The child wants to identify himself on the basis of sex. The boy develops 'Oedipus complex'—love towards mother and jealousy towards father. The girl exhibits 'Electra complex'—love to father and jealousy towards mother. Sufficient social pressures are brought on the child to identify with the right sex. Boys and girls should act according to their sexes, boys' tries to identify with father and girls with mother. The children will establish or develops their own groups/gangs.

Adolescence Stage (Fourth Stage)

A physiological and psychological change takes place within the individual. The adolescents are free from parental control, at the same time they cannot completely decide on their own. Parents restrict the adolescent from moving with the opposite sex groups. In the modern society the parents gives freedom for children by allowing them to do their activities independently. Adolescents will have less social control, will learn new social roles, new behaviour patterns internalise with them. Parents advise them in the field of education, occupation, and life-partners.

TYPES CLASSIFICATION

I. Ian Robertson (1977) has classified socialisation into four types

a. Primary Socialisation

It occurs in the early life of the child; family, friends, playmates are primary agencies, through which the language, cognitive skills, cultural norms, values, emotional ties and appreciation of roles and perspectives will be learned. Internalisation of norms is essential aspect of primary socialisation, the process in which the norms of society becomes a part of the personality of the individual. The child acquires the norms by methods of learning, i.e. doing, trail and error, observation, experiencing, and conditioning. The child learns correct desirable and moral behaviour through primary socialisation. They reinforce the childs' learning by means of approval, rewards and punishments.

b. Anticipatory Socialisation

The individual learns his own group culture and other groups' culture also. *Merton* defined, 'A process by which individuals socialise themselves into the culture of a group with anticipation of joining that group is anticipatory socialisation', e.g: Two persons of different religion desire to marry and lead a happy family life. So in anticipation of joining to other group both tries to learn opposite norms. Thus people are socialised throughout their life at different intervals.

c. Developmental Socialisation

It builds on already developed skills and knowledge as the adult progresses through new situations. It requires new expectations, obligations and roles. As learning is continuous new knowledge will be added and make the individuals to adapt to the situations. e.g: Graduate nurse is appointed as clinical nurse in super specialty areas to acquaint with super specialty ward routines and procedures, will like to attend in-service training programmes, workshops, seminars, review discussions in order to develop familiarity and accommodate satisfactorily to the present situation.

d. Re-socialisation

The stripping away of learned patterns and substitution of new ones for them is re-socialisation. It occurs when social role is radically changes or in periods of rapid social mobility, e.g: Two persons of two different continents meet together and desires to lead family life according to the societal norms especially the couple has to change/adapt their roles to different roles according to new situation.

Classification

a. Child Socialisation

It is very easy to mould the personality of the child. Socialisation will starts from childhood, child learns basic social values, develops characteristics, positive attitudes, cultural norms, customs and traditions. It highlights the formal aspects, e.g: Children tend to see their teachers as authority figures. Children will have ideal expectations and free from conflicts and will accept and submit to the authority. Childhood socialisation is more generalised.

b. Adult Socialisation

Socialisation is a lifelong, continuous process, never it ends in between. Adult has to fulfill several responsibilities in life and he should have the ability to form a family of one's own, he should support himself and his family entirely independently. Adult socialisation is easier because adult is self-motivated to win the goals, which he set in his life, internalisation of various roles, which he has to perform. Communication, language are the main socialisation agents during adulthood. If the complex skills has to be achieved by an individual socialisation, which is a difficult and prolonged process, e.g: Rural citizen has to survive in a sophisticated, complicated society. First the individual will face little difficulty and takes time to accommodate himself for the new environment.

The society has to motivate properly so that adults will develop appropriate skills and values by performing adequate social role. Learning is easy if it is anticipatory socialisation. Adult socialisation is more likely to change overt behaviour, e.g: Assuming parental role in adulthood but the basic views about sharing, concern, love, understanding, cooperation were formed in childhood. Adult socialisation stresses the informal nature of social positions like treating the person as individuals. Adults realize the difference between social expectations and ideal behaviour. Adults gain specific skills pertaining to his roles. The norms and attitudes are already established during childhood, if he has to develop new skills and to change the attitudes, it may be a difficult process, e.g: If the individuals marry at correct age it is easy to accept and accommodate themselves for the change in social role and they can mould easily, whereas for the couple marrying at late age face difficulty in adjusting to the new roles.

Socialisation reduces social distance and increases the nearness. Socialised individuals will not perform any anti-social and non-productive activities. Adult socialisation is essential to maintain qualitative life and standards of society.

Agencies

Socialisation is an endless process, it starts from birth continues upto death. The child valued more for, 'what he will be' than for 'what he is'. Socialisation helps the child to become a useful member of the society. It provides social maturity by means of social learning. Certain socialising agents will have direct influence in moulding the personality of the individual. Socialisation is an interaction process whereby person's behaviour is modified and he will perform the social activities upto the ideal social expectations and values, norms and standards that are held by the members of the group, which they belong. There are two sources for child socialisation:

a. Those who have authority over the child.

b. Who are equal in authority to them, e.g: Friends, colleagues, and playmates.

Socialisation should proceed through authoritarian modes. The child must be given the power and command, obedience. The child expresses his personality through social interaction. The child learns morality, cooperation, folkways, secret modes through family, friends as a cooperative effort.

Family and Parents

Family is the primary agency, which socialises the child early in his social life. Mother, the primary caregiver is the first socialising agent, which will have a great impact on the child's personality; child's capacities and abilities will be developed by parental influence. The child learns culture, communication pattern, language, social morality, respect qualities like toleration, self-sacrifice, love, affection and cooperation are developed through family. Child acquires the pattern of establishing good social interpersonal relationship and interaction pattern through family environment.

Family continues to exercise control or influence over the child's life. Family is the significant group and an active, informal social agency. Family members are nearer and closer to the child and are confirmed to the family norms. Child's socialisation has to be controlled through institutional channels.

School

The child gets his education, which moulds his personality, develops ideas and attitudes. Education brings change in the behaviour of an individual. Well planned system of education will produce good citizens and socially defined personalities. It helps in social progress by inculcating the ideas of equality, fraternity, literacy and social justice. It raises societal standards, prepares the individuals to lead a happy and prosperous life. It promotes the work efficiency and capacities of an individual. It paves the way for real democratic living. It develops group feeling, joint planning and good interpersonal relationship. School enables every child to have higher status within the society; recognises the individual differences within the group and encourage the child to develop higher efficiency, good productivity by developing his career. It enhances the standards of living, child acquires and transmits culture within the school.

Teachers

Teacher plays a prominent role in socialising the child. Next to parents, teachers have greater influence on the child's life. Teachers help the child to develop matured personality and child imitates and follows the instructions laid by the teacher. Child tries to identify them with the teacher.

Playmates, Peer Group/Friends

Child learns some informal aspects of facts and facets of culture, finds clues and modes of gratification, e.g: Fashion through his contemporaries. The relationship between child and their friends is based on equality, morality, cooperation and mutual understanding. During adolescence the child will give more importance to the peer group than family and school. 'Peer group culture' will become effective than 'parental culture'.

Religion

It promotes bond of unity and moulds the beliefs and ways of life. Religious ceremonies will shape the ideas of individuals. It controls the behaviour of an individual, determines the course of life and shows the ideals.

Literature and Mass Media

The ideas, public opinion, attitudes, ideologies, tradition and culture are transformed through literature.

State

It is an authoritarian agency and forms laws, rules, norms of society. It lays down the modes of conduct expected from the individuals. Compulsorily they have to follow and adjust their behaviour in accordance with the laws otherwise they will be punished. Thus the state controls the society.

Elements of Socialisation

Three elements plays an important role in the process of socialisation:

1. Physical and psychological heritage of an individual
2. Environment in which he is born
3. Culture—norms, attitudes, role, performance of social activities

Socialisation promotes human welfare and individual gain/ capacities. The improvement of socialisation offers greatest possibility for the future alteration of human culture and society.

SOCIAL INTERACTION

Society is a web of social relationships, which is established through the process of social interaction. Man is a socio-cultural being and society is both natural and necessary for man. Man is gregarious in nature he cannot live alone for long time. He always lives in association with groups. Members of the other group members will affect the behaviour of each individual. The interaction is essential for social life. It establishes mental relations among the persons and the individuals tend to be influenced by the ideas, achievements and emotions of others. It is reciprocal, mutual in nature and is influenced by inter-stimulation and response. Social interaction is communicative in nature and is a simple form of social process by which the individual attempts to do certain action and establish common reactions. Thus interaction is the basic ingredient of social relationships. Society is deep rooted in social interaction.

Definition

- 'The mutual influences that individuals and groups have on one another in their attempts to solve problems and in their striving towards goals'—*Green*
- 'The reciprocal influence human beings exert on each other through inter-stimulation and response'—*Gish NP*
- 'It is a process whereby men interpenetrate the minds of each other'—*Dawson and Gettys*
- 'It is the general process whereby two or more persons are in meaningful contact as a result of which their behaviour is modified, however slightly'—*Eldredge and Merril*

Elements of Social Interaction

Without social interaction there is no group life. It will have definite influence on social relationships. It is of dual in nature. *Park and Burgers* describes two essential **elements** in social interaction.

1. Social contact
2. Communication

Social Contact

It is first phase of social interaction. Strengthens by physical contact, establishes through the medium of some sensory organ. Any object can be perceived by the sensory stimulation and causes communication with that sensory organ. Hence the means of communication (mass media, language, script, gestures, symbols, telegraph services, SMS, MMS) are essential adjuncts of social contacts. Social contacts may be temporary (contact with colleagues) or permanent in nature. Social contacts can be positive (cooperation, association, assimilation) as well as negative (hatred, jealousy, conflict). Human interaction is essentially communicative interaction.

Communication

Without communication social interaction and socialisation of individual will not take place. The society cannot conceive the ideas without communication, communication is the process, by which ideas, facts, impressions, feelings, information, etc. facilitates through the process of social interaction. Communication is the process for transmission of ideas to other persons. Communication facilitates desirable response and is a two way process both vertically and horizontally in a spirit of 'give and take' or 'send and receive'. Communication is a basic instinct of life, fundamental social process through communication individual shares their experiences with others.

It is a process by which two or more people exchange ideas, facts, feelings, impressions in ways that each gains a common understanding of message. Sender and receiver tuned together for a particular or series of messages.

Principles of Communication

Clarity, consistency, adequacy, timing and distribution, acceptability, adoptability, uniformity, conviction, appropriate, applicability, objective, purpose oriented, intention, attention, perception, active participation, credibility, context, continuity, compatibility, contact, familiarity, utilisation of available facilities.

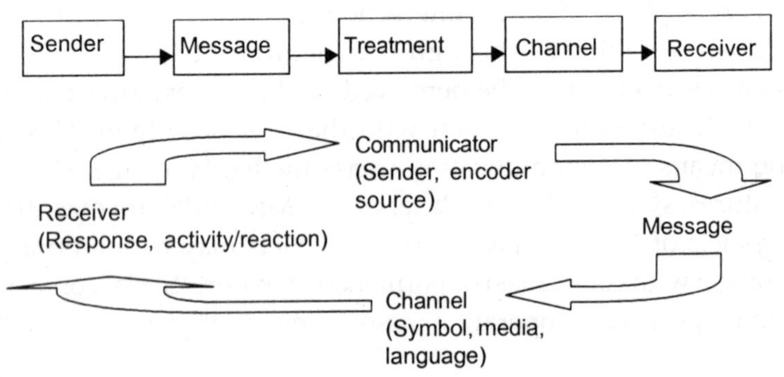

Communication Process

Sender

Sender starts the process into operation and decides what message to send, how to treat it, what channel's to use and which receiver or audience to reach. If the sender does not make the appropriate choice, then communication fails.

Message

Informal package and the content relevant to the topic.

Treatment

The way, in which the message is handled before placing it in the channel, the message should be clear, understandable, realistic in nature.

Channel

Language is the powerful medium of communication through which the message is send.

Receiver

The person who receives the information/message.

Types of Communication

- One-way communication, e.g: Letter writing
- Two-way communication, e.g: Phone
- Interpersonal communication, e.g: Communication between two or more persons
- Serial communication
- Mass communication, e.g: Communicating with a huge population
- Face-to-face communication, e.g: Interview
- Verbal communication, e.g: Language
- Non-verbal communication, e.g: Body gestures, symbols

- Formal communication, e.g: School
- Informal communication, e.g: Family, friends
- Mechanical communication, e.g: Internet
- Physiological communication, e.g: Communication between different parts of the body.

Importance of Social Interaction

The entire society is based on social interaction. It helps the individual to understand various forms of social relationships and to make necessary adjustments. Social interaction forms the ground in which culture arise and ensures its continued existence. Without social interaction man cannot lead social life. It is essential component in individual's life. It moulds the personality of the individual. Individuals ambitions, desires, fulfillment of needs, exchange of information will take place through the process of social interaction and the person develops bondages and leads effective social life. He tries to understands, adopts, accommodates to the changing societal needs. Social interaction plays primary role in the socialisation process of an individual. Inter-stimulation and response are the main ingredients of social interaction. One stimulates the actions, thoughts or emotions of another person and responds to the similar behaviour of others. Interaction increases the mental activity, fosters comparison of ideas, sets new tasks, discovers and accelerates the potentialities of individuals. Thus social interaction is a basic condition for society's existence. Social structure develops and individual performs social activities according to social expectation and fulfills their roles and norms by means of social interaction.

Previous Years University Questions

1. Role of socialisation in health care. (5 m, RGUHS, 2001)
2. Define socialisation. (2 m, RGUHS, 2000, 01, 02)
3. What is direct socialisation. (2 m, RGUHS, 2001)

4. Meaning of socialisation. (5 m, RGUHS, 1997)
5. What is socialisation. (2 m, RGUHS, 2002)
6. Agencies of socialisation. (5 m, RGUHS, 2003)
7. Socialisation. (2 m, RGUHS, 2001, 03, 04)
8. Explain the process of socialisation. (10 m, RGUHS, 1999, 2000)
9. What is social interaction. (2 m, RGUHS, 2003)
10. What is socialisation? What are the stages in the socialisation of an individual. (10 m, RGUHS, 2002)
11. Process of social interaction. (5 m, RGUHS, 1999)
12. Write short notes on socialisation. (NTRUHS, 1985, 87, 89)

MGR University Question Papers

1. Agencies of socialisation in personality development. (5 m, MGRU)
2. Socialisation. (5 m, MGRU)
3. Socialisation and personality development.(5 m, MGRU)
4. Socialisation and personality. (5 m, MGRU)

CHAPTER SEVEN

Social Process

INTRODUCTION

Society has its structure, which consists of groups and institutions and also society is a dynamic organisation constantly changing and presenting variety of behaviours under different circumstances. Social process deals with functional aspects of human association.

Social process is the fundamental ways in which the man interacts and establishes relationships. It is a repetitive form of behaviour, which is commonly found in social life. Interaction is subtle, complex and dynamic. Man's behaviour is not totally identified with in social process. It is a combination of activities, which are complicated in nature, mainly based on social interaction. Society is a system in action, in which moral norms, defined statuses are in action. Individuals try to attempt to solve the problems by performing social activities. Social interaction discloses the concrete results of striving behaviour on which roles, statuses and moral action will be held. Thus social process is mainly depends upon social interaction. Social interaction changes the state of relationship one to another, directed in different directions, i.e. positive, negative, upward or downward directions leading to integrated or disintegrated behaviour.

Definition

- 'The manner in which the relations of the members of a group once brought together, acquire a certain distinctive character'—*Maciver*
- 'Various modes of interaction between individuals or groups including cooperation and conflict, social differentiation and integration, development, arrest and decay'—*Gansberg*
- 'Ways of interacting which individuals can observe when they meet together and establish system or relationships or what happens when changes disturb already existing modes of life'—*Gillin and Gillin*
- 'The characteristic ways in which interaction occurs'—*AW Green*
- 'Repetitive forms of behaviour commonly found in social life'—*Horton and Hunt*
- 'Any social change or interaction in which an observer sees a consistent quality or direction to which a class name is given. A class of social changes or interactions in which by abstraction a common pattern can be observed and named'—*HP Fairchild*

Concept of Social Processes

Society is complex in which various individuals or group members forms specific social relationships with one to another to perform social activities. Social relationship represents the facts and functional aspects of society. It consists of reciprocal obligations, statuses in mutual contact. Hence sociologists felt the need to classify, analyse the social relationships to systematise its thoughts. Social interactions are interrelated and repetitive. Society is an expression of different social process. An aggregation of individuals forms society by forming a complex network of social relationships. To understand social phenomena the knowledge of social process is essential.

Essential Elements of Social Process

- Sequence of events
- Repetition of events
- Relationship between the events
- Continuity of events
- Special result.

Forms of Social Process

- Conjunctive/associative social process, e.g: Cooperation, organisation, adjustment, accommodation, integration, and assimilation.
- Disjunctive/disassociative social process, e.g: Conflict, isolation, competition, differentiation, disintegration and contravention, war.

Social behaviour is classified into different forms based on intrinsic nature, inherent drives, instincts, interests, desires, purposes of the individuals and their observation. Interaction occurs in the form of social process. Society contains cluster of social relationships. It is difficult to study each type of social relationships. So in general the relationships will be classified and studied.

ASSOCIATIVE SOCIAL PROCESSESS COOPERATION

It is the most common social process existing in human society. It is derived from two Latin words:

'Co' means 'together' and 'operan' means 'to work'. Join together or working together to achieve a common objective/ reward/interest. Cooperation is an essential element for group life. Either small group, e.g: Family, or big group, e.g: Educational institutions.

Cooperation consists of two elements, e.g: Common end and organised effort. It is an integrative activity. Several drives will enforce the person to cooperate, e.g: Desire for organisational and individual benefits, desire to give and share, devoted their time and pursuit for common purpose, target for large goal at an end, thus it exhibits certain ego-centered drives. Without cooperation to exist or to survive in society is a difficult task. Thus it is a universal and continuous phenomena. Cooperation is apparent and widen in human and animals. Individuals learn the concept of cooperation first in the family. Collective goals can be achieved only through cooperation. Team spirit, contentment, devotion are needed on the part of individuals to achieve institutional goals. The total needs (biological, physical, mental and even the spiritual needs) of the person will be fulfilled and satisfied when they are working together and agree to cooperate with fellow members. It promotes higher standards of living. Mutual cooperation starts in rearing of progeny, provision of protection and food. It is a psychological and social necessity cooperation is needed at every stage of life. The achievement of science and technology, agriculture, industry, transport, communication, etc. it helps in solvation of problems.

Definition

- 'It is a form of social interaction where in two or more persons work together to gain a common end'—*Merrill and Eldredge*
- 'The process by which individuals or groups combine their efforts in a more or less organised way for attainment of common objective'—*Fairchild*
- 'It is the continuous and common endeavour of two or more persons to perform a task or to achieve a goal, i.e. Commonly cherished'—*AW Green*

Importance of Cooperation in Social Life

Cooperation is a joint effort in pursuit of common goals or shared rewards. To enjoy the social life, cooperation is necessary element, which everybody has to follow. It is a psychological, biological and social necessity for man's continued existence. Common interests can be shared with group efforts. Sufficient time, sharing intelligence, self-control, united action delegation of authority, etc. is the elements of cooperation. Cooperation is a motivation to seek common goal. Group members should possess knowledge of the benefits of cooperative activity. It requires some kind of education, as cooperation is not in-born tendency. If the group has familiarity, favourable attitude towards sharing work and the rewards involved; they will equip themselves with the skills that are necessary for cooperative plan work. *Prince Kropotkin* called cooperation as 'mutual aid'. The principle of survival for existence is essentially the principle of cooperation. Social progress can be attained through united action. For democratic society, cooperation is a necessary condition of people's collective life and activities. Cooperation is required everywhere, in all the means, that's why it is a universal and continuous phenomena. Cooperation suggests solution for social problems, thus society advances through cooperation. It implies a regard for the wishes, needs and aspirations of other people. Groups may cooperate for self-centered gain, self-protection, self-advancement, mutual cooperation and group welfare. Thus cooperation is an indispensable requisite of human existence in all societies. The performance of common task encourages group activities, competitive spirit of individual or groups with which one has to cooperate without an alternative. Cooperation is the sense of oneness for the achievement of common interdependence of interest, like-minded persons with cooperative spirit will work for group welfare. Cooperation implies group harmony, peace and integration. Cooperation is needed for economic life; division of labour and specialisation are examples for economic cooperation, in economic matters like production, consumption, exchange and distribution cooperation is essential.

Characteristics

- Conscious process—Members are conscious of each other's presence and efforts.
- Universal process—Observed in almost all groups and nations.

- Continuous, life-long process.
- Personal process.
- Exist when two or more persons or groups are involved.
- Common goal.
- Members work together for group welfare and achieves organisational goal and group interest.

TYPES

I. AW Green has classified cooperation into 3 types

Primary Cooperation

Found among primary groups, where close, long-lasting association exists. No distinction between the aims and means of group. All the group members will work together for their achievement, e.g: Playing, worshipping, celebration of festivals, functions, ceremonies, etc. face to face and close contact are stimuli and performance of activity to achieve the goal is a response, which leads to group satisfaction; at the same time individual fulfils their needs also. Cooperation found out of love, concern and affection.

Secondary Cooperation

The formal cooperation found among group members. It exists in secondary groups, e.g: Educational, economic institutions. Individuals within this group will work together for their organisational goal but each other has their own specialised functions. Secondary cooperation is based on 'division of labour'. It requires specialisation of skills and functions. This interest cannot be achieved if the individual strives for themselves in their own capacity.

Tertiary Cooperation/Systemic Cooperation

It is a social interaction between big and small group. It leads to mutual adjustment and adaptation of these groups to each other. The attitudes of the cooperating practice are purely opportunistic, fragile and loose in contact. One group is forced to cooperate with the other due to circumstances, e.g: After the war, the defeated country is forced to accept and follow the terms and conditions of winning country.

II. Maciver and Page Classified Cooperation into two types

Direct Cooperation

Group members work for common goals knowingly. It involves all the people in the same kind of activity, i.e. identical in function, e.g: Harvesting crops, workers activity in industry, studying together. Identical functions can be performed by face-to-face contact, e.g: Primary groups. People performs the activities in the company with other members in a joint effort is a stimuli which leads to social satisfaction.

Indirect Cooperation

Members cooperate unknowingly. It is based on 'division of labour and specialisation function'. Seen in secondary groups, e.g: Industry, state, research, recreation, etc. individuals are not directly related to each other. Group members conform to social norms for the maintenance of social order. Persons work individually and perform the unlike tasks towards a similar end. The present technological age requires specialisation of skills and functions.

III. Cuber Classified Cooperation into Five Forms

1. Behaviour, which have loyalty or adherence to a common, e.g: Building up of organisation religious sanctions, social welfare activities.
2. Antagonistic cooperation. Two conflicting groups come to an agreement, paradoxical expressions, opposing interests are resolved by settlement which ensures cooperation, e.g: Property disputes settlement.

3. Cooperation is the result of unavoidable mutual dependence of individual and groups, e.g: Working environment, the relation between employees.
4. Division of labour is an unconscious cooperation in mutual economic interdependency of modern society. It stimulates competitive spirit of the individuals, e.g: Organisation of educational institutions.
5. Cooperation may result from superior power of individual or groups with which one has to cooperate without an alternative, e.g: Compulsorily one has to work to feed himself and his family, the person has to work under the superior where the ethical values of the employee and employer has conflicts.

ADJUSTMENT

Introduction

To fulfill individual's total needs and to lead a happy social life, the person purposefully applies efforts and energy to accommodate perfectly to the society and to the environment. The individual follows the *Darwin's* principles, the survival of the fittest, and struggle for existence. Social heritage makes organic adjustment less rigid and more flexible. Adjustment is highly selective and a specialised process. Members are unable to adjust with all kinds of environment. The adjustment of civilised man is less stable and more dynamic. However, he is capable of readjustment with new environment and there is remarkable mobility in the process of adjustment.

The meaning of adjustment is 'to fit, make suitable, adapt, arrange, modify, harmonise, correspondence with'. Whenever we make an adjustment between two things, we adapt or modify one or both of them to correspond to each other. Sometimes we may not be able to change the factors then the individual has to be modified in some way to suit the other, e.g: Wearing of clothes according to season wise to suit the environment and to make comfortable.

Continuous struggle between the needs of the individual and the external forces exists since ever long.

Definition

- 'Any operation whereby an organism becomes more favourably related to the environment or to the entire situation, environmental and internal'—*Warren (1934)*
- 'A continual process in which a person varies his behaviour to produce a more harmonious relationship between himself and his environment'—*Gates and Jersild (1948)*
- 'Adjustment means the modification to compensate for or meet special conditions'—*James Drever (1952)*
- 'It is the establishment of satisfactory relationship, as representing harmony, conformance, adaptation, etc. '—*Webster (1951)*
- 'The process of finding and adopting modes of behaviour suitable to the environment or the changes in the environment'—*Cater V Good (1959)*
- 'An individual's adjustment is adequate, wholesome or healthful to the extent that he has established harmonious relationship between himself and the conditions, situations and persons who comprise his physical or social environment'—*Crow and Crow (1956)*
- 'Adjustment is psychological survival'—*Vonhaller (1970)*
- It is the interaction between a person and his environment. The process of adjustment which he adapts depends upon his personal characteristics and circumstances of a situation.

Nature of Adjustment

The ways and means to help the individual to meet the demands of changes conditions by adapting or modifying his previous ways of doing or facing the things. Individual has to face the problems than running away from them.

If the individual cannot be able to change the situation, has to make some means to adjust to the environment, which is non-modifiable. Then only he feels comfortable and satisfaction. Harmonious relationships between individual their needs and the environment is required.

The individual either can change the environment to his needs or will change himself to suit the environment. Human needs are vital, indispensable and urgent to meet, sometimes the individual restricts the needs and as a result he may feel satisfied with the limit of his environment. Thus, he tries to maintain a balance his needs and its fulfillment with the environment.

Adjustment is a continuous process; individual from birth to death has to adjust one-way or other. The individuals who are able to adjust themselves to changing situations in their environment can live a harmonious, happy and contented life. Adjustment is a satisfactory adaptation to the demands of day-to-day life. Adjustment will help the individual to change his way of life according to the demands of the situation and gives strength and ability to bring about the necessary changes in the environmental conditions. The individual should maintain balance and adjust to their demands and societal demands too.

Process of Adjustment

Process is in the form of some attainment or achievement, fulfillment of life's ambitions, desires will be done by the process of adjustment, e.g: The student wants to complete higher studies with that he will get promotion, higher status within his society, for that he has to adjust and adopt himself to the rules and regulations, skill, attainment, hard work, etc. binded by himself, achieves his ambitions by acquiring higher degree. An individual's adaptation to himself and his environment by using certain coping strategies. It is a constant interaction between a person and his environment.

Adjustment is a two way process as it is a process of fitting oneself into available circumstances, but also the process of changing the circumstances to fit one's own needs. In majority of the cases adjustment is a compromise between two extremes.

Areas/Components of Adjustment

- Personal
- Environmental

According to *Bell*

- Inventory
- Home
- Health
- Social
- Emotional
- Occupational

Arkoff (1968) enumerated

- Family
- School
- College
- Vocation
- Marriage

Joshi (1964) and *Pandey* described individual's adjustment consists of :

- Heath
- Physical development
- Finance
- Living conditions
- Employment
- Social and recreational activities
- Courtship
- Sex
- Marriage
- Social psychological relations
- Personal psychological relations
- Moral
- Religions

- Home and family
- Future
- Vocational
- Educational
- Adjustment to school and college work
- Curriculum and teaching

Thus adjustment of a person includes harmonious relationship between his personal characteristics and the environmental demands, both factors work along with each other in bringing harmonious, happy and contented life.

Measurement

The adjustment of behaviour, the adaptation to changes circumstances involves both conscious and unconscious level.

Testing Techniques

To assess the individual's characteristics at the conscious level.

Projective Techniques

To assess the individual's characteristics at the unconscious level.

Sociometric Techniques

Used to measure social relationships and provide clues to the level of social adjustment.

Scaling Techniques

Options are collected from some other person about the adjustment pattern of a particular individual known to the respondents.

Inventory Techniques

They have many advantages when compare to other technique.

Types

- Adjustment inventory—*Hugh M Bell*
- Personal preference schedule—Psychological corporation, New York
- Personal adjustment inventory—*Joseph C Heston*
- Problem checklist, etc.

Characteristics of Well-adjusted Person

- A well-adjusted person knows his capabilities, strength and weaknesses, limitations
- Has self respect and respects others as individuals
- A well-adjusted person has his level of aspirations according to his own strengths and abilities. According to his abilities only he will select the activities
- He feels reasonably secure and maintain his self-esteem by satisfaction of his basic needs
- Has flexibility, adapt himself to changes in environment by making necessary changes in his behaviour
- Has the will and courage to resist and fight the difficulties
- Will have control over his environment, possess the capacity to deal with adverse conditions
- Realistic understanding and perception of the world. He always plans, thinks and acts pragmatically
- Feels satisfied with his surroundings
- A balance or positive philosophy of life.

Methods of Adjustment

An individual should lead a healthy, happy and satisfying life by adopting one or other methods of adjustment or coping strategies.

Direct Methods

Intentionally the individual adopts at conscious level. The person uses reasonably, logically in solving the problems.

- *Improving efforts:* To improve the behavioural process and to solve difficulty situations in the environment he will increase in his efforts to improve his efficiency.
- *Compromising methods:* Individual changes his efforts in a different direction to fulfill his aspiration.
- *Withdrawal and submissiveness:* Accepts his own defeat and surrendering himself to the powerful environmental forces.
- *Making proper choices and decisions:* A person adapts himself to and serves harmony with his environment by making use of his intelligence for the proper choices and wise decisions particularly when faced with conflicting situations and stressful moments.

Indirect Methods

- By using defence mechanisms/coping strategies the individual will try to adopt himself to the changing situation and accommodating new life styles.

ACCOMMODATION

Introduction

In life, an individual has to face a large number of conflicting situations, as the change is the law of nature. Man has to adjust and accommodate himself to meet the changes in needs and demands of the life. It is the process of getting along with differences and a way of social arrangement, which will help the people to work together whether they like it or not. It is the process of harmony with the environment. It is less rigid and more flexible. Social adjustment is a cultural process. The social environment is highly complicated and it has manifold aspects and contains diversifies in the process. Adjustment resolves rivalries or conflicting situations. It is a systematic handling of rivalries situations.

Organised forms of accommodation are: Courts, tribunals, commission, panels, state boards.

The philosophy of live and let live, give and take is a strong support of accommodation. All forms of accommodation are devices and cultural process. It is the culture that determines, which rivalries are not accommodative. Even in family situation, interpersonal social interaction takes place where members live by sacrifice and tolerance. Accommodation is usually an outcome of conflict, after conflict and tension, to relieve of stress and to have a peaceful existence accommodation is the way out.

Through accommodation, social order arises. Social organisation is fundamentally the result of an accommodation of conflicting elements. Throughout life man has to face a number of conflicting situations, adjustment of individuals to the situations is nothing but accommodation. It is the process of getting along inspite of differences. It is a way of inventing social arrangement, which helps the people to work together whether they like it or not.

Definition

- 'Permanent or temporary termination of rivalries interaction that permits the rivalrous parties to function together without open hostility at least in some respects'—*Cuber*
- 'The process in which man attains a sense of harmony with his environment'—*Maciver*
- 'The process of adjustment of hostile individuals or groups'—*Ogburn and Nimkoff*
- It is the sequence step by which persons are reconceived to changed conditions of life through the formation of habits and attitudes made necessary by the changed conditions themselves.
- 'It is the form of social process in which two or more persons or groups interact in order to prevent, reduce or eliminate conflict'—*Joseph Fitcher*
- 'It is the process by which competing and conflicting individual and groups adjust their relationship to each other

to over come the difficulties which arise in competition, contravention or conflict'—*Gillin and Gillin*

- 'The adjustments, which people in groups, make to relieve the fatigue and tensions of competition and conflict'—*Lundberg*
- 'It is a process of developing temporary working agreements between conflicting individuals or groups'—*Horton and Hunt*
- It is a non-violent response or adjustment:
- To a stubborn situation that cannot be changes
- 'To a situation, which has changed as a result of violence and hostility or as a result of new rules and requirement'—*HT Mazumdar*
- 'It is the process by which those once in conflict can work together in common enterprises'—*Sutherland and Others*
- 'It is the achievement of adjustment between people that permits harmonious acting together in social situations'—*Anderson and Parker*
- 'It is the condition in which equilibrium between individuals and groups and it is a process in which the conscious efforts of individuals to develop such working arrangements among themselves as well suspend conflict and make their relations more tolerable and less wasteful of energy'—*Mack and Young*

It is a natural resolution of conflicts; the antagonism of the hostile element is for the time being regulated and conflict disappears as overt action although it remains latent as a potential.

Methods

1. *Yielding to coercion:* It involves use of force or threat of force for making the weaker parts to accept the conditions. When parties of unequal strength are staying together, powerful party pressurises the weak party to accept its own terms, e.g: The country, which won the war, put forth demands on the loser country.

2. *Compromise:* Combatants are of equal strength, none can prevail over the other. Under such circumstances compromise is the only way to overcome the situation.
   a. *Arbitration:* Mediator will solve the problem, e.g: In property disputes among the families, relatives or friends will try to arbitrate between two groups and tries to avoid the conflict by giving a decision or judgment which is binding for both.
   b. *Mediation:* The mediator has no power to settle the conflict. He will advise the situation and try to find an amicable solution.
   c. *Conciliation:* The conciliator persuades the disputants to develop friendship and to come an agreement.
3. *Toleration:* When the conflicts are not solved or differences are not resolved, but the parties tries to avoid each other, deliberately avoiding conflicting situations. It is based on 'live and let live; policy, e.g: In working situation, if conflict occurs between employees and employer or among employees themselves, they will try to avoid the situation, which may aggravate the issue.
4. *Conversion:* When difference of opinion occurs between two individuals or two parties, one is convinced that they are wrong and tries to accept the viewpoint of other voluntarily, e.g: In family, we usually notice the conversion pattern, if couple have difference of opinion, one will understand their mistake and accept the view of other spouse voluntarily. It involves sudden rejection of one's beliefs, convictions and loyalties and adopting others views or policies.
5. *Rationalisation:* Instead of accepting one's faults and shortcomings, the party tries to justify their own behaviour, e.g: Certain individuals will not accept their mistakes, instead they will try to justify their actions with their own rationales. Instead of accepting one's defects and asking plausible excuses or explanations for one's own behaviour, one will blame others for their own faults.

6. Super ordination
7. *Subordination:* In family, father's authority is accepted and all other family members subordinate to it. Leaders' (with power and authority) views will be followed by subordinates or followers.
8. Sublimation.

Characteristics

- It is the natural result of conflict.
  An individual cannot experience conflicts throughout his life continuously, has to make temporary or permanent adjustments in the form of accommodation
- Accommodation may be conscious or an unconscious activity
  To accommodate in a society, the individual, in conscious and unconscious manner learns morals, traditions, etc. from birth to death to adjust and accommodate to the needs and demands of society. Accommodation becomes conscious when the conflicting individuals and groups makes a deliberate and an open attempt to adjust to the surroundings and lead a happy life
- It is universal, it is observed in all societies and in all fields of social life
- It is continuous, accommodation is observed in childs' life from birth to death. Accommodation is not fixed for any particular situation of social life, applicable in almost all areas of life, in various situation of life, but it may vary according to circumstances.

ASSIMILATION

Introduction

The process by which, individuals and group come to live in, and share attitudes, values, patterns of thinking and living. It is a form of social adjustment. It is concerned with absorption and incorporation of one culture by another. Like socialisation accommodation is a gradual process. Initially there may be conflict between group members, but as the time passes, if compulsion exists to stay together, the differences may be obliterated and the two sides become united in their views, attitudes, ideals, sentiments and total behaviour pattern.

For example: Aryans came to India as invaders, but they have become a part of the Indian society in due course of time.

For example: When marriage occurs between two persons of different religion, culture setup (total background) though in the beginning adjustment problems may arise, later as the time passes the couple will share their cultural pattern and leads a conducive happy environment, if each possess mutual understanding with one another.

Integration of individuals and groups in terms of common interests, attitude, tastes, outlook and standards. It denotes social acceptance cultural diffusion facilitates accommodation process. Some time two cultures merge into a third culture where both groups' characteristics will be present. New interaction may resolve the differences or they may create new difference on the background of their original culture, certain times accommodation results when the admixture of races results.

Definition

- 'It is the process of interpretation and fusion in which persons and groups acquire the memories, sentiments, attitudes of other persons or groups and by sharing their experiences and history are incorporated with them is a cultural life'—*Park and Burhess*
- 'It is a process whereby attitudes of many persons are united and thus develop into a united group'—*Bogardus*
- 'Social process whereby individuals or groups come to share the same sentiments and goals'—*Biesanz*
- 'It is the process whereby individuals or groups once dissimilar become similar and identified in their interest and look'—*Ogburn and Nimkoff*

- 'It is a process of dual adjustment through which culturally different groups gradually obliterate their differences to the point where they are no longer regarded as socially significant or observable'—*Lundberg*
- 'The process whereby persons and groups acquire the culture of another group'—*Samuel Koening*
- 'It is a gradual process whereby cultural differences tend to disappear'—*Cuber*

Characteristics

- Fusion of two distinct cultural groups into one. It is not limited to single field alone
- Placed easily in the background occupational skills, e.g: The immigrants skilled in profession, they are better placed in the respective societal groups; for instance the people of rural background are better placed in agrarian societies
- Increase in numbers among groups
- Differences in physical traits are common, which may lead to adjustment of problems, group frictions, inferiority complex and undesirability
- Cultural differences are common; language, customs, beliefs, habits and religion are major constituents in culture. If immigrants belongs to different cultural pattern adjustment problems may arise and they may hinder accommodation
- Formation of semi-community, they settle in compact colonies, where they continue to practices native folkways, which enable the new comers to identify themselves with their fellow men and adjust in the new environment easily.
- It is slow and gradual process. The process of accommodation quickens when continuous, direct contact exists among the group members.
- It is an unconscious social process as within the groups, individuals unconsciously discard their original cultural heritage and substitute it with the new one.

- Accommodation is a two-way process, acculturation is a preliminary step towards assimilation. It takes place when one cultural group is in contact with another, other cultural elements incorporates them into its own culture.

Promoting Factors

- *Toleration:* If persons and groups are possessing tolerance towards cultural differences accommodation can result. Tolerance promotes close contact and establishes the relationship among the group members, actively participates in common social and cultural activities.
- *Close association and intimate social relationships:* Social contact and communication are the components in establishment of social relationships. If the group members have intimate and close social relationships assimilation automatically results.
- *Amalgamation:* If marriages are performed between different religious amalgamations of various culture results.
- *Cultural similarity:* If similar culture exists among group members, quick assimilation will take place. Similarity in race and religious beliefs and practices. Helpful role of semi-community in making the new comers to adjust to the new situation.
- *Education:* It brings change in the behaviour of the individuals. Public education plays an important role in bringing assimilation among the group members.
- *Equal social and economic opportunity:* If people have enough social and economic opportunity then only they will feel free and establishes good continuous close contact and intimate social relationship.

Hindering Factors

- *Isolation:* It regulates assimilation process
- *Physical or racial differences:* It is a discriminating factor resulting into disintegration of assimilation process

- *Cultural differences:* If no common two elements in culture exists, even they are living together also socially they may remain apart
- *Prejudice:* Dominant group is having prejudice over recessive group unity will not be present
- Lack of proper understanding with one another among the group members leads to disparities
- *Dominance and subordination:* Lack of equal chances and opportunity between the group members will lead to slowing down of assimilation process.

Comparison Between Accommodation and Assimilation

Assimilation	*Accommodation*
Permanent means (It is a form of accommodation more thorough going and permanent method of adjusting inter-group differences)	Temporary means (Depending upon situation different method of accommodation will be adopted)
Slow and gradual process. It occurs only when there is relatively continuous and direct contact present	Sudden and radical process
Intimate and subtle changes occurs	Temporary, formal relationships
Unconscious process	Deliberate, conscious process
Requires more fundamental changes, the individual and groups discard their original cultural heritage and substitute it with the new one.	Need not necessary to involve both groups
Acculturisation takes place	
Involves two way process by implementation of give and take policy; contact between two groups affects both	

Integration

The structural components of society are properly organised through the harmonising or unifying process is called 'integration'. Each component performs certain socially approved functions, all the components have to be organised properly for achieving organisational goals.

Societal members are bound together and dependent upon each other, forms good interpersonal relationships and combines to constitute total functional structure. Certain values have to be accepted as common and institutional agencies preserve and promote their values. The structural units are interdependent and inter connected. 'Strain towards consistency' is an integrative process. Certain common values should be preserved and promoted.

Aims

- To maintain harmonious and active relationship between structural components of society
- For social reform and social construction
- To lead a harmonious social life
- To perform functions effectively in relation to their social values
- To provide good interpersonal relationship
- To promote character building
- To develop orderly social unity
- State
- Religion
- Economic agencies
- Organisation
- Social groups

(State, Religion, Economic agencies, Organisation, Social groups:) Manifests collective behaviour.

Modes

- *Close woven type:* Only one political party holds official hierarchy and controls all organisations (including families) and communication channels. It achieves integration by threat or use of force.
- *Loosely woven type:* Individual varies in their behaviour; they will perform their activities. No rigid social norms that everybody has to follow. Group relationships are not well defined.

For example: Integration becomes difficult for various reasons such as:

- If non-cooperative members exist within the group
- Group members concentrates for personal and individualised activities, self-centered approach
- Complexity of the society, e.g: Institutional patterns
- Unlike-mindedness
- Cultural heterogeneity
- Rapidity of social change
- Resistance to change or tendency of persistence among group members
- Social problems

Social welfare programs have to be organised to bring integration effectively. Social planning makes the people to move in right direction and takes appropriate social measures. It motivates the people to achieve and reintegrate in a complex society where rapidity in social change results.

Dissociative Social Processes

In the social struggle certain factors will operate and determines the positions of individuals within the groups, e.g.: Competition. These processes are universal elements, which are present in human social existence and are interlinked in a wide range of human activities. When the interests and attitudes are divergent indicates dissociative social processes are operating which hampers the harmonious social relationships.

CONFLICT

Introduction

It is a form of rivalry or struggle which is commonly existing within the society in varying degrees, i.e., organised/ unorganised, transitory or enduring; physical, intellectual, partial or total. It is essential part of human growth and development to certain extent. It takes place whenever the person or group tries to obtain a reward by preventing them from effectively competing, rather than by surpassing other competitors. Conflict is a fundamental social trait and is seen in human relations.

Definition

- 'It is a social process in which individuals and groups seek their ends by directly challenging the antagonist by violence or the threat of violence'—*Gillin and Gillin*
- 'A process situation in which two or more human beings or groups seek actively to thwart each others' purposes to prevent each other's interests even to the extent of injuring or destroying the other'—*Sociology Dictionary*
- 'The deliberate attempt to oppose, resist or coerce the will of another or others'—*AW Green*
- 'A process of seeking to monopolize rewards by eliminating or weakening the competitors'—*Horton and Hunt*
- 'It takes the form of emotionalised and violent opposition, in which the major concern is to over come the opponent as a means of securing a given goal or reward'—*Young and young*

It is opposition or struggle involving:

1. An emotional hostile attitude
2. Violent interference with one's autonomous choice—*Mazumdar*

Causes

- Individual differences
- Cultural
- Differences or clash of attitudes, interests within groups and societies
- Social change
- Vested interests
- Limited resources
- The society is cooperation through conflicts

- Frustration
- Insecurity
- Economic crisis
- Unemployment
- Fear of deprivation of love and affection
- Reduced supply of the means of substitute (Malthus view)
- Innate instinct for aggression in mass (Freud's view)
- Social change.

Nature/Characteristics

- It is universal—clash of interest is common in all groups at all the times
- It is conscious action—it evokes the deepest emotion, everyone involved in conflicting reaction are aware of it
- It is personalised—in social struggle to overcome the competition, the individual or groups will overlook others' interest
- It is conditioned by culture— it is affected by the nature of the group and its particular culture.

The objects of conflict may be:

- Property
- Power
- Status
- Freedom of action and thought
- High desired value
- Culture controls and governs the individual behaviour, it modifies conflict; when culture is not able to do so, corporate conflict results, e.g: Race riots.
- Conflict can be resolved through accommodation and assimilation
- Conflict is intermittent. Society cannot sustain with conflict continuously by intermittent itself societal problems exists
- Conflict defines issues in the society, e.g: Naxalite/religious problem in some states

- Conflict is conditioned by culture. In society, conflict will occur in terms of properly, power, status, freedom of action and thought
- Conflict can be resolved by accommodation and assimilation
- Frustration and insecurity promotes conflict within the same society
- Conflicts are potential when the individuals feel disturbed if their goals are not reached, like desire for power, position, prestige, status, wealth, money, economic insecurity, unemployment, deprivation of love and affection, etc.

Types

Direct Conflict (Open group conflict)

It results, when an individual or group hampers the other person in the attainment of goal, e.g: Quarreling, litigation, war and revolution.

Indirect Conflict

By imposing restraints, prejudice or ill will on the efforts of another to attain his ends. By competition, individuals or groups will compete with each other to win their goals. People will try for winning their goals indirectly. For achieving the objects of desire competition interferes with other's success.

Negative Conflict

Difference or aversion (emotional hostility) or disapproval, divergent of opinions may leads to negative conflict.

Positive Conflict

Healthy competition in achievement of common goals will cause positive conflict among the individuals.

Conflict of interpersonal ideas—conflict carried by an individuals not for themselves but for an ideal.

Feud—intergroup conflict between persons. It may arise due to injustice alleged to have done by one group to another.

Gillin and Gillin's Classification

- Personal conflict
- Racial conflict
- Class/caste conflict
- Political conflict
- International conflict

Other classification:
- Latent conflict
- Overt conflict
- Corporate conflict, e.g: A large section of the society is involved in communal riot.
- Personal conflict, e.g: Few persons are involved.

Latent Conflict

Long before conflict occurs in hostile action leads to social tension and dissatisfaction.

Overt Conflict

When hostile action occurs when one side or the other feels strong and wishes to take advantage of the fact.

Class Conflict

Arises between social classes, which have opposite or hostile interests, e.g: Clash against rich and poor.

Racial Conflict

Due to the physiological differences seen among different sect. of people, e.g: Conflicts between white and Negroes in America.

Caste Conflict

Conflict between social castes, e.g: Conflict between scheduled castes and forward castes.

Group Conflict

Occurs between two or more groups of any type, e.g: Political, social, economic, religious groups.

International Conflict

Between two or more countries or group of nations.

End Results of Conflicts

Positive/Integrative effect	*Negative/Disintegrative effect*
Point out issues, promotes group stability	Creates bitterness
Uses non-violence methods to resolve problems/crisis situations, alliance with other groups and a new consensus, registers progress through social conflicts	Leads to blood shed, destruction, inter group tensions and causes social disorder, chaos and confusion
Keeps group alert	Disrupts normal channel of cooperation
Upholds group morale and promotes solidarity of the group	Disrupts social unity by lowering the morale and weakens the group
Expansion of winning groups, promotes group unity and oneness among the group members	May destroy the lives and property
Keeps alert leadership and its policies upto date	Damages the mental peace, looses moral/ human values
Relative change in status of conflicting parties	Decreases in productivity, men may become idle
Promotes greater cooperation and continuous social relationship by proper understanding	Leads inter-group tension
In personal conflict the individuals can rise to a higher level	Disrupts the normal channels of cooperation
Foster social progress	Negative effect
Promotes group stability and solidarity	Evokes strongest emotions causes material loss
Forms upto policies and promotes alert leadership	Lowers the morale causes psychological damage
Enlargement of victory group	Diverts members attention from group objectives
Leads to alliance with other groups	

Differences Between Conflict and Competition

Conflict	*Competition*
Involves contact between persons and groups	Contact between the parties is not essential
Is a conscious activity	May or may not be a conscious activity
An intermittent process	A continuous process
Violence or threat of violence may be involved	Does not involve violence
Disregard social norms and regulations	Is in accordance with set of norms, rules and regulations
Personalised	Impersonal
Eliminates rivalry by overtaking all rivalries	Process of seeking to monopolize a reward
Universal	Universal
	Brings positive and negative results as healthy competition results social progress; negative competition causes disharmony in social relationships

Differences Between Cooperation and Conflict

Conflict	*Cooperation*
Process of seeking to monopolise a reward by weakening or destroying others	Is a joint effort in pursuit of common objectives or shared rewards
Conscious, deliberate act	Conscious or unconscious
Related to deepest and strongest emotions	Requires sympathy, identification, kindness, consideration of others
Universal and intermittent	Universal, continuous
Brings mostly negative results, destroys social progress	Brings positive social results
Society can permit without conflict	Is basic to social or group life

COMPETITION

Introduction

Modified form of social struggle. It is a natural result of universal struggle for or a commodity, goal or value. All people cannot satisfy their (limited) desires. Competition results whenever insufficient or limited supply of all things those individuals require for the fulfillment of their desires. It is a basic human drive. It is the recognition of one person or one group to have the claim for participation and success.

No society can exist without cooperation and competitions. Competition is a less violent form of opposition in which two or more persons or groups struggle for some end or goal. If competition becomes personal it may turn into conflict, and competition does not have any restriction.

Definition

- 'The form of social action in which we strive against each other for the possession of or use of so limited material or non-material goods'—*Anderson and Parker*
- 'The striving of two or more persons for the same goal, which is limited so that all cannot share it'—*Beisanz and Beisanz*
- 'It is an impersonal, unconscious, continuous struggle between individuals or groups for satisfaction because of there limited supply, which all may not have'—*Woodward and Maxwell*
- 'It is the struggle for possession of rewards, which are limited in supply, like goods, status, power, love anything'—*Horton and Hunt*
- The process of seeking to monopolise a reward by surpassing all rivals
- 'Competition is an interaction with or without social contact'—*Park and Burgers*
- 'A contest to obtain something, which does not exist in a quantity sufficient to meet the demand'—*Bogardus*
- 'Impersonalised struggle among resembling creatures for goods and service, which are scare or limited in quantity'—*Majumdar*

Nature of Competition

- Competition is impersonal struggle it is not oriented to against to an individual or any group
- Competition arises in a scarcity condition, e.g: If inadequate resources and more number of people competition exists in interest of achieving the goals. People compete for the positions of these limited resources
- To achieve fulfillment of basic needs, power, status, positions, name and fame, wealth, competition will result

- Competition is dynamic, continuous, as it is never ending process. Individuals try more and more to achieve higher ends
- Competition leads to social change. It compels the people to adopt new forms of behaviour which finds the way for inventions and innovations which naturally brings about social change
- Competition may be healthy or unhealthy, destructive or constructive, may produce negative result or positive results, personal or impersonal, comprehensive or narrowness
- If two or more competitors tries to win only at the expense of the others is destructive competition, but constructive competition is helpful and stimulating and contributes to the welfare of all at large, e.g: Students want to achieve higher goals and position they will work hard and compete with others knowingly or unknowingly.
- Competition is universal found everywhere and in all societies, e.g: Fields of business, cultural, social, political, education. Also seen in plant, animal kingdom, etc.
- Competition may be conscious or unconscious, e.g: Between students is unconscious, between two institutions is conscious
- It stimulates achievement, lifts the level of aspiration from lower level to higher level
- Competition always governed by norms, standards and are expected to use rules and regulations/norms to reach the other end and to regulate, channelise the competitive spirit of the individuals.

Characteristics

- Universal; seen in all fields
- Impersonal or personal
- Continuous
- Limited goals
- Huge number of competitors, efforts are needed by the total members

- In modern society the rate of competition is high
- Competition is socially restrained
- It is formed within a culture based on interests and attitudes among its members
- Competition is dynamic stimulating factor.

Effects

Positive Effect

- Competition performs more useful functions in society. Healthy competition is always required
- Brings about social progress
- Promotes quality of productive life
- For 'survival of fittest' in society competition is essential
- Helps in personality development of group members
- Encourages hard work among people
- Assigns and enhances status, position for the individuals in the social system
- Competition is a source of motivation for the individuals. It increases individual's efficiency improves the talents, capabilities, inspires the individuals to perform the activities in a better manner
- Social mobility and freedom to move any where and everywhere is possible only through competition
- Promotes general interest of the community as a whole
- Provides better and newer experiences, opportunities for the individuals to improve themselves to reach higher status and recognition
- Brings experimental change
- Stratifies some desire of the competing individuals or groups' community at large. It focuses attention on alternatives, well qualified people can be selected to perform special group functions
- Stimulates economy, efficiency and investiveness
- Enhance one's ego
- Prevents undue concentration of power in an individual or group of individuals

- Creates respect for the rules and regulations
- It is a source of motivation.

Negative Effect

- Uncontrolled competition is always dangerous and it is undesirable as it facilitates insecurity, fear, conflict, instability, panic, neurosis, tension, frustration, corruption, various types of social disintegration and the individual fails in competition, he may try to end his life.
- May lead to monopoly
- May create emotional disturbances
- May develop unfriendly, unfavourable negative attitudes towards one another
- Unethical and violent practices.

Forms or Types

Social Competition

Competition is acute in societies, where individual's abilities, capacities, performance, merits, talents, intellectual levels are recognised. Individuals always compete with each other for higher status and position. Democratic or open societies will encourage healthy competition.

Economic Competition

The main components of economic sphere include production, distribution and consumption. Individuals will compete in all means for employment, profit, wages, increments, promotions, and wealth to achieve a higher standard of living. Economic competition will be seen in every aspect of everyone's life both at individual and group level.

Political Competition

Political power will have more influence over the individual's life within the societies. High competition is observed in political field. Certain times political power will exercise pressure over one another.

Cultural Competition

It may take place between two or more cultural groups or racial groups.

Distinction Between Cooperation and Competition

Competition	*Cooperation*
Individuals try to compete with each other to obtain rewards or achieve the goal	Two or more persons work together to gain a common end
At group level and at individual level competition exists to fulfill their aspirations	Based on joint efforts of the group members to achieve satisfaction
Can bring positive result or can cause damage or loss to the parties and persons involved	Brings about positive result, loss to the individual is rare
Has its own limitations based on norms, rules and regulations	Boundless and less limited. One can go any extent to help the other
Unregulated competition may cause destructiveness and much harm to the individual	
Requires qualities like self confidence, desire, aspiration, spirit of adventure, readiness to suffer and struggle	Requires kindness, sympathy, concern, mutual understanding readiness to help others
Gains positive effect such as satisfaction, happiness etc, at times negative effect also	Brings satisfaction and contentment lessens the internal group conflicts

Contravention

A dissociative social process intermediate between competition and conflict. It is a sort of uncertainty in the beginning, later it converts into aversion, dislike or doubt without necessarily converting into conflict.

Process

- Rebuffing
- Repulsing

- Working against
- Hindering
- Protesting
- Restraining
- Upsetting another plans

Simple Contravention Technique

- Public denying
- Ridiculing and slandering
- Humiliation
- Snubbing
- Ignoring
- Blaming
- Reproaching
- Challenging
- Disapproving
- Expressing contrary views

Intensified Contravention Action

- Inciting to programs
- Exposing

Secret Contravention

- Circumventing
- Denouncing secretly
- Thwarting
- Betraying
- Using secret measures

Tactical Contravention

- Harassing
- Annoying
- Perturbing

Previous Years University Questions

1. Assimilation. (5 m, MP, 2004)
2. Define conflict and distinguish between war and conflict. (15 m, MP, 2004)
3. Co-operation. (5 m, MP, 2003)
4. Conflict. (5 m, MP, 2000, 03)
5. Define caste, Discuss merits and demerits of caste. (15 m, MP, 2002)
6. What do you mean by social process? Discuss the role of competition as social process. (15 m, MP, 2002)
7. What do you mean by caste? Explain its characteristics. (15 m, MP, 2000)
8. What do you mean by social process? Discuss any one process in detail. (15 m, MP, 1998)
9. Explain the importance of co-operation in social life. (15 m, MP, 1997)
10. Types of cooperation. (5 m, RGUHS, 2000, 02)
11. Importance of cooperation in society. (2 m, RGUHS, 2001)
12. Examine the functional significance of cooperation, competition and conflict as a social process. (10 m, RGUHS, 1997
13. Define assimilation. (2 m, RGUHS, 2000,02)
14. Define social process. Explain the functional significance of cooperation, competition and conflicts as social process. (10 m, RGUHS, 2003)
15. Mention associative social processes. (2 m, RGUHS, 2003)
16. Differentiate the social process – competition and conflict. (5 m, RGUHS, 2004)
17. Accommodation and assimilation. (2 m, RGUHS, 2002,04)
18. Types of accommodation. (2 m, RGUHS, 2001)
19. Explain specifically the health problems of the different social classes and that of the backward castes. (10 m, RGUHS, 2002)
20. Write briefly the important social processes and their significance in the social system. (5 m, RGUHS, 2001)

21. Cooperation and conflict. (2 m, RGUHS, 2001,02,03)
22. Functions of competition. (5 m, RGUHS, 2000)
23. Explain assimilation. (2 m, RGUHS, 2000)
24. Enumerate the social processes and their uses in society. (5 m, RGUHS, 2002)
25. What is social interaction and compare the social process of accommodation and assimilation. (10 m, NTRUHS, 1995)
26. Distinguish between associative and dissociative social process. (NTRUHS, 1989, 10 m)
27. Explain the dissociative social process. (10 m, NTRUHS, 1987)

MGR University Question Papers

1. Social process. (5 m, MGRU)
2. Co-operation. (5 m, MGRU)
3. Conflict (5 m, MGRU)
4. Dissociative social process. (5 m, MGRU, Nov-01)

CHAPTER EIGHT

Social Change

The basic fact of today is the tremendous pace of change in human life.—*Jawaharlal Nehru*

Change refers to evolution, progress or adaptation.

Change is the law of nature. The word, 'change' denotes a difference in anything observed, over a period of time. Society is a web of social relationship, therefore observable differences in any social phenomena over any period of time may be observed. Social relationships include social processes, social patterns and social interactions. It is a change in the institutional and normative structure of society and human relationships.

Definition

- 'Variations in or modifications of any aspect of social processes, social patterns, social interactions or social organisations'—*Jones ME*
- 'Large numbers of persons are engaging in activities that differ from those which or their immediate forefathers engaged in some time before'—*Merrill and Eldredge*
- 'Modification in ways of doing and thinking of people'—*MD Jenson*
- 'Alterations as occur in social organisations that is structure and function of society'—*Kingslay Davis*

- 'Social changes are variations from the accepted modes of life, whether due to alterations in geographical conditions in cultural equipment, composition of the population or ideologies and whether brought about by diffusion or invention within the group'— *Ellin and Ellin*
- 'Some change in social behaviour and in social structure'— *B Kuppuswami*
- 'Whatever may happen in the course of time to the roles, the institutions or the orders comprising a social structure, their emergence, growth and decline'—*Derth and Mills*
- A change in course of time in the activities of the people.
- 'Society is a complex network of patterned relationship in which all the members participate in varying degrees. These relationships change and behaviour changes at the same time'—*Merill*
- 'A new fashion or mode, either modification or replacing the old, in the life of a people or in the societal operations'— *Majumdar HT*
- 'A process responsive to many types of changes in man made conditions of life, attitudes, beliefs of men and to the changes that goes beyond human control to the biological and the physical nature of things'—*Maciver and Page*

From these definitions, we can explain social change briefly in the following manner:

1. Social change is a modification in any aspect of social process. It occurs in:
   Geographical environment
   Cultural means
   Biological (physical) level
   Ideological plane
   Structure and function of society.

Nature

1. *Universal phenomenon:* Society exists in universe. No society remains static. The speed and extent of change may

differ from society to society. Some may change rapidly, others slowly.

2. *Community change:* It does not refer to the change in the life patterns of several individuals. It is a change which occurs in the life of the entire community.
3. *Speed is not uniform:* Social change in urban is faster than in rural areas.
4. *Nature and speed of social change is affected by time factor:* It differs from age to age. In India the speed of social change after 1947 is faster than before 1947.
5. *Occurs as an essential law:* Change is the law of nature. It may occur either in the natural course or as a result of planned efforts. Our needs kept on changing to satisfy our desire and for our changing needs, social change becomes a necessity. The enthusiastic response of change has become almost a way of life.
6. *Definite prediction is not possible:* Our attitudes, ideas, norms and values cannot be predicted.
7. *Shows chain reaction sequence:* A society's pattern of living is a dynamic system of inter-related parts. Therefore change in one of the parts usually reacts on the other and those on additional ones bring change in the whole, e.g: Industrialism has destroyed the domestic system of production. It brought women from the home to the factory and to the office.
8. *Modification and replacement are the key factors:* Modifications in living style, social relationship, attitude towards women's rights, religious pattern, etc.

Social change is continuous, never ending process; each moment in our life we have to under go or adapt ourselves to the changing modalities. It takes place in the environment, i.e. geographic, physical or cultural context and involves the human aspect results from interaction of a number of factors. Social change may be planned or unplanned brings immediate results or long time to show its results. The study of social change involves no-value judgment, ethically neutral.

Influencing Factors

Cultural Factor

Changes in culture are accompanied by social changes. It influences social relationship; culture give speed and direction to social change and determines the limits, beyond which social change cannot occur. Any change in the culture in the form of learning is called as 'Cultural change'. It may be materialistic or non-materialistic. Changes in culture occur by acculturisation and diffusion, which are indicative of social change, e.g: Invention of gas stove, TV, pressure cooker, refrigerator.

Biological Factor

Will have indirect influence upon social change, e.g: Aspect of the population related to heredity and mutation like *Darwin's* principle of survival of fittest, struggle for existence.

Population Factor

Factors that determine the number the composition, the selection and the hereditary, quality of the successive generations. The human elements in society are always changing. Every individual is having a different distribution of qualities and potentialities. Each new generation is a new beginning.

For example:

1. If we compare ourselves with our parents we will know that we are different from them in make-up, ideas and in most other things.
2. Growth of population has given birth to a great variety of social problems like unemployment, child labour, wars, competition, standard of living, poverty and moral degeneration.
3. There is a close relationship between the growth of population and the level of physical health and vitality of

the population as there are many mouths to feed which lead to malnutrition, apathy and lack of enterprise.
4. Increase in population may add to social problems. This also creates a demand for more medical and health services.

Geographical/Environmental Factor

Any change in the nature of geographical or environment will have its impact on human society, e.g: Flood, earthquake, and draughts. Physical environment is alone responsible for the growth of human society and social relationship.

Psychological Factor

The cause of social change is the psychology of the man himself. Man is by nature, a lover of change. He is always trying to discover new things in every sphere of life and is always anxious for novel experience. As a result of this tendency the mores, traditions, customs of every human society are perpetually underlying change. He is always attending to what is new and unique and to preserve old ones. The form of social relationships is constantly changing in the process of interaction between these two tendencies. New customs and methods that replace the old traditions are respected but time demands change and adaptation to changing conditions, when change does not occur at the appropriate time.

Technological Factor

The process of application of new innovation is technology.

Technology discloses man's mode of dealing with nature and the process of production by which he sustains his life and thereby lays the mode of formation of social relations and of mental conceptions that flow from them—*Karl Marx*

Technology affects the society by changing our environment to which we in turn adapt. The change is usually in the material environment and the adjustments we make with changes often modify customs and social institutions—*Ogburn*

Technology is a systematic knowledge, which facilitates the use of machines or tools. Technology affects society greatly. Variation in technology causes a variation in some institution or custom. The present age is often called 'The age of power' or 'The scientific age' is a tool for man in his behaviour towards nature. Technology is the means of economic production, which is an end.

Technology is constantly developing and with its development the structure of society is also changing. Increased divisions of labour and higher degree of specialisation are the result of a constant development in technology. It played a major role in the development and progress of human civilisation.

Main Technological Factors

Introduction of Machines in Industries

Some fundamental changes have occurred in social structure due to the introduction of machines.

1. *Birth of factory system:* Mechanisation is the replacement of the system of individual production by the factory system. The invention of machines has led to the creation of huge factories, which employ thousands of people and where most of the work is performed automatically.
2. *Urbanisation:* Industrialisation and birth of factories led to urbanisation and big cities came into existence. With the advent of industrialisation many labourers migrated to the sites of work and settled around it. Establishing market centres, schools, colleges, hospitals, recreation clubs, etc. fulfilled their needs.
3. *Evolution of new classes:* Urbanisation and industrialisation transformed the structure of society. It is divided itself into classes, e.g: Capitalist, labour classes, middle class.
4. *New conceptions and movement:* All factors culminated in the generation of new currents in the prevalent thinking. Trade union movements came into favour as the socialistic

and communist thoughts gained in popularity. Lockouts, strikes, processions became the stocks in trade of those who wanted to promote class interests and are regular features of economic activity.

5. *Improvement in the condition of women:* The burden of work in the family, which falls to the woman, has been decreased by the increasing use of mechanical appliances. With the domestic work being facilitated, they were left with adequate time for occupational and recreational activities and they too competed with men in the economic field.

Thus our attitudes, beliefs and traditions have crumbled before technological advancement. The spirit of craftsmanship, the divine ordering of social classes, traditions regarding the spheres of the sexes, the prestige of birth have affected by mechanisation, e.g: Status of women in the industrial age, has destroyed the domestic system of production, brought women from home to factory, office and distinguished their earnings. It created a new social life for women.

Development of the Means of Communication

The introduction of machinery into industry led to the development of large-scale production, which necessitated communication between traders situated far apart. In this connection much benefit is reaped through postal service, telephone, newspaper, radio, TV, helped to bring news from every corner of the world right into the household. They also facilitated the spread of new principles and became propaganda machines for political parties. They show uniformity and diffusion of culture, recreation, entertainment, transport, education, dissemination of information. Communication is an important factor in determining our social life. Its techniques definitely limit the kinds of organised life that the people can have. Changes in the means of communication have also affected social relationship and social life greatly, however, the changes in the means of communication depend upon the technological advancement.

The primary techniques of communication are speech and gesture, since these provide the base upon which all other modes of communication are built, e.g: Writing is a graphic form of speech, radio is the transmission of speech through space.

Cultural and linguistic differences are the significant deterrent to the growth of intimacy and understanding between people of different societies and groups. Secondary techniques of communication have been encouraged by technological changes. It facilitates the invention and diffusion of cultural elements, e.g: Invention of printing press influenced education, politics and trade.

Development of Means of Transport

It is an important factor in the determination of spatial aspect of social relationships. As the means of transportation have changed, the spatial relationship of the members of the group has also changed. The rapid means of transportation has to be encouraged, the growth of inter-continental trade and the interdependence of the countries. The development of cycle, motor, railway, ship and aeroplane made transportation of commodities much easier. As a result, national and international trade made unprecedented progress. The intermixing of people belonging to various countries led to the removal of misunderstanding, feeling of hatred and jealousy were replaced by sympathy and cooperation. Feeling of benevolence prevailed between different races and nations. This assisted in the progress of the sense of universal brotherhood.

There is a greater mobility of population today in which the modern rapid means of transport have played an important part, broken the barriers of cultural isolation and paved the way for cultural uniformity. The new mode of transport have played significant role in the diffusion of cultural elements. The transportation development has played a vital role in the economic integration of the people of regions, of nations and of the world at large and leads to social integration.

Development of New Agricultural Techniques

An important factor in technological advance is the development of new techniques in agriculture. Changes in the agriculture techniques have affected the rural community, which increased production and thereby increasing the standard of living in the rural people. Fewer people are now needed for agriculture, consequently, many agricultural labourers have shifted to factories and devoted themselves to trade on cities to find employment. In India, the effect of technology is most apparent in this direction because India is eminently an agricultural country and its future depends upon the progress in agriculture. The technological sate of a society determines the economic and political structure.

Social Effects of Technology

The technological changes have affected social values and norms. There is a movement away from family and community loyalty, to a movement towards individualism. They have also intensified social and psychological uprootedness. They have promoted hedonism (believes that pleasure should be the main aim in life). Individualism has supplemented traditionalism. Bureaucracy has grown in number and power. Human relations have become impersonal and secondary.

- Extension of economic limits the areas of states
- Formation of new classes in society
- Development and progress of democracy
- Spread of fashion
- Urbanisation
- Introduction of novel thoughts
- Formation of associations

Had profound effect on the beliefs, thoughts and tendencies of human beings.

The old values been completely changed. Wealth is being accorded almost the highest respect and a measure of prestige. Moral values are no longer in the respect they were once held. Religion has come to be regarded as a private affair. Stress is being laid on secularisation of social relationships. Importance is now given to quantity instead of quality. The fundamental elements of culture are being disregarded in the face of ostentation and pretension. Human relations are becoming personal and secondary. On all sides one is confronted with

'Human machines' which possess:

Motion but not sincerity.

Life but not emotions.

Heart but not feelings.

Every one is running, no one has the time to look to another.

Effects of Social Change on Social Institutions

On Family

Many of the family activities are being mechanically performed. As a result, the women folk have more spare time. Family control is on the decline, signs off disintegration also being observed. The number of children is becoming less, the invention of birth control devices has reduced family size. Disintegration of joint family system. The employment of women in factories and offices has changed the form of husband-wife relationships and affected the family structure and functions in several ways.

On Marriage

Along with the family ties, the bonds of marriage are also becoming ineffective since marriage is no longer a religious ritual but a social contract which can be broken at any time. The sphere of choice in marriage has increased and more emphasis is being placed on love. Love marriages, inter-caste marriage, late marriage are common. The number of divorce is on the increase.

On Economic Life

- New type of economic organisations like factories, agencies, stores, banks have come up.
- Has led to the concentration of industries, which led to packed cities.
- Promotes a higher standard of living.
- Division of labour and specialisation are the product of technology, results in economic depression, unemployment, industrial disputes, accidents and occupational diseases.

On Social Life

- Has led to the decline of community life and poor housing pattern and formation of slums are promoted.
- Recreation has become commercialised.
- Has changed basis social stratification and social values and narrowed the gap of caste system.
- Man has become a machine social contacts have become secondary. Warmth of relations has been reduced.
- Worth of man is judged by what he has got, than by what he is.
- Has grown psychic conflicts and diseases. Modern man suffers great mental strain, emotional instability and economic insecurity.

On State

- The idea of social welfare state is an offshoot of technology, more stable government was found.
- Scope of state activity has been promoted.
- Influence of pressure-groups over the state has been increased.
- Democracy has become the common form of government, and has led to a shift of functions from local government to central government.

On Religious Life

- Superstition, pseudo beliefs are reduced and higher tolerance for religious activities is observed.
- Religious institutions are no longer force.

On Urban Life

- Absence of communal feeling
- Impersonal social relations
- Increase in the number of diseases
- Absence of family control
- Low level of morality
- Increased prevalence of social disorganisation
- Increased facilities for leisure
- Promotes self-confidence.

Pattern of Social Change

Social Invention

Graham Bell invented telephone, *Wright brothers* invented aeroplane.
Mechanical inventions necessarily affect social inventions. However, social inventions spring from the perception of some adjustment need and brings about social change, e.g: The invention of language is greatest of all the invention.

Bonus to wage earner brings about a higher standard of living to workers.

Discovery

It is shared human perception of a fact or human relationship which already existing. The result is social change, e.g: *Columbus* discovered America.

Diffusion

Spread of cultural traits or information from one group to another.

Why people oppose social change

Desire for Stability

The individual must feel secure in his future life. Any change will disturb the existing equilibrium and are apprehensive about their future. They may have fear of unknown or new things. Instead of opting the new and better environment they prefer to cling to the status quo as they feel that the new environment may be painful than the present. This type of individuals is conservative in nature.

Inadequacy in Invention

The consumer will oppose the newly invented product, if that product does not fulfill the needs.

Ignorance

It usually takes a considerable time for a newly invented product to be understood.

Habit and Tradition

Individuals do things mostly by habit and customs. Adaptation of an invention requires the substitution of a new habit for an old one. It is a difficult task, especially for the older people whose habits are fixed.

Traditions are reverence for the past and individuals believe in supernatural check, they will be away from adapting new methods, e.g: People oppose to utilise the contraception devices.

Sentiment

For the acceptance of inventions, a seculiarised environment is necessary which can be produced by cross-cultural fertilisation. Sentiments will affect individuals by not accepting the new inventions.

Economic Cost

To launch an invention, costs money. Thus for adoption of national compulsory health insurance large sum of money may be needed.

Vested Interest

The people who feel that social change endangers, their vested interests fight every proposal when their rights are threatened. For example: Zamindari abolition was opposed by the people who derived great advantage from that system.

Intellectual Laziness

Inertia and intellectual laziness leads man to oppose any change. He would much rather borrow than invent, and will go along the way he is going, than try for a new path.

Theories of social change

The theories of social change will describe the direction and cause of social change.

Deterioration Theory

According to some sociological thinkers, man originally lived in a perfect state of happiness in a golden age, then deterioration began with the result that man reached an age of comparative degeneration.

According to Indian mythology, man has passed through yugas—Satya yug, Treta yug, Dwapara yug and Kalyug.

Cyclic Theory

Human society goes through certain cycles. Society has a predetermined life cycle. (Birth, growth, maturity and decline)

History repeats itself, society after passing through all the stages returns to the original stage then the cycle again begins, e.g: In Hindu mythology Satya yug will again start after Kalyug completes—*Specular's view.*

All the civilisation (Egyptian, Roman, Greek) says that man will pass through birth, maturity and death—*Spengler's view.*

According to Vilfredo Pareto's view, the society consists of two groups.

1. Rentier—one who like to follow traditional ways.
2. Speculators—one who like to change for attaining their ends, e.g: Political institution.

According to Stuart Chaplin's View

The concept of accumulation is the basis for social change. Cultural change is 'selectively accumulative in time and cyclical in character'. The whole culture will be in a state of integration, synchronise. If they do not synchronise it is in disintegrative condition.

According to Sorokin's view

1. *Ideational type of civilisation:* Reality and value are conceived in terms of 'supersensory and super rational God'.
2. *Sensory type of civilisation:* The whole way of life is characterised by positive and materialistic outlook. Reality and value are merely what the senses perceive and beyond perception there is no reality.

According to Arnold J Toynbeo (English historian) view

The history world civilisation consists of:

Youth—response to change.
Maturity—time of troubles.
Decline—gradually degeneration.

Linear Theory

According to this theory—society gradually moves to an even higher state of civilisation and that is advanced in linear fashion and in the direction of improvement.

August Comte—postulated 3 stages of social change.

1. *Theological stage:* Man believed that supernatural powers control and designed the world. He advanced gradually from belief in deities and facilitated to monotheism.
2. *Metaphysical stage:* Theological way gives way to metaphysical stage, during which man tried to explain the phenomena by resorting to abstracts.
3. *Positive stage:* Man considers the search for ultimate causes hopeless and seeks the explanatory facts that can do empirically observed. If man adopts a positive attitude in understanding the natural and social phenomenon, social progress will result.

According to Herbert Spencer

Man compares society to an organism, it is gradually progressing towards a better stage.

1. *Primitive stage:* The state of militarism society is characterised by merciless struggle for existence.
2. *Industrialism:* Greater differentiation and integration of its parts. The establishment of an integrated system is possible for the different social, economic and racial groups to live in peace.

According to Mikola K Mikhalovisky

1. *The objective anthropometric:* Man considers himself as the centre of the universe and is preoccupied with mystic beliefs in the supernatural manner.
2. *The eccentric:* Man is given over to abstraction to real situation.
3. *The subjective anthropometric:* Man comes to rely upon empirical knowledge he exercises more control over nature for his own benefit.

Deterministic Theory

There are certain a social, economic, natural force brings social change, e.g: Material condition of life, effort and rational planning, economic factors (production, distribution and exchange), political evolutions.

Social Welfare Planning in India

Any measure taken for the benefit of the weaker and vulnerable sections of the society. Welfare is a dynamic aspect, preliminarily the meaning is 'Helping the others', e.g: Poor, orphans, widows, physically and mentally handicapped children. The welfare measures like provision of health, education and housing services, legislation for the protection of the working class, social security are provided. All collective measures or interventions to meet specific needs of the individual or to serve the wider interests of society, e.g: Food, clothing, shelter, normal satisfaction of family life, enjoyment of physical and mental health, opportunity for the expression of skills and recreations abilities, active and pleasurable social participation.

Social welfare has grown out of, and is constantly influenced by, evolving social, economic, political and cultural trends to meet new situations. It is the central responsibility of the state, i.e. the provision and maintenance of an acceptable standard of social and economic well-being for the entire population, which cut across the fields of health, education and labour.

Social welfare is the organised system of social services and institutions, designed to aid individuals and groups to attain satisfying standards of life and health. It aims at personal and social relationships, which permit individuals, the development of their well-being in harmony with the needs of the community.

Social work is a professional service, based upon scientific knowledge and skill in human relations, which assists individuals, alone or groups to obtain social and personal satisfaction and independence. It is usually performed by a social agency or a related organisation.

Social services, 'Those organised activities that are primarily and directly concerned with the conservation, the protection and the improvement of human resources'.

Social welfare was the result and social work was the process employed to secure it. Social workers were the people working through social work for social welfare.

If the process was understood the attendant skills were appreciated, the information on subjects of direct concern and on allied fields together with the necessary relevant background material was carefully compiled and presented and the social policy makers, social planners, social administrators, professional and lay social workers were properly equipped, the quality of social welfare services would improve and expansion of social welfare programmes and services would be less difficult more economic and efficient—*Smt Durgabhai Deshmukh*

The five-year plans suggests that 'The object of social welfare is the attainment of social health, which implies the realisation of objectives, e.g: Adequate living standard, the assurance of social justice, opportunities for cultural development through individual and group expressions and readjustment of human relations leading to social harmony'.

The aim of social service in the past was essentially curative and efforts were directed towards relief for the handicapped and the uplift of the under privileged sections of society. It is now essential to maintain vigilance over weakness and strains in the social structure and to provide against them by organising social services.

For a long time, society has remained apathetic to these conditions; but with the awakening of political consciousness and the enthusiasm of organisations and workers to improve social conditions, there is possibility of developing programmes, which could gradually remedy the present situation. The economic programmes of the five-year plan will mitigate these problems to some extent, but the gains of economic development have to be maintained and consolidated by well-conceived and organised social welfare programmes spread over the entire country. Family welfare includes taking care of the people who are divorced, deserted, treatment of maladjusted members of the family.

Objectives

- To determine the social needs
- To arrange for careful and conscientious planning to meet the needs of the population
- To mobilise the forces of the community in the best way to achieve this goal.

Welfare activities—goals

- Economic development
- Full employment
- Equality of opportunity for the young
- Social security
- Protected minimum standards—nutrition, housing, health, education
- Provision of social services, recreation facilities
- Nationalisation of civil liberties
- People's participation
- Rehabilitation of the injured or diseased persons
- Social investment in the young
- Prevention and cure of sickness
- Moral guidance to the needy individuals
- Welfare of backward classes.

Steps in Organisation of Social Welfare

1. Assessment of resources and the needy of community (Community diagnosis).
    - Priorities has to be fixed by preference ranking method, to achieve certain objectives
    - Targets are to be laid down to achieve and to avoid wastage and overlapping.

2. Planning at all levels—central, state, regional, district, block and village levels.
   - Planning has to be done with the consent of the people
   - Planning in consonance with overall planning.
3. Implement the process into activity.
4. Evaluation of programme.
5. Modification to achieve set objectives.

Social welfare services are specialised service meant to enable handicapped and maladjusted individuals and groups to reach their full potential like:

- Establishment of schools for physical handicapped children
- Home for the destitute
- Certified institution for the delinquents
- After care of discharges prisoners
- Rehabilitation of women rescued from moral danger
- Provision of education and health services
- Providing adequate financial assistance for water supply, family planning, sanitation, urban development to increase efficiency
- Programmes relating to social defense, social and moral hygiene and after care services, foster-care, adoption services
- Welfare projects, night shelters, holiday homes for children, technical guidance to aided institutions
- Meeting the needs of destitute children
- Counselling or advisory service
- Prevocational training
- Programme of social defense like
  - Prevention and treatment of juvenile delinquency
  - Probation
  - Suppression of immoral traffic in women and girls
  - Eradication of certain problems like beggary.
- Basic health services—maternity care, child care
- Distribution of cooperative credit for weaker sections.

COMMUNITY DEVELOPMENT PROGRAMME IN INDIA (PEOPLE'S PROGRAMME)

Definition

The process by which the efforts of the people themselves are united with those of governmental authorities to improve the economic, social and cultural conditions of communities, to integrate community with nation and to enable them to contribute fully for national progress.

Philosophy

- Maximum utilisation of main resources available (manpower)
- Self help of the people to build a nation
- People's programme dedicated to the well-being of the people
- A programme of the people
- A programme by the people
- A programme for the people
- Capable of inspiring the people with the will to better living trough their own effort.

Objective

1. To develop more than 5 lakh village communities with the help of villagers themselves.
   It is an external organisation for it develops channels between all higher centres of information and villages, develops varied personnel to carry technical knowledge to villagers in the scientific fields, e.g: Agriculture, health, education, economic development, social justice, democratic growth.
2. To stimulate and promote conditions for social, cultural, economic progress by coordinated methods, which involve a emphasis on responsibility and action at the local level.

Principles

- Activities undertaken should be initiated in response to the felt needs of the people
- Multi-purpose programmes should be established and concrete action to be taken
- During an initial stage of development changed attitudes, material gains should be considered as equally important

3. The community should be encouraged to actively participate in their own programmes so as to become independent in local self-government by trained leadership.
4. Encourages participation of women and youth in community projects.
5. Tap the resources like voluntary, non-governmental organisations.
6. The self-help projects of the community must be encouraged by intensive and extensive assistance from the state.

Aims

1. Rural population will be promoted to full employment and increased in agriculture production.
2. The largest possible extension of principle of cooperation by making rural families credit worthy.
3. Increased community effort for welfare of to the total community as a whole, e.g: Roads, schools, wells, children's park.

Methods Used

Assessing of community needs and motives for action by:

- Survey of community needs, e.g: Preference ranking method
- Discovering the community's material and human resources
- Holding of systematic discussions
- Arriving at decisions on effective implementation of the projects undertaken.

Selection of appropriate channels of communication with the community.

- To stimulate
- To recognise the importance of acquiring facilities through 'self help', which were carefully selected and utilised.

INCEPTION OF COMMUNITY DEVELOPMENT PROGRAMME (CDP) IN INDIA

The planning commission was established in March 1950 by Government of India. Its main responsibility is to formulate a plan of action for the most effective use of the country's human and material resources.

The commission laid down, Community Development Programme on October 2, 1952. The technical and monetary assistance was provided by USA.

Initially 55 community projects located in selected areas in different states of India. Each project consists of 300 villages with the area of about 500 square miles and a population of 2,90,000. Each project was further divided into 3 development blocks, each consisting of 100 villages a population of 90,000 to 97,000. Each group of 10 villages was the filed of operation for a village level worker, called 'Gram Sevak'.

Community Development—Five year plan

Community Development Programme is an integral part of our five-year plans. The five-year plans aim at bringing about an all-round development of the country in a planned democratic manner, while the community development is to take care of the rural sector of development.

- Initiating a process of transforming social and economic life to the villages
- To provide the setting in which the national plan approaches the needs and aspirations of the country-side
- Promotes the diversification of the agricultural economics and increase agricultural production through the operation

of land reforms, strengthening of village organisations, building up of local leadership and growth of the cooperative movement.

CDP should become 'a positive force in bringing about both an integrated rural society and an expanding rural economics'.

Development of CDP

Financial provision is made at this stage to do work primarily in the agricultural field/health/educational fields to promote the growth of Panchayat and cooperatives.

Stage I

After a year, the block enters the first stage when full staff is given and the development of block is planned over a 10-year period (Stage I—five years, Stage II—five year)

During the first stage the state and central Government provide Rs. 12,00,000/- as budget provisions towards development inclusive of what may have been spent in the earlier period.

Stage II

Rs. 5,00,000/- is allocated. The local people have to contribute an equal amount in work, materials and money. Since 1958, the CDP is responsibility of the block development office and the Panchayat raj, the local Government.

Administrative set-up

At National level—administrative in-charge or the block development officer

↓

At State level—development commissioner (Secretary of planning department of state government)

↓

At District level—district collector

↓

Personal assistants (block development officers)

↓

For example: Town panchayats, village panchayat, audit, loans, establishment, inspection cell, stamp duty, survey, land records.

↓

Taluk level—tahsildar (mandal development officer)

Deputy tahsildar

↓

Assistants, revenue inspectors, junior assistants, village level worker.

Community Development and Health Services

Health is an integral part of community development because standards of health are closely linked with economic and social structure of the community.

Health care in the community development areas is an integrated pattern, combining preventive and curative services with emphasis on the preventive aspect, as per the recommendations of the health survey and development committee. This integrated health care is provided in rural areas through primary health centres.

Role of Nurse in Community Development

At district level, district public health nurse (DPHN) will keep herself informed to the key persons about activities of C.D.P, such as the president of zilla parishad and its other members.

- District public health nurse (DPHN) take part in all relevant discussions of district coordination committee concerning the nursing services of the district through the district medical health officer who is the member of the committee
- DPHN will interpret the needs of nursing services to the zilla parishad, through the district health officer and will attend the health committee meetings for betterment of the services

- When DPHN goes for supervisory visits to PHC and sub-centres, she will try to meet the Taluk development officer for maintaining good relationship for the success of the health programme
- All the block head quarters, the DPHN officer, MPHW (F) will keep in touch with the block development workers and with the village leaders for the villages, which falls within their jurisdiction
- At the sub-centres every MPHW (F) must be acquired with the village officer and sarpanch of the village, which fall within the area of her work and also with other community workers, e.g: Gram sevika, president of mahila mandal, youth mandals, social education organiser.
- MPHW (F) must become a member of that mandals, so that the village people feel that she is an equal member of the village community. It will help greatly in popularising her services being rendered.
- The nurse must keep constant contact with teachers as they are great asset for health services
- Increase students' awareness on health related issues to become healthy citizens
- Immunises the children against preventable diseases
- Promote the village community for better follow-up services
- Nurse can also get to know the important members of the village cooperatives, since they usually hold the village-purse. These persons therefore will be useful in helping for betterment of health amenities in the village, e.g: Arranging for provision of safe water supply by converting open wells into closed wells; construction of gobar gas plants.
- Nurse can completely change the outlook of the village, by building a healthy village community.
- She can be proud of her achievements and the villagers in return will look up to her as a source of constant inspiration and guidance.

The CDP is collaborated effort of all agencies and institutions of the people with the people themselves recognising the importance of 'self-help' specially at village level as the villagers play a vital role in preserving social cohesion, cultural values and stability.

According to Pandit Jawaharlal Nehru:

A panchayat—deal with political affairs of the village.

A cooperative—deals with the economic affairs

A school—deals with education

The health centre—deals with health aspects of individual, family, community, are necessary for stronger foundation for any nation. The healthy individual, who can build the country on a strong foundation.

COMMUNITY DEVELOPMENT

Project and Planning

In the community development programme, we aim at a comprehensive and all-round development programme of rural people. It can be understood as a 'Movement designated to promote better living for the whole community with active participation—both at levels of Government and community. The planning commission, Government of India has defined community, development as 'An attempt to bring about a social and economic transformation of village life through the efforts of the people themselves'.

Aims

- Integrated development of rural community covering social, cultural and economic aspects of rural life
- Fullest development of available material and human resources
- Development of a sense of responsibility and awareness among the villagers
- Development of initiative among the villagers
- Development of agriculture, animal husbandry and cottage industries

- Development of social life by providing better communication, health, sanitation, housing, education
- Women and child welfare.

The Pattern of Programme

The community development programme was launched in 55 selected projects on October 2nd, 1952, each project covering an area of 300 villages with a population of about 3 lakhs. The pattern was revised in 1958, according to this; a block covered an area of 400 – 500 sq. kms; 100 villages and a population of 60 – 70 thousand. The block has two active stages of operation; first stage of 5 years, followed by 2nd stage of 5 years. Then the block enters the post-development phase. A financial assistance of Rs. 12 lakh for the first stage and Rs. 5 lakh for the second stage is provided.

Achievements of the Community Development Programme (CDP)

In the first five years plan, more than 900 crores of rupees have been spend on CDP. In the VI plan another 160 crore rupees were spent. At present, every block in a span of 5 years will receive an assistance of Rs 35 lakh.

Previous Years University Questions

1. Social welfare. (2 m, RGUHS, 2000)
2. Discuss the factors of social change.(5 m, RGUHS, 1997)
3. Bring out the aims of social welfare planning. (5 m, RGUHS, 2002)
4. Define social change. Discuss briefly various factors of social change with suitable examples. (10 m, RGUHS, 2003)
5. Legislations and social change. (5 m, RGUHS, 2003)
6. What is social change? Examine the different factors of social change. (10 m, RGUHS, 2004)

7. Social welfare and the important measures. (5 m, RGUHS, 2004)
8. Nursing and family health care. (5 m, RGUHS, 2004)
9. Child guidance clinic. (2 m, RGUHS, 2004)
10. Social welfare. (2 m, RGUHS, 2001)
11. Community development. (5 m, RGUHS, 2002)
12. Technological factors of social change. (5 m, RGUHS, 2003)
13. Community development programme. (5 m, RGUHS, 1999, 2003)
14. Family's role in health of the children. (5 m, RGUHS, 1999)
15. Define social change. Discuss the theories of social change. (10 m, RGUHS, 2001)
16. What is community development? What are the important community development programs in India. (5 m, RGUHS, 2001)
17. Social change. (2 m, RGUHS, 2001,02)
18. Consequences of social change. (5 m, RGUHS, 2000)
19. Explain social planning. (2 m, RGUHS, 2000)
20. Briefly examine the social welfare panning in India. (5 m, RGUHS, 2002)
21. Write a short essay on family in health care. (5 m, RGUHS, 2002)
22. Factors of social change. (5 m, RGUHS, 1999, 2003)
23. Explain the impact of community development programmes of India's villages. (10 m, RGUHS, 2002)
24. Barriers to social change in India. (5 m, RGUHS, 2002)

MGR University Question Papers

1. Examine the causes and consequences of social change. (15 m, MGRU)
2. What do you understand by social change? What are the factors of social change? (15 m, MGRU)
3. Social change. (5 m, 2 m, MGRU)

4. Explain the factors influencing social change. (15 m, MGRU)
5. Consequences of social change. (5 m, 15 m, MGRU)
6. Define social change and discuss the factors and consequences of social change with illustrations. (15 m, MGRU)
7. Social legislation and social security measures for the disabled (5 m, MGRU)
8. Social planning. (2 m, MGRU)

CHAPTER NINE

Social Control

Control of society over the individual, where the undesirable or harmful tendencies of the man will be reduced by emphasising self control. It keeps on changing, in accordance with changes in the society.

Definition

- 'It is the way in which entire social order coheres and maintains itself, how it operates, as a whole or as a changing equilibrium'—*Maciver and Page*
- 'It is a social process by which the individual makes group responsive and by which social organisation is built and maintains'—*Lane*

Meaning

It is a system of measures, suggestions, persuasions, restraints, cohesion and physical codes by which a society brings into conformity to the approved behaviour and influence may be exerted through various agencies or by society or the group.

The effectiveness of each agency depends upon the circumstances. It is exercised for promoting the welfare of the group as a whole. The person is influenced throughout in the interest of others rather than in accordance with his individual interest. Social control is exercised for some specific aim or goal. The individual is made conscious of others existence and their interest and adheres to the appropriate social ways. To make the individual as a social being, whereby he found to conformity with the typical pressure of social control.

Need of Social Control

1. *To maintain the old social order:* Members in the society behave in accordance with social order. Although enforcement of the old order in a changing society may hinder social progress, yet it is necessary to maintain continuity and uniformity in the society, e.g.: The old age people in the family enforce their ideas over the children.
2. *To establish social unity/Social cohesion/Social solidarity:* To regulate behaviour in accordance with established norms which brings uniformity of behaviour and promotes the unity among the individuals.
3. *To regulate or to control individual behaviour:* No two individual are alike in his or her attitudes, interest, habits, ideas. Every movement of them is a possibility of clashes, conflicts between them. As man become too self-centered social control is necessary to preserve the social interest and satisfy commands.
4. *To provide social sanction:* If the individual violates the social norms, he is compelled to follow certain measures to control his behaviour.
5. *To check cultural maladjustments:* Society is subjected to change for every movement. New inventions, new discoveries, new philosophies continue to take origin in the society.

The individual has to adjust himself for meeting the changing needs of society. But all the individuals cannot adjust themselves to the changes, which may lead to cultural maladjustments and the people may violate the social norms. It has to be justified in the name of progress called 'social reform'. Effective social control is necessary, as India is passing through the transitional period.

Types of Social Control

I. *Karl Mannheim* classified social control

a. Direct Social Control

It is the control exercises upon the individual by the reactions of the people who are living within the proximity, e.g: Family, neighbourhood, and playgroup. Individual is deeply influenced by the opinion and views of their parents, colleagues, neighbours, and those who work with them. Individuals' behaviour is controlled or determined by the criticism, degradation, praise, suggestion or persuasion of colleagues, parents, etc.

b. Indirect Social Control

The control is exercised upon the individual by the factors like customs, laws, opinions, which affects the entire social system, e.g: Secondary group, traditions, institutions, customs, rationalised behaviour.

II. *Kimbell Young* Classified Social Control

a. Positive Social Control

Rewards and incentives has an immense value upon the activities of the individual. Everyone desires to be rewarded by the society, consequently they have to confirm to the traditions, mores, values, ideals, accepted by the society, e.g: Rewards, fame, respect, recognition, positive or constructive criticism.

b. Negative Social Control

A person is prevented from doing something wrong by threat of punishment. The society encourages the people to indulge in certain types of activity of promising rewards, also discourages and prevents people from many activities by fear of punishment. Fear of these punishments helps the people to prevent from violating the socially accepted customs, traditions, values and ideals, e.g: Verbal punishment, defamation, negative criticism.

III. Informal/Formal Social Control

a. Informal Social Control

Socially desirable behaviour will be performed, where the individual will follow the norms, standards formed by the society. The primary group will formulate the controlling measures, e.g: Mores, traditions, customs, etc.

b. Formal Social Control

They are specifically designed for control. Secondary groups like social institution formulates the norms, rules and regulating to control the people's behaviour within the society, e.g: Law, police, army, code, custody.

IV. According to Hayes

Control by sanction, e.g: Awarding the obedient and punishing the miscreant. Control by socialisation and education.

Formal Agencies of Social Control

Law

The society grows in size and complexity consisting of number of organisations, institutions and structures. Informal means of social control are no longer sufficient to maintain social order and harmony. Therefore the law provides uniform norms, rights, responsibilities and penalties throughout a social system. Laws are prominent means of social control, laws are formulated by legally authorised bodies or agencies to control the deviated behaviour and to develop desired behaviours.

Functions of Law

- To follow the rights and to act cooperatively. Laws will protect the society and contributes for its welfare. Thus law controls the conduct of the people of the state, grants everyone the opportunity to progress.

Education

Education is a process of socialisation, it prepares the child for social living and reforms the attitudes wrongly formed by children already. It corrects the belief and removes the prejudice. It teaches them the value of discipline, social cooperation, tolerance and sacrifice. It instills in the individual the qualities of honesty, fairness, sense of right and wrong. Thus education makes the people polite and what they ought to be. Education teaches man the use of various capacities, abilities, intelligence, etc. it gives him the ability to succeed in his struggle for existence. It is an art of adaptation. The child learns to respect the opinion and advice of others, hence education is a necessary condition for the proper exercise of social control.

Coercion

It is the use of force to achieve a desired end. It may be physical or non-violent. It is the ultimate means of social control, when all other means fail. In the coercion physical way of doing things such as bodily injuries, imprisonment and penalty should have immediate effect upon the offender but it does not have enduring effects. Society has to protect its own citizen.

Informal Agencies of Social Control

Growth within the society, and no special agency is required to create them. It is exercised through customs, religion, traditions, folkways, mores. It prevails in all aspects of man's life. The individual wants praise, appreciation, honour and recognition by the society. The child through the socialisation process confirms to the norms of the group. A person with socialised attitudes will not commit socially harmful activities.

Beliefs

It is a conviction, that a particular thing is true. Beliefs influence human action and they are vital for human relations. They define the purpose, interests for the individual and control his choice of means.

a. *The belief in the existence of unseen power:* It leads man to perform right actions because he believes that his actions are being watched by an unseen power.
b. *The belief in the theory of reincarnation:* It keeps the man away from the wrongful acts because he believes that in order to have a good birth in the next life, he must do good deeds in the present life.
c. *The belief in the nemesis (The Goddess of Vengeance):* This regulates mans' behaviour as he believes that he will be punished whenever wrong act is done.
d. *Belief in the existence of hell and heaven:* Individual believes that heaven is full of luxuries, fairs and romance and hell is full of terror, miseries and tortures. If one does good deeds and actions will attain heaven after death is the common belief.
e. *Belief in the immorality of the soul:* It leads man to avoid such actions as it causes pain to the souls of the ancestors.

Social Suggestion

It indirectly communicates the ideas, feelings of others, to follow influence upon the individuals to perform good deeds.

a. Following the great individuals life goals, e.g: Celebration of anniversaries of great leaders.
b. Through literature, e.g: Books, journals and papers. It may inspire the people heroic deeds and develops communal conservation.
c. Through education. The curriculum should prescribe the norms, laws, rules and regulations to learn the desired social behaviour and to make the individuals as disciplined citizens.
d. Through advertisement. It depicts the advantage of visiting certain places suggesting the prestige attached to these places. Thus suggestions may be conscious or unconscious either international or national.

Ideologies

There are powerful dynamic forces of contemporary social life. They express the vital interest of social group and desire the design for a scheme of social betterment. They stimulate action and provide a set of values, which are meaningful. Completeness and coherence influences the ideology.

Interprets the social reality to process the correctness and correlate to these ideas in their social activities, e.g: Gandhism; it influences the social life to a deep extent, Leninism; influences the social life of Russians, Hitler's life influences Germans, they began to regard themselves as a supremacy in the world.

Communal Codes

The laws of community by means of which the community exercises its control over the individual.

Customs

These are the long established habits and uses of the people. They persisted for long time and have passed from one generation to another. There is no constituted authority to declare, to apply or to safeguard them. They are accepted by the society, followed because they have been followed in the past. Customs are so powerful that no one can escape their range. They regulate social life to a great extent. Binds men together, controls purely selfish impulses and compel the individual to confirm to the accepted standards. They act as storehouse for human experiences determining and controlling human behaviour, acts as guardian of social solidarity, stimulating the social change and violation of customs is regarded not only a crime but also a sacrilege. In Hindu societies customs are powerful means of social control but in modern times their forces has loosen. It is a kind of social necessity. Disobedience of custom brings social disgrace.

Folk Ways

They are recognised modes of behaviour, which arise automatically, spontaneously and unconsciously within the group. These are socially approved and have some degree of traditional sanction. They are foundation of group culture and are developed in the society unaided by the law of trial and error. If an individual does not follow them he may be socially boycotted by his group or the society look upon such behaviour as degenerate and ridicule it. The fear of social ridicule acts as a large measure of control on the conduct of the individual, e.g: Greeting each other.

Mores

The standardised means and related to the fundamental needs of the society directly. They express a sense of light and conducive, which is essential for the welfare of the group, e.g: Marriage pattern. They incline a value judgment and moulds the behaviour and restrains the individual from doing antisocial acts. Conformity to mores is regarded as necessary behaviour, contrary to it is not permitted by the society.

Morals

These are the laws concerning concepts of goodness and badness. It is a force of the conscience. They change according to their context, current ethical concepts govern the social behaviour of the individuals, e.g: Non-violence, truth, justice and equality.

Rituals

These are the forms of socially accepted behaviour, which are important in times of festivals and religious celebrations. These rituals are to be followed as a matter of duty.

Religion

It is an attitude towards super-human power. It is having several forms like superstitions, animism, totamism, magic, ritualism. It pervades protectively all the societies. It influences man's behaviour. It explains certain laws and makes the people more benevolent, charitable pervading of all the religions. It emphasises truthfulness and more trusty and used as a tool to make the people content, obedient to their rules. The base of religious laws is the fear of divine displeasure and sufferings coupled with love and respect for some power. The individual feels the pressure of this belief even more than the pressure exerted by the state or family or the society.

For example:

1. Children should obey their parents, and should not tell lies or cheat others. Women should be faithful to men.
2. Men should limit their desires. These are some of teachings of religion, which influences the individual behaviour. Sometimes it may deny the freedom of thought and may favour poverty, exploitation, idleness, encourages certain practices like cannibalism, slavery, untouchability and communalism. It is a powerful agency, which controls the society.

Art

Influences the imagination and exert control on human behaviour. It may arouse a feeling of sympathy, affection and hatredness. There is a close relationship between the art of person and national life style. The civilisation of any specified time can be judged by an examination of his art. An artist is called as 'an agent of civilisation'. It controls the behaviour of the man, e.g: Painting, sculpture, folk songs, music, dance, rhymes.

These have their effect on man's emotions and sentiments. It is a pleasant social control and its influence is universal and communal songs and dances enhance community feeling.

Literature

It possesses high quality, which makes life worthfull. Good literature work for great social values, e.g: Ramayana, Bible, Koran, Bagavad Gita. Bad literatures have its own effects like criminal and delinquent behaviour.

Humour and Satire

It often serves to relieve a sense of tension or tensed situation. It is also used to gain a favourable response. Human being controls his behaviour by supporting the sanctioned values of the society in the form, e.g: Light in spirit but effective in control. Satire is used with a bad intension to deflate others without a reason, e.g: Laughing at others.

Public Opinion

The influence of public opinion as a means of social control has its effect in simple societies. In a village the people are known to one another personally, and it is very difficult for the villagers to act contrary to the public opinion of the that village. It is a power body as it controls the government, even the powerful government has to resign, if the public opposes it. Opinions are formed through propaganda, newspaper, and radio. An individual is more concerned with the reaction of people than with the wrath of God.

It is the fear of disgrace in the society, which keeps a check on the behaviour of the people. Opinions are difficult to contradict. It controls the conduct, behaviour, ways of living and methods. It greatly influences human actions, for fear of public ridicule and criticism, human beings will not indulge in immoral or anti-social activities. Every individual wants to win public praise and avoid public criticism. The desire for recognition is a natural phenomenon.

Family

The first place where an individual socialised, is the family. He learns various methods of living, behaviour, conversion, obedience and respect for others. The control of parent upon the child is the control of society upon the individual. It is a basic form of society. It forms certain rules and laws, which are enforced lovingly and effort is made to make the individual to understand them. The child is taught to behave in a fashion, which conforms to the standards of behaviour of the people. Infringement of the rules of family brings punishment in its wake and the child learns to accept the pressure of law. It initiates him to take a value judgment and differentiate between good and the bad. The communal ideas, values and thoughts control the behaviour. The family educates the individual to accept and obey social control.

Recreation Group

A person under goes specialisation and learns the methods of behaviour towards other people. Games are based on laws without following them games cannot be played. In this way, games instill in man the habit of remaining in control and obeying the law. Games make a person pliable and teach him to obey the orders of the leader and cooperate with other people as a result the sense of group responsibility is awakened in the participants.

Leadership

The leaders show the way for the masses to follow the path taken by great men of the past. The path influences the religious, political and other fields to the fellow men.

Fashion

In civilised society, the determinant in the field of thought, conduct, deeds, belief, opinions, recreations, ornaments influences to a greater range. Fashion is constantly changing but the people are ever desirous of changing with it. Fashion controls the individual's thoughts, ideas, attitudes and behaviour.

Previous Years University Questions

1. Define fashion. (2 m, RGUHS, 2000)
2. Explain the role of fashion in modern society. (5 m, RGUHS, 2002)
3. Informal means of social control. (5 m, RGUHS, 2003)
4. Formal means of social control. (2 m, RGUHS, 2001)
5. What is social control? Enumerate the important social control measures in society. (5 m, RGUHS, 2001)
6. Describe the social control methods in the society. (5 m, RGUHS, 2002)
7. Social control mechanism. (5 m, RGUHS, 2000)

MGR University Question Papers

1. Social control. (2 m, MGRU)
2. Agencies of social control in regulating the human behaviour. (5 m, MGRU)

3. Goals of social control. (5 m, MGRU)
4. State the different agencies of social control. Explain with suitable examples. (15 m, MGRU)
5. Write an essay on the different methods of social control. (5 m, MGRU)
6. Social control. (5 m, MGRU)

CHAPTER TEN

Social Stratification

It is a social process in which the society is divided into various groups, which will have their own characteristics, status and roles. The relationship to one another is determined on the basis of stratification. It continuously undergoes change. It is the division of society where they are linked with each other by the relationship of superiority and inferiority.

Definition

- 'Social stratification is a horizontal division of society into higher and lower socials units'.
- 'It is a division of society into permanent and temporary groups or categories. The groups are interlinked with each other by the relationship of superiority and subordination'.
- 'A group of people who possess particular social status or position by virtue of which they possess some privileges, responsibilities and powers'.

Social class is determined on the basis of certain acquired characteristics, e.g: Economic condition, individual attainments.

As a result of class system, the people have different roles and social statuses. It means, that the members in a particular class have a status attached to them and have to play a role in relevance to the society.

Thus a social class is an aggregate of persons giving essentially the same social status in a given society.

Characteristics

- Social
- Ancient
- Ubiquitous
- Diverse in its forms
- Consequential
- Differentiation, evaluation, ranking, rewarding.

FACTORS OF SOCIAL STRATIFICATION

Difference in Human Being

Individuals will differ with each other based on biological factors and socio-cultural factors. Hence the individual is placed into various groups to discharge their obligations towards their society in a proper manner.

Biological Group

1. *Sex:* In matriarchal society, the women are considered superior and have control over the political and social institutions. She will be the decision maker in the family. Where as in patriarchal society, men hold domination superiority and power.
2. *Age:* The society is divided into children, adolescents, youth, middle age, and old age. In these societies others respect old aged people.

Birth

If a particular person is from a particular caste, he is considered as superior or inferior, e.g: Indian caste system—Brahmins are considered as superior, Sudra is considered as inferior group.

Based on Race

People belong to a particular race and possessing racial characteristics, they are considered superior to others, e.g: In America, whites are considered as superior than black people. They have separate quarters, places of recreation, congregation, etc.

Socio-cultural Basis

Based on factors such as

1. Economy: Higher class, middle class, and lower class.
2. Religion: Hindu, Muslim, Christian.
3. Caste: Forward, backward.
4. Occupation: Professional, administrator, and class IV group.
5. Need for different functions: Teachers, doctors, engineers and cook.

Equilibrium

Every society should have proper organisation, and they should possess social equilibrium. If the society is divided into various groups based on functions, they are mutually dependent and maintain balance within the society.

Forms of Social Stratification

Racial Stratification

There is a hierarchal order or in the superiority of one class in relevance to the other is determined on the basis of membership of a particular race. It is not possible for people to leave one race and join the other.

Class Stratification

Every society has many classes. Each social class has a status in the society. In accordance with, it receives social prestige. The members of all classes have some special benefits and facilities, which are bestowed upon them due to class status. Class-consciousness is generated in by differences in the social status.

Basis for class stratification

- Economic factors
- Occupation

CASTE STRATIFICATION

Indian Caste System

Three basic pillars of Indian social system are: Joint family, caste and village system. As a form of social stratification and inseparable aspect is peculiar to Indian society where unity among diversity is found. Latin word 'castus' means 'pure'. The Portuguese used caste word to denote the Indian institution. The factors influencing caste system in India are: The geographic isolation of the Indian peninsula for a long time; influence of Hindu religion, they believe caste system is looked upon as a divinely ordained institution, karma siddhantha, fatalism, beliefs in reincarnation; existence of many races in the country; rural social structure, no uniform laws and standards existing in the system, illiteracy or lack of education, hereditary, occupations, ideas of exclusive family, ancestor worship, beliefs related to sacrament, clash of races, prejudice, conquest, etc. contributed to the growth of caste system in India.

Caste is derived from Spanish word, 'caste' which means break, race, strain, a complex and hereditary qualities. Indian society has castes such as forward caste, e.g: Brahmin, vysya, backward caste like scheduled caste and scheduled tribes (dalits).

Definition

- 'A caste is an aggregation of persons, whose obligations and privileges is fixed by birth, sanctioned and supported by religion'.
- 'An endogamous unity with a more or less defined rituals status and some occupation traditionally linked to it'—*SC Dube*
- 'A system of stratification in which mobility up and down the status ladder, atleast ideally may not occur'—*AW Green*
- 'Collection of families bearing a common name, claiming a common descent, from a mythical ancestor, human and divine, preferring to follow hereditary and regarded as a homogeneous community'—*Herbert Prisely*

Characteristics

- Determination of membership is by birth
- Each caste should possess certain rules and regulations
- Definite occupation
- Endogamous group
- Rules concerning status should posses the superiority and inferiority status
- Caste is a segmental division of society. Castes are groups with a well defined boundary of their own
- The membership and status is determined by 'birth' hence it is unchangeable, unacquirable, unattainable, and non-transferable
- Each caste will have certain customs, traditions, practices and rituals
- Caste Panchayat in certain areas regulate the conduct of members
- It is a hierarchal division of society. A sense of 'superiority/ higher or lowness or inferiority' is associated with gradation or ranking, e.g: Brahmins are treated as superior and scheduled caste are treated inferiorly

- Restrictions on food habits, e.g: Brahmins and Vysyas are vegetarian in nature; and will not consume garlic, onions
- Restrictions on social relations and marriages, e.g: Higher caste people should not interact with low caste people in early days
- Certain low caste people are still suffering with social and other religious disabilities.

Merits of Caste system
(Conditions favouring Caste system)

- Geographical isolation
- Static society
- Rural societal structure
- Aggregation of people
- Influence of religion
- Difference of races
- Lack of education
- Formation of trade unions
- Spirit of cooperation
- Economic pursuits
- Racial purity
- Intellectual make-up
- Integration of the country
- Cultural diffusion
- Separation of social life from political life.

Demerits (Unfavourable factors)

- Modern education
- Urbanisation, modernisation
- Industrialisation
- Wealth consciousness
- Movements of social emancipation (mixing)
- Means of communication
- Political agitation
- Appearances of new social classes

- Denies mobility
- Retarded solidarity
- Wrong men in occupation
- Obstacle to national unity and social progress
- Undemocratic

Difference Between Class and Caste

Class	*Caste*
Membership is based upon objective facts, e.g: Status, occupation, standard of life, wealth.	Membership is based upon birth (Subjective phenomenon).
Open stratification, a person can change his class dynamic.	Closed stratification of table, unchangeable.
Class consciousness.	Subjective consciousness.
Does not hinder democracy.	Hinders democracy.
Individual will have greater freedom.	Rigid with more restriction.
Less social distance.	Greater social distance.
Endogamous group.	Endogamous group.
Flexible restriction.	Rigid restriction.
No ethnocentric feeling.	Ethnocentric feeling.
External similarity is maintained, e.g: Dress, language, customs.	No external similarities.
Internal similarity maintained, e.g: Thinking, ideas.	No internal similarity.
Elastic nature. Easy social mobility.	Close, rigid stability
Secular origin.	Divine origin.
No fixed order of social prestige.	Fixed order of social prestige.
No restriction on interaction food drinking pattern	Restrictions on eating, drinking and mixing with others.
Achieved status.	Ascribed status.
Temporary association flexible, based on need membership is attained.	Durable relationship.

Changes in Traditional Features of Caste in Independent India

- Caste is recognised by social and secular meaning than a religious interpretation
- Restrictions on food habits and occupation choice was relaxed
- Inter-caste marriage are legally permitted

- Constitutional provisions were revised to overcome the handicappedness of low caste people, e.g: Reservation facility in education, employment, etc.
- Caste continuous to ascribe social status
- Caste panchayats become disappeared or weakened
- Social interaction and social relationships has been establishing in the society without seeking the caste background
- Ritual status on caste system was changed
- Caste has lost its hold over social usages and customs practiced by its members
- It is not dictating individual's life or its freedom, it is not barrier for the individual's progress
- Industrialisation, urbanisation, westernisation education, etc. changed the role of caste system.

Causes for the Changes in Caste System

- Uniform legal system: For removing untouchability, Indian law made provision in articles 15, 16, 164, 225, 330, 332, 334, 335, 338 to enable the low caste people to come up to the level of upper caste.
- Impact of modern education: Educational facilities has extended to all castes, relaxation in admission riles made for the provision of more education facilities for lower social groups.
- Industrialisation, urbanisation, westernisation, technological advancement, improved transport and communication system, etc. made weakened the caste system, different categories of people have started to work together, stay together in all areas like factories, offices, workshops, etc. migration of manpower is not having any bar because of advanced transport system.
- Democracy and social legislations, reforms movements' uniformity among the individuals.

- Threat of conversion to other religions made relax in caste rigidities
- Improvement in the status of women, evolution of new social classes, division of labour relaxed the rules of caste system.

Interdependence of Caste System (Jajmani System)

Caste system is having stronger influence in the rural society. It provides rules of society behaviour, which cannot be violated and maintains control over its members. Even though castes are socially segregated, on several situations, one caste has to secure the services of other caste. Such dependency among the caste is called, 'Vertical unity'/'Jajmani system' in which each group of village is expected to give certain standard services to the other castes. It is based on economic interest and fulfillment of needs and requirements, e.g: Brahmins will perform various religious ceremonies for the welfare of all castes.

- *Kumharas* will prepare earthen pots for storage of drinking water during summer.
- Barber plays a role during several religious occasions like death ceremonies.
- *Darji* stitches clothes to all caste people.
- *Bania* sells the daily used utensils on cash or credit basis.

Jajmani relations are permanent, hereditary, based on Barter system. It provides occupation and removes exploitation of lower castes, but in modern India, Jajmani system decreases and forces an individual for exploitation of the lower caste, who is helpless in terms of wealth and power. Due to urbanisation, improved transportation, communication facilities, awareness of resources and services, etc. are the contributing factors for the disintegration of Jajmani system. But in villages interdependence of caste system is still prevailing.

Health Among Under Privileged Sections of Society

Due to poverty, social stigma, over crowding, illiteracy, ignorance, beliefs, traditions, cultural barrier, living in slum area and under developed communities, poorer sanitation, low standards of living etc., predisposes to the occurrences of communicable diseases and low standards of living.

Previous Years University Questions

1. Define social stratification. (2 m, RGUHS, 2000)
2. Difference between class and caste.(5 m, RGUHS, 2002)
3. Changes in caste system. (5 m, RGUHS, 2001)
4. Explain the difference between class and caste. (2 m, RGUHS, 2001)
5. Social stratification. (5 m, RGUHS, 1997)
6. Explain the features of Indian caste system. Write a note on the future of caste system in India. (10 m, RGUHS, 2002)
7. Mention the forms of conflicts. (5 m, RGUHS, 2002)
8. What is meant by class. (2 m, RGUHS, 2002)
9. Write a short essay on Indian caste system. (5 m, RGUHS, 2004)
10. Class and caste. (2 m, RGUHS, 2000,04)
11. List out the characteristics of the caste system. Explain the changes that have taken place in the caste. (10 m, RGUHS, 2002)
12. What is meant by casteism. (2 m, RGUHS, 2002)
13. Changing trends of caste system in India. (5 m, RGUHS, 2003)
14. Characteristics of caste. (5 m, RGUHS, 2000)
15. What is varna system. (2 m, RGUHS, 2000)
16. Explain the adverse effects of caste. What are its consequences on health. (10 m, RGUHS, 1999)
17. Define caste. Critically examine the Indian caste system. (5 m, RGUHS, 201)

18. Briefly describe social stratification. What are the difference between social stratification and social classification. (5 m, RGUHS, 2001)
19. Adverse effects of caste. (5 m, RGUHS, 2000)
20. Define class and caste. Discuss the caste system in India. (10 m, RGUHS, 2002)
21. Describe social stratification and show its peculiar nature in India. (5 m, RGUHS, 2002)
22. Describe basic characteristics of Indian caste system. (10 m, RGUHS, 2003)
23. Origin of caste. (5 m, RGUHS, 2002)
24. Bases of social stratification. (5 m, RGUHS, 2002)
25. Explain Jajmani system. (3 m, RGUHS, 2002)
26. Caste in Today's Indian society. (5 m, RGUHS, 2000)
27. Health among under-privileged sections of population. (2 m, RGUHS, 2000)
28. What is social stratification and discuss any one of them. (19 m, NTRUHS, 1998)
29. Diseases common in slums.(5 m, SVIMS, Tirupati, 2003)

MGR University Question Papers

1. Social stratification. (5 m, MGRU)
2. Changing trends in caste system. (5 m, MGRU)
3. Features of caste system. (5 m, MGRU)
4. Describe the origin, evaluation and characteristics of caste system. (15 m, MGRU)
5. Caste system. (5 m, MGRU)
6. Define caste. Describe briefly the salient features of the Indian caste system. (20 m, MGRU)
7. Explain the characteristics features of the caste system in India. (15 m, MGRU)

CHAPTER ELEVEN

Social Institutions

INTRODUCTION

Satisfaction of value oriented interests through association of individuals grouped together in organisations. Individuals in institution will have their own specific status and role. Everyone in the organisation will work together to achieve the common goal. They coordinate the group activities in the interest of achieving/satisfaction of the specified objectives. The collective efforts of group members to reach the common interests or said goals. Structural mechanisms are intended to regularise the behaviour of people, specifically carried out for proper functioning of society. 'Institution' will set-up clearly defined methods to attain the goals. 'Institutions' are essential for smooth functioning of the society. It outlines its purpose, it may continue with new goals. The varied interests of people like religion, education, government or state, art, cultural economic, etc. find expression through social 'Institution'. Aims, functions and activities are listed in the form of constitutions leading to formal structure. The social institution may be oriented towards mutual benefit/business type/client-centred/public interest. It influences human behaviour. Rituals help in the continuity of institutional practices. Human beings obtain a large part of their material, social and cultural satisfaction. Objectives, values of life are emphasised in social institution. It functions through a complete structure of reciprocal roles that prescribes the individual's behaviour in his institutional capacity. Institution has its followers, it has an inseparable part of our collective life. Thus institutions are structured processes through which people carry on their activities.

Definition

- 'A concept (the ideas, notion, doctrine, interest) or a structure (framework or apparatus) and a number of functionaries set to cooperate in prescribed ways at a certain conjuncture'—*Graham Summer*
- 'A system of patterned expectations defining the proper behaviour of persons playing certain roles, enforced both by the incumbents own positive motives for conformity and by the sanction of others'— *Parsons*
- 'A social institution is 'an organised behaviour/structure in a recognised established pattern oriented towards the satisfaction of fundamental, human needs and the fulfillment of basic social function necessary for the maintenance and preservation of the social order'
- 'Recognised and established usages governing the relations between individuals and groups'—*Ginsberg*
- 'An organised cluster of folkways and mores centred around a major human activity'—*PB Horton and CL Hunt*
- 'Established forms or conditions of procedures characteristic of group activity'—*Maciver and Page*
- 'A set of inter-woven folkways, mores and laws built around one or more functions'—*Kingsley Davis*
- 'The social structure and the machinery through which human society organises directs and executes the multifarious activities required to satisfy human needs'—*Barnes HE*

- 'The habitual ways of living together which have been sanctioned, systematised and established by the authority of communities'—*Ellwood CA*

Society accepts the rules and considers them binding. It brings moral restraints on individual's behaviour and most people accept them as right. Through institutionalisation is meant the development of orderly, stable, socially integrated forms and practices. It consists of the establishment of definite rules, which assigns position, status and role functioning in connection with such behaviour. It is a set of folkways, mores, laws built around one or more functions. It is an organised form of customs and procedures. These are focusing on the fundamental social function and the behaviour is structured in the process of fulfillment. The major social institutions are the family, economic, political, educational and religious institutions.

Structure of Social Institution

It refers to the ways human being behave and the mechanism they employ in the process of fulfillment of the basic social function and the realisation of social values.

The institution structure includes:

1. Personnel: The members of society as they play the social roles related to the various institutional functions, e.g: In the institution of family the social role like siblings and grand parents will exist.
2. Equipment: All the apparatus through which the personnel functions.
3. System: It refers to the pathways in which the personnel and equipment are arranged under a set of organising principles, which give direction to their behaviour, e.g: In family-monogamy, polygamy, patriarchal and matriarchal types are followed.

Each institution will have a normative structure (cluster of mores, expectations, rules, procedures, which may be written or unwritten, formal or informal). In some institutions the procedures are highly standarised like army.

Types

Primary institutions: The most basic institutions formed even in primitive societies, e.g: Family, religion, marriage.

Secondary institutions: To meet the secondary needs of people, e.g: Educational institution, banks, legislation, constitution, business.

Summer classified: Social institutions as:

Crescive institution: The institutions, which are developed naturally, unconsciously and spontaneously, e.g: Primary institution.

Enacted institution: Consciously and purposefully in a planned manner established are referred to by him, e.g: Secondary institution.

Functions

Need fulfillment: In economical institutions fulfillment of basic needs like substance and need for survival, i.e. production, distribution and consumption will be met. In family, need for birth, security, love and affection and companionship is being fulfilled.

In political institution, maintenance of social order and exercise the authority over the human beings. Provision must be made for the unanswerable questions for human existence, for propagation and seeking to manipulate the supernatural power for the formation of a system of ritual action.

It is common for the major social institution to perform a variety of social activities or functions to meet the organisational goals and they are often overlapping, e.g: In religious institution apart from the functions mentioned above, the teaching, education is rendered as a charitable service.

As institutions are socially organised established and pattern of behaviour they have normative pattern and they reflect social order, which is right, legitimate and expected modes of relating and acting. Thus social control will be maintained.

Social continuity is preserved since institutionalised patterns are transmitted from one generation to the other. The character, structure and other personality traits, which emerge and crystallise, reflect the desirable character, structure and personality trait. Institution pressures are exerted to elicit appropriate character in house, school, religious institution and on the job. Institution contributes to unity and uniformity within the society.

Institutions are socialised. The character and other personality traits, which emerge to reflect what the institution complexes prescribe as desirable character, structure and personality traits. They will be compatible with the maintenance and preservation of institutions, e.g: Family tends to cultivate affection, love with mutual respect and loyalty.

Economic institution tends to cultivate faith, devotion, compliments, ambition and punctuality. Religious institutions tend to cultivate faith and devotion. Political institution tends to cultivate sub-ordination, patriotism, obedience and loyalty. It fulfills the manifest function and latent functions of the society. The manifest functions of institution include social importance and preservation of internal position, e.g: In army the manifest function is protecting the country. Latent functions are discipline, defining nation character, training the youth and making them physically fit for holding any responsibility.

Characteristics

- Institution have some definite objectives
- There is a symbol of every institution, which can be either material or non-material, e.g: National anthem and *vande matarum* are symbols of our nation.

- Every institution has some rules, which must compulsory carried out by the individuals
- Institution has definite procedures based on dogmas, principles and norms
- Institution depends upon the collective or group activities of man, but not individual, thus it is social in nature
- Regular and repetitive forms of social relationship will be established and they are essentially interlinked
- Institutions are ubiquitous in nature, exist at all stages of social development thus universality is observed
- They are means of controlling the individuals behaviour
- They are most stable than any other means of social control
- They are the means of fulfillment of primary needs/basic needs, e.g: Self expectations, self preservation, self expression.

Process of Institutionalisation

Institutions emerged as planned products of social living. The people search for practical ways of meeting their needs. They find pattern, which passes through repetition into standarised customs as time passes these patterns acquired a body of supporting folkways, which justifies and sanction them. Thus the institutions are arised. Institutionalisation consists of the establishment of definite norms, which assign status, position and role function in connection with such behaviour.

Our social relationships gets institutionalised by:

- It directs the behaviour of people in their manifold activities
- Acceptance—large number of social group accept the norms formed by the societal leads.
- Institutions are formed to regulate the behaviour of society
- Permits sanctions and norms. All the members are guided by social sanction.
- Essential for proper functioning of society in order to achieve the goals.
- Satisfies varied needs and interests of the people.

Each of the institution has its peculiarity as they maintain the loyalty of their participants. Assign authority to different functionaries formulate standards of behaviour and develop methods of dealings with others. These are called as institutional traits, which are peculiar to that institution only. Similarly role, which is a set of behaviour expectations. All the institutions develop symbols, which is a short hand remainder of the institution, e.g: National flag is the symbol of the Country. Parliament Bhavan indicates President's role and the place where the functions of Government will take place.

Codes of Behaviour

Each institution has to prepare their members to carry out the roles assign to them. They should feel responsibility and accountability. Those roles are often formal codes such as oath. The formal codes of behaviour are only the part of total behaviour that makes an institution.

Importance of Institution

According to *Maciver,* it transfers cultural norms from generation to generation. It involves unity in human behaviour and controls a conduct and guides man according to circumstances. The following considerations deserve mention with regarding to importance of social institution. The society morals, ideals, knowledge and forms of behaviour are transferred from one generation to other through the medium of institution. It helps to the younger generation in its solutions of problems. Institutions indicate the right path to man and imposes control upon his activities. The society by means of the institution compels people collectively to work in conformity with in the social framework.

MARRIAGE

Introduction

Marriage is an important social institution. It is changing in its form according to the change in its culture. It is an institution, which permits or admits man and women for family life. It is more or less durable condition between male and female, beyond the mere acting of propagation (birth of off-spring). It is an approved social institution where by two or more persons forms the family. There has been mutual attraction due to certain biological and psychological causes resulting in the establishment of intimate relationships. From the biological view point the sexual inter-course is necessary for physical satisfaction and the birth of the progeny. It also leads to mutual help in times of need, psychologically they have so many traits, which are mutually complementary.

Definition

- 'Marriage is a ritual, which creates the family and in the form of husband and wife. It is a ceremony of uniting marital partners'—*Stern*
- 'Marriage denotes unequivocally sanctioned unions, which persist beyond several satisfactions and thus come to unduly family life'—*Robert H Lowie*
- 'It is socially approved way of establishing a family of procreation'—*Gillin and Gillin*
- 'The more or less durable connection between male and female lasting beyond the mere act of propagation'—*Edward Westermarch*
- 'A contract for the production and maintenance of children'—*Malinowski*
- 'A socially sanctioned sexual relationship involving two people of the opposite sex, whose relations is expected to endure beyond the time required for gestation and the birth of children'—*Duncan Mitchell*

It involves the social sanction generally in the form of ritual or religious ceremony authorising two persons of opposite sex to engage in sexual and other consequent and correlated socio-economic relations with one another. It includes the following characteristics:

- It is a result of civil as well as religious ceremony
- Means of contact of persons of opposite sex
- Right of mutual relationships in biological, psychological, social and economic spheres of male and female
- Establishes family building activity and a house hold activity
- 'Procreation and providing care of off-spring'—*DN Majumdar and TN Madan*
- Universal institution
- Requires social approval
- Creates mutual obligation; it imposes certain rights and duties between husband and wife, both are required to support each other and their family.

Thus marriage is a more or less permanent association of one male with one female for the purpose of giving social sanction to progeny, satisfaction of biological and social need and fulfillment of Dharma.

Importance of Marriage

- Regulates sex life and sex relations of the individual
- Puts restrictions on the premarital and extramarital sex relations
- Establishes family formation. Sexual satisfaction offered by marriage results in self perpetuation
- Marriage insists the couple to establish family by procreation. Marriage determines the descent of the newborn individual. Inheritance and succession follow the rule of descent
- The partners of marriage distribute and divide work among them and perform them. The couple works outside the

family to earn more income, provides economic cooperation in order to elevate their economic status

- Marriage develops intense love and affection towards each other and deepens emotions, strengthens the companionship between the two
- Marriage helps intellectual cooperation among both of them
- Minimises the social distance between groups and strengthen their solidarity.

Selection of Mates

The life partners may be selected by parents or by elders or the choice left to the wishes of the individuals concerned. Marriage is institutional arrangement made by society according to which the individuals establish marital or making relationships among themselves.

Types

- *Endogamy:* Within the same group or caste
- *Exogamy:* Outside the group or caste
- *Polygamy:* Marrying more than one spouse
- *Polygyny:* Many wives
- *Polyandry:* Many husbands
- *Consanguineous marriages:* Endogamy among blood relationships.
- *Group marriage:* Marriages are held in a common place by a group of brides and grooms.
- *Syndesmian marriage:* The pairing of male and female is temporary and not controlled by any rules and regulation.
- *Patriarchal:* Male dominate system; a male can marry several women who would live separately to each other, e.g: Hypogomy and polygamy.
- *Monogamy:* One male marries a female at a time and lives with her until legal separation.

- *Matriarchal:* Female dominated.
- *Bigamy:* Man marries two women.
- Inter-caste marriage.
- Inter-religious marriage.
- International marriages.
- Inter-continental.
- *Hypergamy:* To enforce celibacy, early signs of female, variety to have more children as a social prestige and economic necessities hypergamy takes place.

Marriage Problems in India

- Lack of trust
- Unstability
- Change in relationship between man and woman
- Sex laxity
- Economic imbalance
- Sexual heterogeneity
- Decline of religious control
- Decline of family control
- Decline of moral
- Divorce, separation
- Dowry system
- Impact of western family system
- Inferiority and superiority complexes.

Legislations Related to Marriage

The laws enacted in India related to marriage are:

- Age at marriage
- Field of mate selection
- Number of spouses in marriage
- Breaking of marriage
- Remarriage
- Dowry to be given and taken.

Prevention of Sati Act (1829)

The glorification of the deal of 'pativratya' had led to the inhuman practice of 'sati'. Widows are often forced to make a vow or sankalpa to die after their husband's death. Sri Rajaram Mohan Roy took up the cause of women and impressed upon. Lord Bentinck, the British Governor General of India brings out a legislation prohibiting the practice of 'sati'. The formation of Sati Act, 1829 includes saving the lives of widows, and punishing and fining those instigates the practice of 'sati'.

Hindu Widow Remarriage Act (1856)

Through prevention of Sati Act, even though widows were saved, but they were subjected to exploitation and humiliation. To remove the deplorable condition of Hindu widows, Pandit Ishwara Chandra Vidya Sagar brought pressure on the British Government to make legal provision for widow remarriage.

The Civil for Special Marriage Act (1872)

The legislation treated Hindu marriage as a civil marriage, provided legal permission for inter-caste, inter-religious and registered marriages. It was modified in 1954, Special Marriage Act for register marriages in which the would-be couple has to inform the marriage officer a month before the scheduled marriage and two witnesses has to be present during the time of marriage.

The Hindu Marriage Act (1955)

This Act is applicable for the total India except Jammu and Kashmir. The word 'Hindu' in the Act includes Jains, Sikhs, Buddhists and the scheduled castes.

Conditions for Valid Marriage as Provided under this Act

- Prohibits polygyny, polyandry and child marriage and concedes equal

- Neither party has a spouse living
- Neither party is a lunatic
- The bridegroom must have completed 21 years of age and the bride 18 years of age
- Provides for equality of sex, i.e. equal rights for men and women in marriage
- Both parties should not be 'sapindas' of each other unless the custom permits such a marriage
- Given permission for inter-caste or inter-religious marriages.

Conditions Under which Divorce as per this Act

- The spouse must have been impotent at the time of marriage and continuous to be so even afterwards
- Lunatic at the time of marriage
- Consent of the petitioner or of the guardian was obtained by force or fraud
- The wife was pregnant by some person other than the petitioner at the time of marriage
- The dissolution of marriage may be obtained on the grounds of cohabitation not resumed after 2 years after judicial separation; adultery; unsound mind; renunciation; conversion of religion; sexual transmitted disease; leprosy; desertion for 7 years.

Dowry Prohibition Act (1961)

It permits exchange of gifts for not more than Rs. 2000/-. It prescribes the penalty of 6 months imprisonment or a fine up to Rs 5000/- or both for the violation. The Act got amended in 1986 and there after its rules became still more stringent. It does not apply to Muslims.

Child Marriage Restraint Act (1929)—CMRA

This Act was in force from April 1st, 1930. According to this Act boys under 18 years of age, girls under 14 years of age, if gets married is an offence. Later the Act was amended in 1978 to 21 years of age for boys 18 years of age for girls. Violation of the Act prescribes penalty of 3 months imprisonment and Rs. 1000/- fine.

Divorce According to Muslim Law

Divorce can be obtained directly in two ways without the intervention of the civil court.

Khula or Kohi and Mubarat

Divorce by mutual consent by 'khula' and 'mubarat'. In 'khula' divorce is initiated at the instance of the wife and in 'mubarat' both the parties desire separation, initiation is either by husband or by wife.

Talaq

The husband has the right to dismiss his wife by repeating the dismissal formula thrice. The talaq is effected by orally or by making some pronouncement or in writing by presenting 'talaq nama'.

1. *Talaq-e-Ahasan:* A single pronouncement of talaq followed by a period of conjugal abstinence till the completion of 'iddat'.
2. *Talaq-e-Hasan:* Three pronouncements of talaq made during three successive menstrual periods and no sexual contact in this period.
3. *Talaq-e-ul-Bidat:* Talaq pronouncement takes place to any one of the following ways:
   - In a single sentence 'I divorce the thrice'
   - In separate sentences, i.e. 'I divorce the'
   - In a single but clear pronouncement.

Divorce According to Shariah Act 1937

Three forms of divorce provisions are available:

Illa

If the husband swears by God to obtain from sexual relations with his wife for a period of four months or more or for a specified period. He is said to Illa. If he sticks onto his words, then marriage gets dissolved.

Zihar

The husband with sound mind declares in the presence of two witnesses; the person will see his wife as his mother to him. Based on this the wife can go to court on this ground.

Lian

The husband accuses his wife of being guilty of adultery. It gives an opportunity for the wife to go to court insisting on her husband either to withdraw such an allegation or prove the same.

Provisions for divorce as per the dissolution of Muslim Marriage Act (1939)

A Muslim woman to seek the dissolution of her marriage on the following basis:

- Husband whereabouts not known for four years
- Failure of husband to provide for her maintenance for two years
- Imprisonment of husband for 7 years or more
- Impotency of husband since the time of marriage
- Failure to fulfill marital obligations for three years
- Insanity of husband for a period of two years
- Husbands' incurable diseases.

The Hindu Adoption and Maintenance Act 1956

It provides provision for childless women the right to adopt a child and to claim maintenance from the husband if she is divorced.

The Suppression of Immoral Traffic of Women and Girls Act 1956

Protects the women from being kidnapped or compelled to become prostitutes.

Medical Terminal of Pregnancy Act 1971

Legalises abortion conceding the right of a woman to undergo abortion on the ground of physical and mental health.

Criminal Law Amendment Act 1983

Prohibits the women against crimes.

Family Court Act 1984

Provides justice to women who get involved in family disputes.

DOWRY SYSTEM

In the Vedic age dowry system was unknown, since women enjoyed equal status with men; in those days, marriage was popularly known as, 'kanyadana' indicated that it was far from the evil of dowry. At the time it was of solemnisation of marriage, the parents will give gifts and presents to the bride and groom to express their love, affection and respect. 'Vara dakshina' is not a dowry; in-laws should not demand even the 'stridhan' as a right. 'Stridhan' refers to 'the gifts given to a woman by her kith and kin or by her husband at or after wedding and the money she inherits from her parents or earn by personal efforts'.

In ancient times, women regarded with dignity and respect by all regions, their role in society was well defined, treated as equal citizens. Parents will give gifts as a token of love and affection for the newly married couple, who were forming or starting a new life. Marriage is a sacred bond between two individuals. Gifts given at the time of marriage are intended to help them to set-up house.

Religion, customs, age-old prejudice, etc. have kept Indian woman in a exploitable, lack of economic independence, value bias operating against them have resulted in the women being dependent on men folk and on the family, neighbourhood and larger society. Women are unaware of their rights and they do not have easy access to justice. Women in India have a long way to go in concretising the constitutional goals into reality. Education and gainful employment do not make women equal to men in matrimonial matters.

Mahatma Gandhiji, the father of nation, believed that the dowry system is 'nothing but the sale of girls' (1958) Dowry started as an innocent custom, a symbol of love from parents to their daughters on the eve of the marriage. In the recent years, it has grown into a social evil. Dowry has gained social acceptance as a normal marriage procedure, throughout the country. It has become a status symbol for both the parties. Father, who is quite willing to part with a lot of money as dowry at the time of marriage is hesitant to give a share of his property to his daughter. Even though the Hindu Succession Act has given property rights to women; they themselves are probably are not ready to got to court to seek these rights.

Bride's parents and other siblings are deprived of their minimal comforts, nutritious food, proper education, etc. to save enough for dowry. Many married women and prospective brides have been forced to end their lives to escape from the clutches of the system. The situation is worse when the birth of the female child is considered as a curse and female foeticide has become the fashion and trade of the time.

Definition

- 'Property or money brought by a bride to her husband when she marries him'—*The Oxford Dictionary*
- 'Any amount of money, property or valuable securing offered and given in connection with the marriage of the said parties, before, at the time of or any time after the marriage'—*Section 2 of the Dowry Prohibition Act, 1961*

- Money, gifts, clothes, ornaments or wealth or contributions estate that wife brings to her husband in marriage; on the basis of contribution given by the parents
- 'The property which a man receives from his wife or her family at the time of marriage according to the capacity and wish giving'—*AX Radis*
- 'It is the property that is given to the women at the time of her marriage'—*Encyclopedia of Britannica*
- 'Gifts and values received in marriage by the bride and bridegroom and from his relatives'—*Ram Ahuja*

The dowry is considered as a social evil

- Dowry is causing suffering of the people and parents
- It is the corruption and bribe in the society
- It has deteriorated the status of women
- Results in dowry death, suicide, homicide, etc.

Dowry is not to be confused with the concepts of 'kanyadan' and 'stridhan'.

Dowry system is considered to be a prestigious issue the demands become unaffordable in certain caste and communities but practiced by all most all castes. The dowry plays a major role in marriage irrespective of their status. In our country, marriages are fixed by the elders in the family and they demand money, jewels, and other household items.

Factors responsible for dowry system are:

- Caste system
- Social custom
- Inevitability of marriage
- Physical handicaps
- Aspiration to money in rich families
- False notion of social status
- Vicious circle

The amount of dowry is regulated by factors like:

- Brides and bridegroom's salary and service
- Social and economic status of the girl's father
- Social prestige of the boy's family

- Educational qualifications
- Family size of both families.

Dowry Through Ages

If we observe the history of dowry system through different stages we find change in its structure from ancient through medieval period to present India.

In Ancient India

In *Atharvana Veda,* 'royal brides bringing with them the dowry of one crore'. The queens *Drowpadhi, Subhadhara* and *Sita* were also given valuable presents like elephants, acres of land, jewellary from their parents at the time of marriage have been perceived as 'dowry'.

The Smritis

Has recognised eight forms of marriages, in Brahmin marriage only, the father gives gifts for his daughter.

Medieval Times

In earlier society, advanced maidenhood was tolerated, in the medieval times pre-puberty marriages came into existence. Dowry was regarded as dakshina, the gifts offered willingly. Even in Muslim marriages, the girl's father used to give property, money, etc. thus dowry system is followed as a positive evil in 13th and 14th century.

British Period

During this period the educated youths had high rates in marriage market.

Present Period

Dowry has assumed scandalous proportion. It has become a kind of a bargain. The prospective economic position of the young boys belonging to high classes will make them to attract for marriage. His price in the marriage market has automatically increased and this has heightened the difficulty of the parent, who has to give their daughter to such young men.

Sociological Implications of Dowry System

Certain specified castes and rich classes wants to retain and continue in one or other form. They specified the advantages of dowry system are:

- Provides an opportunity for meritorious boys and of poor classes to go for higher education and make their future
- Helps in establishment of new household
- Increases status of women in the family
- Enhances the possibility of marriages of girls with handicapped
- Increases the family status within the society
- Maintains harmony and unity among the family members
- Promotes inter-caste and inter-religious marriages
- Whereas majority of community are treating dowry system as social curse or evil as:
- In everyday life we are witnessing many female deaths due to dowry, suicide, the family members commit suicide; homicides like bride burning
- Promotes for child marriages inorder to escape from dowry system
- Leads to lot of other social evils like alcoholism, bribery, theft and prostitution
- Parents of the girl often commit forgery, misappropriation to arrange for dowry
- When the parents are not able to arrange dowry, they are compelled to arrange for the marriage to a widower or divorcee, old aged person, etc.

In Indian society two types of people are observed:

1. Those who consider dowry as their birth right, they are blatant about giving and taking dowry without any thought about the impact of their actions on society at large. They treated daughters without any intrinsic value.
2. Other group considers it to be a social curse, these people stopped giving and taking dowry but at the same time they have not given their daughters right to property and inheritance. This group is progressive as daughters are neither received dowry nor any other property or share in the inheritance. These people will feel that daughter is a gift of God to the family, she is not a piece of property that she can be gifted away; marriage is not contract, it is a sacrament, sacred bond between two human beings should not be sullied by evil practices.

   Society's attitude towards dowry system is neither consistent nor uniform. Educated generation disfavours it though inwardly they uphold the system citing social and cultural reasons.

   - Families part with their savings and fall into debts their houses and property got mortgaged
   - Promotes marital conflicts, family problems, divorce sometimes sanction social evils like prostitution
   - Family members, daughters suffer with fear, neurotic illness related to dowry system.

Legislation Measures

The Dowry Prohibition Act, was formulated in 1961 and amended in 1984 and 1986.

Section 3 imposes:

- A minimum of 5 years of imprisonment
- Rs 15,000 fine or the equivalent value of the dowry taken, whichever is more for giving or taking dowry
- For demanding dowry, the punishment is imprisonment for a minimum period of 6 months and fine

- If the dowry is actually received by any person other than the bride, the person has to transfer it to her within 3 months after the date of receipt. Failure gives penalty of minimum 6 months imprisonment and a fine not less than the value of the dowry received (section 6)
- Every offence under the Act is made non-bailable, non-compoundable and cognisable for the purpose of investigation
- To escape from the purview of the Act, it must be proved that, the presents were given without any demand being made, they were entered in the list maintained according to the prescribed rules and the said list was handed over to bride or the groom to be preserved as the case may be, after being signed by both of them.

Dowry death (section 304-B of the IPC) by the Criminal Law II Amendment Act, 1983; the essential ingredients which constitute dowry death are:

- Relates to the death of women only
- Death occurs due to burns, bodily injuries, abnormal circumstances
- Must be within seven years of marriage
- It has been shown that the woman was subjected to cruelty/harassment by her husband or his relatives
- Harassment is related or in connection with any demand for dowry.

If the above ingredients are proved, the husband or relative shall be deemed to have caused her death (section 113-B Indian Evidence Act) says, if cruelty or harassment before the death of the woman in connection with dowry demand is proved, dowry death shall be presumed against such person.

Cruelty Harassment (section 498 A of IPC)

- Any willful conduct is likely to drive the woman to commit suicide to cause grave injury or danger to life, limb or health (physical/mental) of the woman.

- Coercing her or any person related to her to meet any unlawful demand for any property or valuable security or an account of failure by her or by any person related to her to meet such demand.

Measures towards Abolition of Dowry System

- Increase public awareness and social understanding about the evil effect of dowry system and law enforcement by conducting mass education, mass media activities and IEC training programmes
- Financial and social independence of woman
- Encourage or motivate the woman to improve the will to safeguard and fight for the their rights
- Initiate youth through propaganda and public enlightenment to change their ideas
- Encourage full freedom for the boys and girls to select their mates.

Adverse Health Effects of Childhood Marriages

Childhood marriages arc observed in the rural societies of India, where many female children gets married below 8 years of age. Immediately after menarche, the child conceives at an early age which leads to high-risk pregnancy, abortions, intra-uterine foetal deaths, still births, affects with minor disorders and complicated labour, premature births, post-natal problems, maternal depletion, anaemia, stunted growth, low-birth weight babies, and the young mother is unable to care the new born child as she herself needs care and attention by the parents. Due to the ignorance/innocence the young couple may not follow contraceptive precautions, which leads to closed birth interval results into childhood morbidity, mortality and large family size, affects the socio-economic status of the family. In maternity cycle the young women needs adequate nutrition and care, which lacks in the case of early child bearing stages.

Health Benefits of Monogamy

- Enhances good inter-personal relationship among the partners
- Establishes effective bondage with love and affection where the partners can plan for family formation
- Single partner leads healthy procreation prevents the occurrence of STD, AIDS
- Internal harmony leads to healthy, happy, stable, conducive environment for qualitative living
- Provides security, support and welfare for the children, which prevents the psychological/social maladjustment.

FAMILY

Introduction

Family is a group of people organised on the basis of natural love and affection. It is the fundamental social unit formed in the society, which provides the safety, security, rearing of children and for fulfillment of certain human needs. It is a primary group in the society to fulfill the function of procreation and nurturing socialising the children and transmits the culture. It is a group of interacting personalities who have definite and specific roles to establish mutual relationship between the family members. Family is a sacred institution deriving sanction from religion and social traditions with myths and legends.

The word family has been derived from Latin word 'famulus' means servant. In Roman the word is denoted by a group of members connected by a common descent or marriage.

Definition

- 'A group defined by sex relationship sufficiently precise and enduring to provide for the procreation and upbringing of children'—*Maciver*

- 'The biological social unit composed of husband, wife and children'—*Eliot and Merril*
- 'A group of persons united by ties of marriage, blood or adoption constituting a single household interacting and intercommunicating with each other in their respective social roles of husband and wife, father and mother. Son and daughter, brother and sister, creating a common culture'—*Burgess and Locke*
- 'More or less durable association of husband and wife with or without child or of man and women with children'—*Nimkoft MT*

General Characteristics

1. The family is a group defined by sexual relationship between male and female, which is sufficiently precise and enduring to provide for procreation and by bringing of children.
2. It is constituted by living together of males with females and their offspring. It establishes a permanent relationship between husband and wife through permanent sexual relationship.
3. A form of marriage or other institutional arrangement in accordance with the mating relationship is established and maintained.
4. Attachment of blood relationship among the family members.
5. It may be real or imaginary.
6. Financial provision or some economic provision shared by the members of the group to fulfill the economic needs associated with child bearing and rearing.
7. A system of nomenclature involving a mode of recognising descent.
8. Common habitation.

9. There is a cultural variability in the family forms, e.g: The different forms of mating relationship, selection of mates.
10. Universality.
11. It fulfills emotional needs of the individual.
12. It is a formative agency of socialisation.
13. Will have limited members.
14. It controls the activities of the members with in the society.
15. It may be permanent or temporary in nature.
16. The family members will have certain responsibilities, duties and obligations; the happiness in the family depends on how best the members' discharge their responsibilities in coordination with the other individuals of the family.
17. The family is peculiarly guarded both by social taboos and by legal regulations.

Functions

- Fulfills the biological function
- Replacement of species through the propagation of progeny
- Social repetition where the sex relations are controlled and regulated
- Family is a medium or sex excretion and its regulation
- Provision of food, housing and clothing, which are necessary to the existence of human life.

Psychological Function

The affectionate bond, love and belongingness, intimate relationships will gain importance as the major factor in the family life. The psychological function includes affection, sympathy, love, security, attention and emotional satisfaction of responses. The affectional activities in the family include the care of offspring, sexual relationship, companionship, intimacy and romantic fulfillments.

Educational Function

Home is the first institution of the child and mother is the first teacher, who gives primary care. Child receives the earliest knowledge and experience in the family, which lays foundation for the child's personality and character formation. Family exercises profound influence on the body and mind of the child, which automatically moulds the personality of the individual.

Protective Function

It has to protect the interests of the child. It gives security in all the dimensions of healthy behaviour.

Recreational Function

The family provides entertainment for its members. The love between couple, elders and children serves to create an atmosphere in which every one of us will find an object, which can develop positive interest in the child.

Religious Function

The family has to provide some religious instructions to child to develop thoughts, kind-heartedness and fulfilling fellow feelings.

Maintains Status

Social, cultural values are to be developed to train the child. Family is a miniature community. The child learns honesty, truthfulness, traditions, cultural pattern and role model activities.

Cultural Function

Family keeps the culture of the society alive. It moulds its members according to the social culture. The family creates such an environment and educational functions in the matters of contact, thinking, religion and ethics. Family serves as an instrument of culture transmission and cultural continuity of the society It transmits ideas, ideologies, folkways, mores, customs, traditions, beliefs and values from one generation to another.

Social Function

To establish status. It is a socialising agency maintains social control. Accumulation and transmission of social heritage and social contact with all the members is established. The functions of family are divided into essential functions are (retained, which cannot be changed)

1. Satisfaction of sexual stable relationships; procreation regularity and stability that all societies recognise as desirable. Thus family introduces legitimacy into the act of reproduction by fulfilling it. Family has made it possible to have the propagation of species and the perpetuation of human race.
2. Production and rearing of children.
3. Provision of home.

   These three are interlinked.

   The non-essential functions, which can be transferred and specialised to other institutions:

1. The Government or State agency.
2. Religious functions, e.g: Church, Temple and Masjid.
3. Economic function—banks, financial corporations, insurance offices.
4. Educational—school.
5. Recreational—cinema hall, clubs.
6. Care of sick—hospital.

Family as a Social Institution and Basic Unit for Health Services

Family is a primary socialising agency and basic institution, which moulds the personality of the child. Family fulfills the basic needs of total family members, which includes health needs also. Family is a fundamental unit of society where the psychological, emotional, social needs of child will be met through family members. To protect the health and welfare of family members; the elders in the family will be working. Sacrifice, affection, binding, caring, looking after, welfare, etc. are the some of the basic functions of society. 'Health is Wealth', every member in the family will try to maintain total family health status. If any one is sick, entire family functions will be altered, strenuous relationship, alteration in family living pattern is observed. But at the same time the needy individual will feel comfort by the presence of family members and it promotes safety and security of the affected one. Family lays emphasis on kinship patterns. Elders in the family teach the ways of behaviour in an accepted manner and performance of the individual within the society.

Types of Family

1. On the basis of authority
   - Patriarchal family: The father is the most powerful and unquestionable authority (Supreme authoritarian)
   - Matriarchal family: Mother plays dominant role in the family.
2. On the basis of residence
   - Matrilocal family: The husband lives in the wife's home.
   - Patrilocal family: The wife lives in the husband's home.
   - Changing residence: Husband and wife alternate continuously change between each other's residence, e.g: One year husband lives in wife's residence, next year wife lives in husband's residence.
3. On the basis of ancestry
   - Matrilineal family: Mother is the basis of ancestry.
   - Patrilineal family: Father is the basis of ancestry.
4. On the basis of marriage
   - Polygamy family: One man marries many women and lives in a family with his wives and children.

- Polyandrous family: Woman marries many men and lives in a family with all of them or with each of them alternatively.
- Monogamous family: One man marries only one woman and establishes a family.

5. Based on dominance
   - Matronymic: Family/ancestry is the name of the mother.
   - Patronymic: Family is named after the father.
   - Immediate: Consists of mother, father and their children.
   - Conjugal family: Husband and wife lives together.
   - Extended family: Besides the couple, other relatives also live.
   - Consanguine family: Blood related will together.
   - Nuclear family: Husband and wife with their offspring live together.
   - Joint family: Couple with their children's family lives together.
   - Extended family: Husband, wife, children and other dependents like brothers, sisters' stay together.

Importance of Family

Family is the first institution in the history of man, belongs to primary group and fundamental unit of society where face-to-face contact of the members will be established; relationships are intimate, long lasting. It meets the total needs of the individual. In the modern age many functions of the family had shifted to other institutions but which cannot fulfill without a family. Man is a social being in which man can't live without a family. It is the nucleus or major part of man's activity. It maintains social organisation and develops the characters of the members of the society. It lays emphasis on kinship pattern. A person is socialised in a family where an enduring association of parents and children will take place. It socialises the child and teaches the accepted way of behaviour. The child learns about the roles of adults in the family. The child acquires sincerity, honesty, sympathy, self-esteem, character formation and consciousness of responsibility. The child gets an opportunity called free expression of thoughts and development of his entire personality. The child's first school is his home and family. It is the family, which impart practical education to the child concerning the customs in society, conduct, culture, conservation of health, love, sympathy and cooperation. It moulds the character and personality of the individual. It is a conveyance of tradition.

Social Control in Family

Society is a web of relationship and a system of rights in order of duties and responsibilities in an organised manner to maintain their relation properly, which avoids conflicts between members of society and allows them to develop as compromise to each other. The child learns the process of sympathy towards others, to carry out some times single ways of occupation and it educates the individual in cultural conduct, behaviour, custom, religion. Loss of thinking, ideals, values, occupation, fulfillment of responsibilities and use of authority. It pays desirable attention to all the dimensions of the health of the child. It encourages blossom of interest. It provides opportunity to the education of child according to their desire and urge. Provides religious education and cooperation in character training. Helps in the intellectual development of child and fulfills economic needs and confines political will of the society.

Problem Confined to Family

1. Problem of adjustment between the couple
2. Problem of social adjustment
3. Marriages are based on love
4. Problem of broken marriage
5. Problem of working women
6. Laxity of family control

7. Family conflicts and strive
8. Lower birth rate
9. Dowry system

Modern Family

Meaning

The individual nuclear family is universal social phenomenon. It can be defines as 'a small group composed of husband and wife, immature children which constitutes a unit apart from the rest of the community'.

A nuclear family is one which consists of husband, wife and their children, soon after the marriage, the children leave their parental home and establish their separate autonomous unit free from the control of the elders. Thus a nuclear family is a characteristics of all the modern industrial societies. The American family is typical example of the modern independent nuclear family.

Structure

This gives rise to two kinds of nuclear families:

a. The family of orientation
b. The family of procreation
   i. The family system in which the nuclear family is relatively independent.
   ii. Systems in which the nuclear family is incorporated in or subordinated to a larger group, that is to the polygamous or the extended family.

Recent Trends in Modern Family

The family has undergone some radical changes in the past half a century. Its structure has changes, its functions have been altered and its nature has been affected. Various factors—social, economic, educational, legal, scientific, technological, etc. the following important changes are:

1. *Industrialisation:* The consequent birth of the factory system of production affected the economic functions of the family. Family transferred its economic functions to the factory and because more a consumption unit than a productive centre.
2. *Urbanisation:* Industrialisation and urbanisation very often go together. Family is cut in size. Families are the smallest and ties are weakest.
3. *Democratic ideals:* Democracy assures equally and provides liberty to all, to women too, women now play not only domestic roles but also economic and political roles.
4. *The decline of the influence of:* Mores and the religious beliefs and the spread of secular attitude.
   Morality and religion are slowly losing grounds. Family members' have become more secular in outlook. The religious functions of the family have diminished.
5. *The spirit of individualism and romantic love:* Today individualism and romanticism are widespread. Individualism has affected love-making and marriage. Romanticism has encouraged the idea of free choice of mates on the basis of love. Marriage has become as easily dissolvable as it is entered into by a mutual consent of the partners.
6. *Economic independence of women:* The women have become the earning member. She now works in offices, colleges, banks, hospitals, schools, etc. The economic independences has increased her status, but affected her attitude.
7. *Emancipation of women:* Women are now liberated from the chains of traditionalism. They stand on an equal footing with men. They are demanding more rights and liberty for women.
8. *Decline in birth rate:* The size of family is becoming smaller. Joint family is fairly uncommon. The birth rate

is adversely affected. Absence of children is a glaring feature of the western families.

9. *Divorce:* Today more stress is laid on romantic love. 'Love is no more sacramental' now. In the west, love at first sight and divorce is next is common. Instance of divorce, desertion and separation are mounting in the west. Marriage has become a civil contract.
10. *Parent-youth conflict:* Inter-personal conflicts in the family are increasing. An unusual amount of conflicts between parents and their adolescent children are taking place. This is often denoted in terms of the generation gap.

Problems of Modern Family

Lack of trust: In almost all the modern families there is a lack of trust between the husband and wife, also between parent-children.

Unstability: Now many of the modern families are unstable, the relationship between husband-wife is temporary and unstable, lack of permanency is character of present families.

Change the relationship between man and woman: The relationships between man and woman in present families is totally changing; very less good or positive characters we find today.

Sex laxity: In the modern families both the partners can have extra-marital affairs and also illegal sexual relations and this has been taken in very common in today's society.

Economic imbalance: Because of the colourful life, more expenses, new fashions, modern style of life and luxurious demands of the family members are forcing the people to earn by illegal means and because of some other reasons also there will be imbalance of economic condition in family.

Sexual heterogeneity: In modern families both husband and wife will have extra sexual relations along with the life partners, so there is no sexual homogeneity of the partners.

Decline of religious control: In olden families all the members use to have lots of religious control, but in modern families there is no value of religion, ideals, values, customs and traditions. So now religions are losing its grip on the individuals.

Decline of family control: In joint families, elder members of each use to control almost all the family affairs but in modern families there is no control by elders, so no proper discipline.

Decline of morale: In modern families there is less value of customs, values, traditions, morals, discipline and folkways.

Divorce: Common is nuclear families marital relations are not so sacred and permanent as comparing to the older families.

Impact of western family system: Present Indian society is affecting because of western style and culture, joint and ideal families are converting into nuclear or single families, so our culture don't have any control on nuclear families.

Dowry system: This is not only a problem but also an obstacle for marriage in an India society, because of which many other problems are taking place in present society.

Disorganisation of Modern Family

- Lack of family unity
- Decrease in family control
- Strive
- Laxity of marital bond
- Conflicts between parents and children
- Lack of security

Causes of Instability in Nuclear Family

- Less social protection in the family wise
- Replacement of domination by cooperation
- Industrialisation

- Lack of control in social relationships
- Idea of romantic love
- Hedonism
- Individualisation

Changes in the Modern Family

Social changes that are affecting in the family, structure, functions and its nature:

- The birth of factory system of production affected the economic functions of the family and became more a consumption unit than a productive centre
- Urbanisation influenced the people to migrate, thereby its size became limited family ties became weak
- Democracy assures equality and provides liberty to all and they can fulfill their rights and use their power significantly
- Decline of the influence of more and religious beliefs; family members become more secular in outlook. Religious functions of the family have diminished. Religious sentiments, beliefs and attitudes are changing
- Reduction in the economic function of family. Many of the economic functions, which were previously performed by family are now transferred and performed by banks, associations and government aid
- Education activities of family, the looking after of the child is transferred and performed by baby-sitting, crèches, and kinder garden schools
- Increase in family recreation with invention of radio, TV, indoor games
- Decrease in importance of blood relationship
- Disorganisation of joint family into nuclear family
- Socialisation function increased
- The status definition, function continuous to change
- Status and economic independence of women increased
- Emancipation of women: Women are liberated from views of traditionalism; enjoying equal status in all spheres along with men

- Inter-personal conflicts in the families are increasing due to stressors; strained interpersonal relationship exists leading to broken family
- Older generation finds themselves lost and lonely due to limited space and expensive housing in urban areas
- Self selection of spouse is increasing among young working men and women in urban areas

Thus we see that changes taking place in family, but the importance of family as a basic unit of society will be continued to provide the emotional, financial and material support essential to growth and development of its member.

JOINT FAMILY

Joint family will have two to three generations and kinship relatives' shares the kitchen and common group. It provides bedrock on which social values and attitudes are built.

Definition

- 'A group of people who generally live under one roof, who eat food cooked at one hearth, who hold property in common, who participate in common family worship and who are related to each other'—*Dr Iravathi Karve*
- 'It is a collection of more than one primary family, the basis being close blood ties, common residence and patrilineal descent'—*CB Mamoria*
- 'Greater generation depth and the members of which are related to one another by property, income, mutual rights and obligations'—*IP Desai*

A joint family is a group of people who are blood related belongs to 3 or more generations generally live under one roof and who eat food from one kitchen and who hold property in common and participates a common worship, work under a common head and are related to each other as some particular type of kind.

Characteristics

- Large in size
- Joint property; provides social security, leisure and recreation
- Antithesis of nuclear family
- Common residence; sharing common roof, kitchen
- Common version
- Cooperative organisation; promotes cooperative virtues
- Productive unity
- Mutual right, responsibilities and obligation
- Authority with head of family
- Self sufficiency—to meet the economic, recreational, medical, educational and other needs of members
- Higher rate of procreation.

Advantages

- Ensures economic progress
- Protection of members
- Division of labour
- Mean of recreation
- Avoids fragmentation of property
- Security in wealth
- Development of good quality
- Cooperative, sharing and economy
- Stable and durable relationship.

Demerits

- Hinders in development of personality
- Encourages litigation or strikes
- Uncontrolled procreations (reproduction)
- Low status for women
- Promotes laziness, idleness
- Lack of privacy and affects adversely socialisation of children

- Rigidity of superstitions and customs
- Poverty
- Damages individual initiative and enterprise; the centre of quarrels
- Limits social mobility.

Factors Causing Disintegration of Joint Family

- Lack of understanding, cooperation and unity
- Individuality
- Employment
- Industrialisation
- Needs are different
- Extension of communication and transport
- Increased cultural contact/social contact
- Influence of technology and others
- Decline of village trades
- New social legislation, e.g: Child Marriage Restraint Act (CMRA), Child Restraint Act.

Family Cycle

Family cycle or the various stages in the development of the family vary from culture to culture.

Maciver and Page Indicates Certain Stages in the Family Cycle

Formative Prenuptial Stage

It is marked by an increasing intimacy of men and women; an exploration and understanding of personality of each other. It is observed in western country.

Stage of Formation (The nuptial stage)

It begins with marriage, when the couple starts to form the family before the arrival of their offspring. It involves the couple to live together; promotes conducive environment to live at home and creates new experiences, establishing positive attitude towards each other.

The Child Bearing Stage

It fulfills the family proper linking the partners to one another through child, introduces newer growing responsibilities.

The Growth Stage

Family size increases with the birth of children; the average family size in India is 3.2 members.

The Maturity Stage

Parents have been fulfilled their responsibilities and children are no longer requires parental care.

The Retraction Stage

The children grown up and leave the family and form their own family, leaving the parents alone.

FAMILY CYCLE

Description	*Beginning of phase*	*End of phase*
Formation	Marriage	Birth of first child
Extension	Birth of first child	Birth of last child
Complete extension	Birth of last child	First child leave home
Contraction	First child leave home	Last child leave home
Completed contraction	Last child leave home	First spouse dies
Dissolution	First spouse dies	Death of survivors

DUVALL'S FAMILY CYCLE, BY LENGTH OF TIME IN EACH OF EIGHT STAGES

Stage

1. Married couples (without children)
2. Child bearing families (oldest child, birth–30 months)

3. Families with young children (oldest child–30 months to 6 years)
4. Families with school children (oldest child 6-13 years)
5. Families with teenagers (oldest child 13-20 years)
6. Families launching young adults (first child gone to last child leaving home)
7. Middle – aged parents (empty nest to retirement)
8. Ageing family members (retirement to death of both spouses).

HILL'S MODEL OF THE FAMILY LIFE CYCLE STAGE

1. Establishment (newly married, childless)
2. New parents (infant–3 years)
3. Pre-school family (child 3-6, and possibly younger siblings)
4. School-age family (oldest 6-12, possibly younger siblings)
5. Family with adolescent (oldest 13-19, possibly younger siblings)
6. Family with young adult (oldest 20 until first child leaves home)
7. Family as launching centre (from departure of first to last child)
8. Post-parental family, the middle years (after children have left home until father retires)
9. Ageing family (after retirement of father).

According to the **Traditional Indian System** four stages of family cycle:

- *Brahmacharya* (Bachelorhood)
- *Grihastha* (House holder)
- *Vanaprastha* (Preparing himself to enter into *sanyasi* life)
- *Sanyas* (Completely detached from society).

Life Cycle of an Individual

- Birth
  - New born—1-7 day
  - Neonate—7 days-1 month

- Infant—1 month-1 year
- Toddler 1–3 years
- Pre-schooler 3–5 years
- School age 5–12 years
- Pre-adolescence 13–15 years
- Adolescence 15–19 years
- Youth 20–40 years
- Adulthood 20–40 years
- Middle age 40–60 years
- Old age above 60 years

PSYCHO-SOCIAL DEVELOPMENT OF AN INDIVIDUAL FROM BIRTH TO OLD AGE

Infancy (0–1 year) Trust *vs* Mistrust

The concept of mutual regulation between mother and infant, especially as it applies to feeding, must be established if infant trust the mother. If this sense of trust is not learned, the reverse, a sense of mistrust is developed.

1st Month

- Totally egocentric
- Complex dependence on caregivers
- Bonding progresses
- Smiles briefly.

2nd Month

- Eye-to-eye contact, smiling, and vocalisation are the evidences of attachment between infant and parents.
- Has learned that crying brings attention.

3rd Month

- The true social smile may appear
- Interested in surrounding.

4th Month

- Shows interest in new stimuli
- Shows eagerness when feeding bottle appears
- Breathes heavily when excited.

5th Month

- Smiles at self, looking at mirror
- Begins to discriminates family members from strangers
- Plays enthusiastically, plays with own feet.

6th Month

- Recognises strangers
- Imitation of others is beginning
- Knows what is liked and disliked.

7th Month

- Responds socially to own name
- Emotional instability–rapidly changes from crying to laughter.

8th Month

- Increases anxiety over loss of parent especially mother
- Dislikes changing clothing and diaper.

9th Month

- Knows what 'no' means
- Beginning fears about being left alone
- Dislikes having face washed so covers face with arms and hands.

10th Month

- Expresses several emotions such as anger, sadness, jealousy, anxiety, pleasure, excitement and affection

- Plays social games with adults
- Attracts the attention of others by pulling on their clothes or fussing.

11th Month

- Becomes frustrated when activities are restricted.

12th Month

- Responds to requests for affection such as a kiss or a hug
- Has established beginning view of self as a separate person 'securing blanket' or favourite by beginning to provide comfort
- Cooperate in dressings
- Drops objects on purpose so some one can pick them up.

Toddler (1–3 years) Sense of autonomy *vs* Shyness, Doubt and Shame

Infants develop from clinging, dependent creatures into human beings with minds and wills of their own. If children succeed in the developmental tasks of this stage in their maturing process, they will have a degree of self-control (autonomy).

If they do not succeed, they will doubt their own worth and that of others and will have a sense of shyness and shame.

15th Month

- Separation anxiety: Coping depends on primary caregiver's presence but can tolerate some separation
- Hugs and kisses parents
- Kisses pictures in book
- Begins to imitate parents doing house-keeping chores.

18th Month

- Autonomous behaviour increasing
- Seeks help from others when in trouble

- Thumb sucking peak especially before or during sleep for comfort
- Awareness of ownership, possessiveness begins
- Awareness of gender identity begins.

2nd Year

- Begins to show early signs of individuality and independency
- Behaves as though other would like to make friend but does not know how
- Sleep resisted overtly; has many demands before bed time
- Upset by changes in routine
- Violent temper tantrums decreasing.

30th Month

- Achieves some self-control based on self-esteem rather than fear
- Ritualistic behaviour peak
- Imitates sex role behaviour of adult
- Knows own sex.

Pre-school (6–12 years) Sense of Initiative *vs* Guilt

Children at this age want to learn what they can do for themselves. They have active imaginations, imitating adult behaviour and wanting to share in adult activities. The positive, maturing outcome of this force with in children is sense of initiative delineated by conscience or super ego.

The negative outcome is a personality overwhelmed by guilt.

3rd Year

- Alternates between reality and imagination
- Tolerates short separation from parents
- Fears the dark
- May have dreams and nightmares.

4th Year

- Tends to impatient and selfish
- Physically and verbally aggressive
- Demonstrates strong attachment for parents of opposite sex
- Jealousy of siblings may be evident, more cooperative in play.

5th Year

- Independent and trust worthy
- Has fantasies and day dreams
- Looks for parental support and encouragement
- Very industrious.

School going (6–12 years) Sense of Industry *vs* Inferiority

Children in this age group have a strong sense of duty. They want to engage in tasks in their social world that they can carry out successfully, and they want their success to be recognised by adult and by their peer.

The danger of this period is the development of a sense of inferiority. If the parents or the school expect a level of achievement that children are unable to attain.

6–8th Year

- Has a 'know it all' attitude insists on being first in everything
- Returns to temper tantrums–may use verbal, physical attack
- Uses of tensional releases wiggling, chewing, nose picking
- Has good days and bad days
- Curious about every thing
- Becoming peer oriented
- Begins hero worship

- Enjoys running around, helping when mother is busy
- Aware of appropriate sexual role
- Sincere, confident, greater self-control
- Respects parents and their role
- Able to control anger.

Early Adolescence (12–17 years) Sense of Identity *vs* Identity Diffusion

Adolescent want to clarify who they are and what their roles in society are to be. Success in this period brings self-esteem, an attitude towards the self that is essential to the normal breaking away from depending up on their parents and to planning for their future.

The danger is identity diffusion for they face in reality and in their dream of the future, a life full of conflicting desires, possibilities and chances.

12–14 Year

- Has intense loyalty to peer groups
- Shows mood swings and extremes of behaviour
- Continues same sex friendships.

14–16 Year

- Ego centrism diminishes
- Hetero-sexual relationships and interests common
- Verbally attacks parents beliefs and norms.

Late Adolescence Sense of Intimacy vs Isolation

After puberty, youths out grow the 'going age' and group their own sex; young people develop a sense of intimacy with individuals of their and the opposite sex and with themselves.

Failure to establish such intimacy results in psychologic isolation.

17–21 Year

- Severs ties with parents
- Has fewer but closer relationship (friends)
- Hetero-sexual relationship are the rule.

Early Adulthood

'People who are in-charge of their own lives'. Developmental tasks in adulthood are: To escape parental control, establishes peer group orientation, developing their independence by making comments to career and family, marriage and career goal; realise the life goals, people accept their lives and past things and develops tolerance. Individuals begin to stabilise their identity. *Erikson* described young adulthood as 'intimacy versus isolation'. Intimacy is characterised by warmth, mutuality of feeling, deep commitment, socio-emotional relationships produce a sense of security, trust and the desire to be close to others. Attachment is a life long process influencing the frequency and quality of interpersonal relationships. Adults tend to have friends and acquaintances. Intimate friendships are more likely based on mutual sharing of feelings.

Middle Adulthood

Erikson's view, 'generativity *vs* stagnation' focus on, 'caring for others'. Intellectual development continues in later adulthood, cognitive skills, e.g: Wisdom and expertise in living crystallised intelligence like vocabulary, general information, social judgment, reasoning ability related to formal, logic and knowledge; crystallised intelligence is associated with the use of principles common to the culture in which one lives. Divergent thinking, i.e. the ability to think of many different ideas appropriate to a situation; originality and the ability to change and transform ideas from one state to another. Preference for complexity is increased.

Senior citizens shows decline in social interaction and social relationships. Friendship and social interaction can be important factors in elderly adjustment. Older people tend to move toward more self-centered positions; they are concerned more with their own problems. They will spend more time in spirituality.

Interdependence of Family Members

Family is a primary group; functional social unit in which members will have long-lasting, direct intimate, good interpersonal durable relationship exists among family members. Family is indispensable unit for the societal members. Mother is a primary caregiver, family is the first socialising agency for the child. The total personality development of the child will be influenced by nature of family members. Good human/interpersonal relationships are essential for healthier relationships; everyone in the family will work for the welfare of other members, they sacrifice their lives for one another. Familial communication is essential to understand each member's feelings, attitudes, emotions of its members. The relationship between couple, parents, siblings, relatives is essential otherwise it may lead to family disorganisation, conflicts. Men and women in the house has to perform different roles and statuses; activities according to their nature of work. If they are unable to cope up it may lead to maladjustments. In the family people will play dependent, independent and interdependent roles. It provides sense of love, affection, sharing, reciprocity, bondage among its members.

Basic Needs of Family

Family is a vital social institutions, fundamental unit of society where the basic needs of the individual will be met; love, affection, bondage, procreation, food, safe water supply, shelter, proper disposal of waste products, sexual regulation, upbringing of children, socialisation, adequate nutrition, socio-cultural needs, psychological and emotional needs, attainment of social status, protective in nature, conveyer of planning, arrangement of income, language development, religious, educational functions, modules the personality of the individual, controls individual behaviour in society, provides psychological security.

Child Adoption Law

To uplift and welfare of destitute children on Indian society, we are encouraging the adoption of children. To provide security, Adoption of Children Bill, 1980 was passed, which has been pending for more than two decades. The Hindu Adoption and Maintenance Act, 1956 allows adoption only by Hindus. In 1984, law was formulated which prevents the export of children in laissez-faire manner. International council of social welfare describes the rules for adoption of children by foreigners, 'before any plans are considered for a child to be adopted by a foreigner, the appropriate authority or agency shall consider the alternatives for permanent family care within the child's own country'.

However, one wishes to adopt two children, they must differ in sex. The adopted child can inherit the property of the adoptive family. Adoption legally establishes parent-child relationship between persons; children are provided with the physical and psychological benefits of family life and caring adults are afforded a chance to become parents and experience growth as family. It improves childcare welfare and more carefully planned families. Child welfare services also have been promoted, e.g: Sponsorship, crèches, balwadies, etc. they will put maximum transit care fee and time limit, as fixed by the supreme Government. Foster care will be providing according to Guardian and Wards Act of 1890.

In 1995, the union Government issued revised guidelines as adoption of Indian children. According to that central adoption resources agency (CARA) can enlist agencies both Indian and foreign involved in adoption process. No objection certificate has to be obtained from CARA by foreign parents.

According to the Supreme Court judgment in December, 1986 inform the social welfare department about the discovery of abandoned or destitute children. Every Indian parent registered with foster homes or recognised placement agencies for adoption of a child will be entitled to information in the consolidated list of children maintained by them. The agency should not take more than one month to decide whether an abandoned or destitute child is legally free for adoption. Government has to publish recognised placement agencies and social welfare agencies in each state every year. The Indian council for child welfare has been given the work of scrutinizing applications for adoption, if asked by court. Adoption of children must become an effective method of rehabilitation of such children so that they grow like any other children and contribute their mite to the main stream of our national life.

Family as a Basic Unit for Health Services

Family is a fundamental social unit, where the individual fulfills/satisfies their physical, biological, social, psychological, emotional and spiritual needs. Man can satisfy his basic human relationships emphasise kinship patterns. As a social institution, family performs the functions off socialisation, it teaches the accepted ways of behaviour for its members. If health personnel wants to bring awareness about health in the society and community, first identify the families who are in need and identify the influencing personalities, provides situational support who can motivate the individuals to inculcate healthier habits, family should encourage the blossoming of the intelligence of children, provides opportunities for the expression of joys, desires, pleasures, urges and familiar with the factual life, religious, ethical education and character training and intellectual development of the child.

Health professional has to conduct domiciliary visits, identify the family needs and meet their needs (felt needs and demand needs) in a holistic approach. Family is a basic social unit, which will have influencing effect to change the behaviour of individual, attitudes, beliefs and to develop healthier practices, which will promote healthier living in the community. Health professionals should show interest, cooperate, coordinate in implementation of health related activities.

Health related facts have to be informed to the public as soil, seed, shower approach (community—soil; health elated facts—seeds; educational approach is like a shower) has to be used in bringing health awareness. Information, education and communication training programs has to be conducted to motivate, mobilise, reinforce the persons to achieve healthier practices in order to improve standards of living.

Advantages of Planned Parenthood

Planned parenthood is essential for qualitative family living development of total family members. It improves family background in specific and community and nation development at large. It raises the standards of living. It facilitates the eligible couple to attain net reproduction rate one or none; reduces fertility rate, morbidity and mortality pattern and changes the outlook of the people, creates a strong motivation to utilise the contraceptive services. If couple follows planned parenthood by having less children, then the parents have to feed less members, provide better education, good health.

Planned parenthood eliminates various social problems like poverty, theft, beggary, unemployment, family conflicts, overpopulation, and increases per capita income thereby increasing national income, increases harmony in the family, reduces stress in the family, promotes intimate and conflict-free environment. Improves economy, better planning and implementation of the funds.

Family Welfare Activities

India is the first country in the world, which launched National Family Planning Programme in 1952, though it is second populous country, birth control clinics started functioning in the year 1930. During the third five-year plan (1961–66) the family planning was considered as, planned development, the clinic approach has been changed to extension education approach, motivating the eligible couple to accept 'small family norm'. In June, 1977 the new Janta Government formulated new population policy, changed the concept of "Family Planning' as "Family Welfare". The acceptance of programme is purely on voluntary basis. In 1977, Government of India launched rural health scheme in which the local people, i.e. trained *dais*, village health guides, opinion, informal and formal leaders were involved at the grass-root level in implementation of family welfare activities. In 1983, the National Health Policy was formulated and, kept an aim of attaining net reproduction rate = 1, implies a two child family norm, the attainment of birth rate of 21 and a death rate of a per thousand population and couple protection rate of 60% by the year 2000 and revised population policy in 2000, to promote family welfare, to provide comprehensive health services and to improve the quality/standard of living. Family welfare services includes sex education, advice on sterility, planned parenthood, counselling, pre-marital consultation and examination, marriage counselling, spacing and limitation of births, screening for pathological conditions related to the reproductive tract infections, home economics, services for unmarried mothers, safe water supply, control and prevention of communicable diseases. Safe disposal of excreta, providing of adoption services, promoting women and child health, RCH programme activities, to raise the living standards of people, measure to improve education facilities, compulsory education for children, conducting IEC campaigns to change the deep rooted beliefs, attitudes and practices related to large family size, raising the age of marriage, increasing women's status, and old age security.

Principles of Family Welfare Programme

- Family welfare services are voluntary
- It will provide comprehensive maternal, child health and family planning services
- Information, education, communication and mobilisation activities to create awareness and effective implementation and utilisation of program.

FAMILY HEALTH CARE

Family is the basic fundamental unit of health care services, where the community health services will be focusing. The health of one family member affects the other members in the family.

The family is affected by all the aspects of community life. Family meets the essential and non-essential needs of its members. It provides love, affection, unity and security. Many families are able to cope up with the difficulties by replacing community health services.

Definition

- It is the continuing ability to meet defined functions with coordination of several sub-systems like education, social, political, economic and health systems.
- Developing the abilities and utilising the resources to fulfill family developmental tasks
- The health problems of the family members are interlocking, e.g: If one member in the family become sick, it affects the total family environment. An interaction between the family members reinforces its members to maintain conducive environment.

Determinants of Family Health

1. External environment
   e.g: Safe water, air, ventilation, housing, biological environment.
2. Internal environment
   e.g: Family size, structure, type of family, inter-personal relationship, cultural factors and social values.

Objectives of Family Health Care

- Assessing the felt needs of family members. Identifies health problems of its members
- Ensure the family members to understand and accept the problems
- Develops competency among the members to implement the activities for uplifting their own health with their own hands
- Utilises various community resources for family developmental activities
- Provides family health education
- Reduction of maternal, infant, child mortalities or morbidity rate
- Ensures planned parenthood
- Improves and meets the total needs of the family members.

Principles of Family Health Care

- Establishment of good inter-personal relationships
- Provide guidance and counselling services for the family members to take care of themselves with their own efforts
- Identifies the problems by priority ranking methods and intelligently provide need based health services
- Improves family members health status
- Health care services should be provided to all the people
- Proper health messages will be carried out and communicated to every family by using mass-media technology.

Reasons for Considering the Family as the Unit of Service

- Family is a basic fundamental unit of society
- Shoulders responsibility for prevention and treatment of health problems for their members
- Promotes the health of total family members
- It provides a crucial environment force
- It focuses health decisions and actions in personal care
- It is a collective enterprise based on relationships defined by marriage and birth
- It provides love, protection, security, bondage, intimate relationships with its members
- The members in the family work together to meet their material needs one member will sacrifice for the welfare of others
- The group process, morale group dynamics are interlocking with each other in family.

Role of the Nurse in Family Health Care Services

Community health nurse plays liaison role between the community and health care agency. Apart from professional training and skills, the nurse has to understand the family ways, traditions, customs, culture, and traditional pattern of living. Nurse has to identify the community resources, which are ready to extend their cooperation in solvation of the community problems. The nurse must recognise and understand the family unity, love, protection, security, form, structure and development aspects of family, interpersonal relationship and pattern of life. Nurses should strength family ties and help them to have sound conducive environment.

Nurse has to conduct domiciliary visit, observational visit in order to identify the problems related to individual (specific) family and community at large.

For effective implementation of health care services in the community health nursing process it's principles and steps has to be followed to help the family to reach and maintain maximum health in any given situation.

Family Assessment

Nurse has to conduct domiciliary visits and continuously develops the contact with the families, establish good interpersonal relationship with each individual in the family in order to collect pertinent information to make adequate plans.

Systematic approach in gathering the data has to be followed. Family assessment includes health assessment (utilises multi-dimensional approach which will be different from each age group), nutritional assessment (clinical examination, anthropometric measurements, laboratory tests, observation of dietary pattern, study of vital statistics, and assessment of ecological factors), non-physical assessment by using family coping index, social assessment where the nurse will gather the information related to cultural history, present practices, rules for acceptable behaviour, economic status, and leadership pattern, interacting system with in the family has to be assessed.

Nurse should collect facts/data about the family by using the techniques like observation, interview, subjective appraisal, communication pattern, reviewing records and reports.

Family History

Type, size, particulars of age, educational status occupational status, income, any history of hereditary diseases.

Environmental History

Sanitation, housing and ventilation, air, water, noise, lighting, radiation, disposal of solid and liquid waste, garbage, facilities for kitchen gardening, presence of domestic animals like cat, dog, etc.

Dietary History

Type of diet, food beliefs, pads, cultural pattern associated with food consumption, cooking practices, food storage.

History of immunisation status of under-five children.

Family planning status, information related to vital statistics like birth, death, marriage, morbidity, mortality, etc.

Any information related to health of the family and community.

Study of community and social factors affecting the health and economic status of the family.

Transport and communication facilities.

Nursing Diagnosis

Identify the felt needs of family, list the family problems, discuss with the family members and prioritise the problems by preferential ranking method. The problems may include family's health needs (current, potential health problems) level of wellness.

Planning

Analyse the facts, classify health problems, discuss the problems with the family to find out what they are doing (or) what they wish to do about the problems. Review the individual and family records. Identify the resources, supportive systems and other positive factors which will make plan of action in easier manner.

Community health nurse has to formulate the family health care plan, setting goals, choose effective resources and set the priority. The goals (short-and long-term) should be in realistic manner and acceptable to the family members where by the family members will utilise the available resources and accomplish appropriate developmental tasks, accepts health problems and tries to implement the activities by using family coping measures and action plan will be made.

Implementation

Interventions are strategies which will help the family members to adopt specific activities to attain the goals in set time. It increases the family members abilities and achieve the health status in all efficient manner.

Evaluation

It is the appraisal of the effects of some organised activity. It involves assessing the progress by comparing the objectives and results. After implementation of specified nursing interventions the nurse has to evaluate whether the family members has achieved their health status or nurse has to identify the difficulties in attaining the goals accordingly modified, suitable strategies can be implemented. Nurse should teach the family members the techniques related to identification of existing, potential health problems, formulation of short and long term goals.

Child Guidance Clinic

The first child guidance clinic was started in Chicago in 1909 with a intention to deal with juvenile delinquent child. Now all forms of child with maladjustments are tackled.

Indication

- Bed wetting/enuresis
- Refusing to go to school
- Family maladjustment
- Ignored/neglected
- Stealing
- Heightened reaction to normal situations.

Team

- Psychiatrist

- Clinical psychologist
- Educational psychologist
- Social workers
- Public health nurses
- Paediatrician
- Speech therapist
- Occupational therapist
- Neurologist.

Services

- Psychotherapy—to restore positive feelings of security in the child
- Play therapy, counselling, suggestion, change in physical environment, easing of parental tensions by diversional therapy, reconstruction of parental attitudes
- Promotion of mental health in childhood, adolescence and up to adulthood.

Role of Community Health Nurses in Child Guidance Clinics

- Setting up of clinics
- Register the children
- Assist the team members in diagnosis and therapy of the client
- Educate the children about family life.

Child Welfare Services

These services are concentrated around in meeting the needs of children, who are unable to avail of services provided by the community, supportive services, assist the family in its natural obligations for the child welfare.

Child welfare services are four fold in nature, i.e. promotive, preventive, developmental and rehabilitative in nature. Attention paid to the children of working mothers, destitute children and handicapped children.

Agencies (National)

- Indian Council for Child Welfare
- Central Social Welfare Board
- Kasturba Memorial Trust
- The Indian Red Cross Society

International

- UNICEF
- FAO
- WHO
- International Union for Child Welfare

These agencies have got branches all over the world and the proposed budgets to Government and other funding agencies to get financial aid and organise child welfare service throughout the country.

Services

Day-care Services

Balwadies, nursing schools, play homes and crèches will be arranged for the children of working mothers. Specially meant for infants and toddlers.

Holiday Homes

For children between the age group of 12-16 years. During vacation, summer camps, sea-side resorts, holiday homes, where the child will be given training in extra-curricular activities, the method of spending their time in recreational activities and provide relaxation to the mind.

Recreation Homes

Organisation of play centres, parks, libraries, bal bhawans, religious education centres, where the child will be oriented towards recreation and relaxation; religious training whereby child will feel secured and oriented towards moral development.

Art as a Social Institution

Art is a skill, which are acquired, modified and strengthened through learning. Art is overtly seen through the activities. It can be developed through established ways in an organised behaviour, it fulfills the fundamental needs, which are necessary to preserve and maintain social order. It exercises control over human behaviour. It fulfills the imagination of the people. Maintenance of calmness and control the mind and activities of individual to ease the emotions and to recognise behaviour patterns with certain situations. Allow a feeling of strength and determine the condition, behaviour of individual. Generates emotional feeling in approved fashion. Meets psychological, emotional, social needs of the individuals through organised efforts.

Political Institution

Political system establishes five characters:

- Universality of political systems
- Universality of political structure
- Universality of political functions
- Multi-functionaries of political structure
- Culturally mixed character of political structure

Social Functions of Political Institutions

- The production of extent of the whole group of political parts of the group
- Preservation of order in the interest of the group of power of the whole population
- Regulates the individual and group behaviour
- To exercise closer regulation of individual and group section than to regulate relationship with the society in which customs and behaviour are not adequate

- Differs new ideas and encourages scientific discoveries and infusion into the society where radically different scientific philosophical religious or economic doctrines may disturb
- Makes the individual to adjust for longer serve
- Creates new regulations between various groups and order the conduct of individuals along time and better adjusted to the new instructions
- Substitutes educational and propaganda methods
- Encourages development of new traditions and customs supporting the new order
- Supplements private and voluntary organisation in regulation and conduct of activity conceived of importance to all the people
- Works for welfare of society
- Controls the property and person that the state may survive in times of danger
- Protect the individual and vital interest and order in the relationships between its citizen and its counter parts.

RELIGION AS A SOCIAL INSTITUTION

Man is a religious or spiritual being; it represents the main social facets of man.

The religion plays an important role in controlling the animistic and selfish tendencies of a person and channeling them in the service of humanity. Thus, the inculcation of moral and spiritual values is as much important for modernisation as are the advancement of science, technology and economic resources. Religion has an important role to play in the economic development and modernisation of a democratic country, but it is an end itself for the development of personality religion institution is essential.

Progress is mainly concerned with the fulfillment of self, the maximum realisation of the various individual potentialities in a socially acceptable way, the harmonious exercise of human faculties and powers. Thus progress consists in exercising the powers of living in their highest form in an attempt to achieve and enjoy relative fullness of life. Religious education should be given to all age groups and to all classes. Moral values like truthfulness, honesty also should be taught. Reorganisation of our religious beliefs so as to inculcate virtues like honesty, tolerance, justice, truth, concern for others, etc. among masses.

Religion is instinctive to man. Man is the only religious being and has looked up to some invisible power for assistance, motivation strength and health.

Definition

- 'Religion is an attitude towards superhuman power'—*Ogburn*
- 'Religion is a relationship between man and some higher power'—*Maciver and Page*
- 'Unified system of beliefs and practices relative to sacred things'—*Durkheim*
- 'Powers superior to man which are believed to direct and control the course of nature and of human life'—*James G Frazer*
- 'To discover a road to spiritual serenity across the perplexities and dangers of daily life'—*Edward Sapir*
- 'A mental faculty or disposition, which enables man to apprehend the infinite'—*Max Muller*

Characteristics or Elements of Religion

- It is a belief in supernatural or super-human forces; human being considers God as omnipotent, omnipresent and omniscient
- Religious activities are considered as sacred
- It involves specific set of practices or rituals
- It motivates the people the right way to live and keeps the individual in right track by following norms and adopting moral codes

Functions of Religion

- Provides opportunity for the individual for attaining religious experience, e.g: Prayer, worship, meditation, man expresses awe, gratitude, reverence, allegiance to the almighty. Individual converses with the divine through prayers. He forgets the worldly life and its problems. Religious experience facilitates personality development, increases sociability and creativeness
- It provides peace of mind, emotional support and maturity
- Promotes goodness and develops good character
- Acts as the healer of life; reduce the grievances in life
- Reinforces the morale, supports established values and goals in life
- Offers inspiration, hope, faith, optimism and courage
- Explains individual suffering and helps to integrate the personality
- Enhances self importance, promotes social solidarity
- Conserves value of life: Moral, spiritual and social values are supported by religion
- Promotes welfare: People who have religious background will have spirit of mutual help, cooperation, sympathetic, merciful and cooperative
- Provides recreation: Through *kirthanas*, drama, dances, music, *bhajans*, lectures, fairs and festivals, art exhibitions.

Primary Components of Religion

- Belief in supernatural power to influence human condition and events
- Man is dependent on these powers. He must adjust himself to them. Consequently each religion provides some outward acts like prayers, *prarthana* or other forms of reverence. Failure to perform these acts regarded as sinful acts
- Each religion defines certain acts, which will destroy man's harmonious relationship with God. Those acts are called as 'sinful acts'.

Method of Salvation

Man needs some method by which he can regain harmony with God for removal of his guilt.

Social Role of Religion

Is a powerful social controlling agency in the society as it rationalises and makes bearable the individual suffering in the known world. Man does not live by the knowledge alone. Whenever man suffers with disappointment from traditions, conflicts, imbalance between hopes and achievements. Man tries to console and compensate himself to the God. Religion gives release from sorrows, worries and fears. It enables the individual to interpret any catastrophe of intermediate and secondary. Helps the man to bear his emotional balance and integrate his personality, enhances self-importance. Man unites himself with the infinite and feels ennobled. Religion assures a greater reward in the after-life to worldly failure than to the successful. A source of social cohesion, the common possession of social values by which individual control the actions of self and others to which society is perpetuated. It gives security and belongingness in society and maintains discipline. Love and service are the great features of religion. It shapes domestic, economic and political institution. Religious rights are performed in many occasions in the individual's life. It is a central element in the life of civilisation, works for social welfare. It acts as an agency of social control and gives rewards or punishments by following approved or disapproved actions. Supports the folkways and customs by playing the powerful sanction of supernatural power behind them. Provides a model for living by up holding certain ideals, values to become moral, discipline and socialised citizens of the society. It controls and affects the economic life. It provides as agency for service and serves humanity through spreading of education; by diffusing education among the members of community. Religion and benevolence—It serves the helpless and sick people as part of worshipping God. It gives economic support to poor people. All religions emphasise sacrifice for bearing morality, honesty, courage and unselfishness. It encourages non-violence activities. Provides place and comfort for individuals troubled by the problems when they get counselling, advice, and condolence. Immoral activities under religious pretext. Dogmatism—religious people do not have courage to break ancient customs and traditions.

Dysfunction of Religion

- Religion is conservative, retrogressive and not progressive
- Promotes evil practices like untouchability, sacrifices either animal or human, cannibalism, slavery
- It creates confusion, contradiction and conflict as it consists of some inconsistencies, it is not a standard of morality as it has supported war and pace, wealth and poverty, hard work and idleness; virginity and prostitution
- It contributes for inequalities and exploitations
- Promotes superstitious beliefs, which causes harmful effects, e.g: Children are the God's gift; chicken pox is due to the mistake committed and the punishment from God
- Causes economic wastes, e.g: People will spend more money for celebrating fairs and festivals sometime it may lead to waste of human labour, energy, wealth and time
- Creates conflicts, promotes war and battle in the name of religion
- Promotes faith without reasoning the reality

Thus religion has been used by the society to serve the humanity and also to exploit the people at large.

STATE AS A SOCIAL INSTITUTION

State regulates the social relationship of man to the society and it is the overall control of the society.

Definition

- 'It is an organisation, which rules by means of a supreme government over definite territory'—*Ogburn*

State is an association, which is acting through laws as promulgate by the government endowed to the end with power to maintain within the community territorially demanded the universal external condition of social order.

Elements of State

Population

The state cannot exist without population. It is essentially a human organisation. It is the result of man's fundamental need to live together. It affects both quality and quantity of the population. The efficiency of a state depends upon personality of the members. Its strength depends upon the number as well as the strength of the people.

Territory

It gives specification for the area of authority.

Government

It is the missionary through which the state functions, e.g: Ruling political party. It includes the officials and departments who are elected appointed to determine, interpret, and carry out the regulations of the state or its sub-divisions.

Sovereignty

It is the ultimate authority there is no appeal, which acts as the supreme authority.

Peculiarity of State

It is an association of people inhibiting a territory and living under sovereign government. It has special attributes, instruments and formals. Its membership is obligatory or compulsory.

Social Function

- Acts as an agency for social control
- Maintains social order
- Exercises power over the behaviour of individual in society
- Moulds the character
- Conserves and develops the personalities in a conservative manner
- Imposes mural and ethical values.

Economic Institution

These are the products of a given culture and are affected by nature, structure, functioning of the elements in the culture, e.g: The historical role of the family in getting and wages of goods even today affects the economic structure and function.

Modern Economic Institution

Property

It includes goods or things own by individual or group of individuals, e.g: Strangible items and instrangible items.

Money Credit

Money is still used as medium of exchange. Our business is transacted in credit basis.

Large Scale Factory Production

The machinery and its power influences over the labour and capital in large units production was on a limited basis.

Corporation

It is development of joined stock company as it has limited liabilities and it is easy means of investment for small-scale industries.

Company

It enables few people with only a fraction of capital involved in the capitalisation of understanding companies to determine policies and distribution of earnings.

The Wage System

With industrial revolution the wage system became as a formally established economic institution.

Contract

To give loyal obedience and to perform certain services and to pay certain economists views.

Competition

It is developed between different crafts men based on the interest upon the general public because it tends to production of goods at least possible price.

Co-operative

It grew out of the attempt of consumer to eliminate the middleman's proportion in the purchase of commodities.

Division Labour

To place the right man in the right place and the worker will become an expert in that area. It saves time and the things will be produced at cheaper rate.

EDUCATION AS A SOCIAL INSTITUTION

The term, 'education' is derived from Latin word, 'educare' means 'bring up'/'bring forth'. It imports knowledge, develops habits and attitudes to face the future successfully.

Definition

- 'A continuous effort to impose on the child ways of seeing, feeling and acting which he could not have arrived at spontaneously, the socialisation of the younger generation'—*Durkheim*
- 'An attempt to transmit the child the mores and learn the approved behaviour'—*Summer*
- 'The sum total of experiences, which moulds the attitudes and determines the conduct of societal members'—*FJ Brown and JS Roncek*
- 'An attempt to shape the development of the coming generation with its own ideals of life'—*James Welton*
- 'Formal conscious training by specialists within formal educational institution to adopt effective social roles'—*AW Green*
- 'The process whereby the social heritage of a group is passed from one generation to another, socialisation occurs, i.e. the child learns the rules of group behaviour'—*Samuel Koenig*

Education has become an eminent need for fulfillment of social needs. It consists of a set of codes, norms, organised behaviour. Education system contains programmed instructions. The non-essential function done by the fundamental unit of society, i.e. families alone previously has been taking care, now it has been transferred to institutions. The joint family system was disintegrated into nuclear families where the people are over burdened with many responsibilities and with lack of personnel equipment and system to meet the needs of non-essential functions such as education, rearing of the children and recreation. The family cannot cope up with changing demands. It was developed to bring a change in a positive way and in acceptable position through acquisition of knowledge, attitude and practice by observation, imitation and formal education. It makes the individual to fit for the adult social life.

Education is the mother of civilisation. A society will be civilised based on proportion of the members are educated in that society, as knowledge is the society, power. The educational institutions have an important role to play in the social progress of any country. Education determines the level of prosperity, welfare and security of the people.

In the modern society where the control of tradition and family is less and freedom is more, the individual has much more discretion than in a traditional society. The individual makes the choice either with reference entirely to his own personal satisfaction or in a spirit of service to the community and to farther the common goal.

In India, the love of learning had early origin or has exercised so lasting and powerful influence. The educational system aimed at the 'building of character, the development of personality and the preservation of the ancient culture of the motherland'.

Function of Educational Institution

- Education encourages the spirit of competition
- Acquires knowledge, skills and forms the positive attitudes towards life
- Brings behavioural modification with in the society whereby individual can modify all domains, e.g: Cognitive, affective.
- Holistic development of personality and good character
- Prepares the individual for adult life
- Maintains social order and discipline; transmits social heritage
- Improves emotional unity
- Develops essence of community feeling
- Protect the individual
- Increases the socialisation, reformation of attitudes of children
- Has its own symbol, which may be materials or non-material (e.g: Emblem)

- Increases the abilities, skills, capacities and modifies, internalisation processes
- Occupational placement – e.g: Professional training; conferring of status.

'The University Education Commission' (1948)

'The Secondary Education Commission' (1953)

'Education Commission' (1962–64) in their reports found out the defects in the present educational systems are:

- No sufficient literacy among children as well as adults in the rural areas
- Illiteracy was more among women than men
- Poor quality of teaching and faulty method of education
- More emphasis on academic and theoretical education, which is not related to every day practical aspects of the world.
- Absence of adequate facilities for technical and vocational education, which forces large number of students to go in for general education than, is justified by the requirements of the society
- Lack of agricultural institutes and universities to import education for agriculture and carry on research work
- A dearth of trained teachers and a high cost of education
- The period of schooling is not suited to the various objectives to be achieved at every stage
- Lack of civic and moral education at various levels
- Indiscipline among the students.

Measures to Remove Defects and Deficiencies

- The expansion of education at all levels to implement the provisions of the Indian constituencies
- Larger emphasis on basic education
- Diversification and comprehensiveness of education at the secondary stage through multipurpose schools
- More provision of training for untrained teachers and training of teachers in basic education, especially for women

- Improvement, in the standards of education
- More facilities for technical and vocational education
- Establishment of rural institute and agricultural universities
- Scholarship to poor students
- Improvement in the service conditions and emoluments of teachers
- Programmes for adult education.

Adult Education

It is the basis of modern way of living. The programme of adult literacy is of fundamental importance for the all round development of the country. Education enabled primitive man to overcome the opposition of natural forces and the problems created by the clash between different social forces and ideas. It must also increase human resistance to enable man to accept innovations from abroad, so long as they contribute to human welfare literacy provides knowledge in some of the basic tools of communication. Literacy is essential for the successful working of democracy. Illiteracy is definitely correlated to working efficiency. Reading and writing are tools by which a man may help himself, without them he is handicapped in partially every undertaking.

Adult education is the programme of educating adults in recent knowledge needs due attention. It must be taken up earnestly and systematically. In the light of the social, technological and economic forces problems of a magnitude unknown to earlier generations. Therefore, a more urgent need for educational provision to help the adult population by recognising the nature of problem, the possibilities and the difficulties inherent in rapid social and technological change, the choices available, and the extent to which adults can get through education and knowledge make wise choices and decisions. This educational assistance is only possible through adult education, recognising these facts, adult education should be recognised by governments at all levels, by educational organisations and by the teaching profession as an essential and important branch of the total national educational system.

Adult education emerged in the period of 1939–1947. In adult literacy concept, the illiterates has to be made to literate. To understand cultural social heritage and to perform national activities the citizens should possess literacy. Later the concept of adult literacy has changed to adult education. It is the education given to adult learners on part time basis with a view to develop total personalities.

Aims

- Promotes adult development by universalisation of primary education
- Shows keen interest in village activities
- Improves their vocational or occupational efficiency
- Train the adults to play dual role as adult citizens shouldering their responsibilities and attaining due statuses
- Improve the productive capacity of the individuals
- Improve Nations' wealth by promoting social contribution
- Individuals can perform effective role based on social expectance and acceptances
- Efficient participation of educated individuals in the national activities will meet the social needs
- To built-up national character.

In 1978, October 2nd National Adult Education Programme and Policy was made. The policy states that, universalisation of elementary education upto 14 years of age and educational facilities must be extended to adult population to remedy their educational deprivation and to enable them to develop their personality. Both adult education and universalisation of primary education are mutually interdependent and enable the masses to play an active role in social and cultural change. Educational deprivation will be removed and potentiality will be enhanced. It enables the masses to play an active role in social and cultural change. It promotes individual's growth and the country's socio-economic progress, the people are involved in development process of the country. Liberation of the people will be raised through literacy, dialogue and action. Adult education emphasises the imparting of literacy skills to persons who are economically and socially deprived sections of the society. It includes follow-up programmes, motivation, providing learning situations to improve living conditions, organising mass-media programmes, advancement of functional capability and meeting development needs of the community. The methods like classroom teaching, group participation and correspondence courses are used in adult education programmes. Developing capability in preparation of diversified and need-based teaching-learning materials, training manuals, and training of personnel at various levels to launch the programme at various parts of the state.

Approaches adopted in adult education programme are:

- Literacy with assured follow-up
- Conventional functional literacy
- Dominant development programme
- Literacy with learning-cum-action groups
- Conscientisation and formation of organisation of poor
- Training for the personnel, who requires training includes
- Key functionaries at National, State, District, Project and Block levels
- Professionals and experts in specific areas, e.g: Curriculum construction, preparation of teaching-learning materials
- Field level supervisors
- Adult education centre instructors
- Instructional responsibility will be given to schoolteachers, students, unemployed youth, ex-service men, and voluntary social workers with adequate follow-up programmes.

Causes for Slow Progress of Adult Education Programme

- Lack of awareness about the needs and immediate gains after the education
- The concept of 'earning while learning and learning for better-living' were not well planned
- Unable to create proper interest among the target group
- Superstition
- Absence of well-planned sincere workers
- Mismanagement and defective organisation.

Social Education

It is process of community uplift through community action aimed at actively associating the adults of a community to solve the social problems. It includes social learning as well as development in the form of social and vocational efficiency. Through social education the production of consciousness of citizens among the people and the promotion of social solidarity will be established.

Aims

- Produce educated individuals with higher intellectual minds
- Through educational activities upliftment of the community
- Train the individuals in the art of life
- Makes community self reliant
- Develop democratic citizenship
- Promotes integrated personalities.

Agencies

- Voluntary organisations
- Religious bodies
- Governmental agencies.

Activities

- Promote the social welfare activities of rural community through imparting education, sports, recreation by fixing convenient time for specific groups like women, youth, girls, boys.

- Organising mass-media activities to carry out recreational activities.
- Publicity department will take active part by arranging dramas, exhibition, fairs and excursions
- Health education programmes have to be carried out specific contents has to be covered, e.g: Health, community hygiene, methods to improve standards of living, methods of cultivation.

Community Education

To bring about the needed socio-economic changes in the community as rapidly as possible.

Non-formal Education

Life indeed, environment oriented, need-based and development linked activities will be planned to improve the learning power of learners.

Functional Education

To meet the needs of the people oriented to their environment based on their lives to improve the community, socio-economic status and enables them to share their responsibilities in the national development through community participation in the developmental activities in their own ways, 6–35 years of age group will be involved in functional education.

Content: Literacy, numeracy, health education, familial responsibilities, understanding of socio-economic cultural changes.

Previous Years University Questions

1. Define marriage and explain its type. (15 m, M.P, 2004)

2. Explain the economic organisation as a asocial regulator. (15 m, MP, 2004)
3. What is marriage? Discuss the aims of marriage. (15 m, MP, 2002)
4. Education. (5 m, MP, 2000)
5. Aims of marriage. (5 m, MP, 1998)
6. Disintegrating factors of joint family. (5 m, RGUHS, 2000)
7. Define dowry. (2 m, RGUHS, 2000)
8. Family disorganisation. (5 m, RGUHS, 2001)
9. Causes of dowry. (5 m, RGUHS, 2001)
10. Functions of family. (5 m, RGUHS, 1997)
11. Advantages of polyandry marriage.(2 m, RGUHS, 1997)
12. Legislation on Indian marriages and family. (2 m, RGUHS, 1997)
13. How does nuclear family differ from joint family. (5 m, RGUHS, 2002)
14. Point the merits of monogamy. (5 m, RGUHS, 2002)
15. Explain various forms of marriage.(10 m, RGUHS, 2003)
16. Experimental marriage. (3 m, RGUHS, 2003)
17. Give an account of merits and demerits of nuclear family in the modern society. (5 m, RGUHS, 2004)
18. Marriage as an institution. (2 m, RGUHS, 2004)
19. Explain the legislations on India marriage and family. (10 m, RGUHS, 2001)
20. Describe the changes in the functions of family in modern India. (10 m, RGUHS, 2001)
21. What are the provisions of Hindu Marriage Act. (2m RGUHS, 2002)
22. Describe the changing trends in modern family and its impact on health and diseases. (10 m, RGUHS, 2003)
23. Benefits of joint family. (5 m, RGUHS, 2000, 03)
24. Explain fraternal polyandry. (2 m, RGUHS, 2000)
25. What are the adverse health effects of child marriage. (2 m, RGUHS, 1999)

26. How women are benefited by Hindu Succession Act. (2 m, RGUHS, 1999)
27. What are the advantages of monogamy. (2 m, RGUHS, 1999)
28. Explain sarroral polyginy. (2 m, RGUHS, 1999)
29. Give a brief account of the different types of family and their salient features. (5 m, RGUHS, 2001)
30. Importance of Hindu Marriage Act of 1955 for women. (5 m, RGUHS, 2000)
31. What is family? Describe the types and functions of family and the changes occurred in the modern family. (10 m, RGUHS, 2002)
32. Explain the functions of modern family. (10 m, RGUHS, 2001)
33. Marriage laws and health of women.(2 m, RGUHS, 2001)
34. Joint family system. (5 m, RGUHS, 2000)
35. Features of modern family. (2 m, RGUHS, 2000)
36. Write the advantages and disadvantages of nuclear and joint family. (19 m, NTRUHS, 2003)
37. Discuss the importance of education in imposing health status of women in India. (19 m, NTRUHS, 2002)
38. Discuss the advantages and limitations of adult education in India. (19 m, NTRUHS, 2002)
39. Define family. What is the impact of family as a social organisation on society. (19 m, NTRUHS, 2002)
40. Explain the term 'family'. List the different forms of marriages and describe one form of marriage in brief. (19 m, NTRUHS, 2002)
41. Discuss the effects of early marriage on women's health. (19 m, NTRUHS, 2001)
42. Explain about the advantages and disadvantages of joint family system. (19 m, NTRUHS, 1999)
43. Describe about the advantages and disadvantages of joint family system. (19 m, NTRUHS, 1999)
44. 'Family is a social institution'. Discuss. (19 m, NTRUHS, 1998)

45. Explain the changes taking place in the functions of modern family. How family influences health status of its members. (13 m, SVIMS, Tirupati, 2002)
46. Child welfare services. (5 m, NTRUHS, 2002)
47. Child guidance clinic. (5 m, RGUHS, 2003)
48. What do you understand by family? Discuss its main functions. (15 m, MP, 1997)
49. Discuss the major causes of family disorganisation. (5 m, RGUHS, 1997, 2004)
50. Demerits of joint family system. (5 m, RGUHS, 2001)
51. Marriage and family problems in India. (5 m, RGU, 2003)
52. Define marriage and family. (2 m, 2001, RGU)
53. What is the importance of adult education in the society. (19 m, NTRUHS, 1999)
54. Functions of modern family give a briet description. (9 m, SVIMS, TPT, 2003)

MGR University Question Papers

1. Social institutions. (5 m, MGRU, Apr-04)
2. Conditions of marriage. (5 m, MGRU, Apr-04)
3. Types of marriages. (5 m, MGRU)
4. Conditions and types of marriage. (5 m, MGRU)
5. Dowry system. (5 m, MGRU)
6. Functions of a family. (5 m, MGRU)
7. Discuss the changing functions of the family in modern period. (5 m, MGRU)
8. Functions of family. (5 m, MGRU)
9. Institution and association. (5 m, MGRU)
10. Importance of marriage in Indian society.(5 m, MGRU)

CHAPTER TWELVE

Social Organisation

INTRODUCTION

Social refers to human beings living together as a group in a situation requiring that they have dealings with one another.

Organisation means a set of differentiated activities serving a common purpose and so correlated that effectiveness of each is increased by its relation to the rest.

Organisation refers to 'the way people relate themselves to one another'.

'Persons and groups making up a society are somehow held together'.

'Any interrelated system of roles and statuses'.

The whole function and structure of society, including man and all the ideas, culture, knowledge, techniques, achievements, traditions, aspirations, fashions, folkways, mores and institutions which have interpenetrated within an existing social order.

Definition

Social organisation is 'A state of being, a condition in which the various institutions in a society are functioning in accordance with their recognized or implied purposes'.

'It is a relative harmony between individual attitudes and social values'.

'The totality of the cultural institutions and their interrelationships together with the body of the organised activities'.

Thus social organisation is the organisation of society. Society is a web of relationships. Social organisation is a system of relationships. The mutual relationships between individuals are controlled and regulated by institutions and associations. The important forces keeping the social organisation in balance and bringing adjustment between the various elements of the society are social control, which consists of folkways, mores, laws, beliefs, attitudes, values and ideologies. By, which the group improves upon the members import a certain consistency and stability to human activities. Complete social harmony implies unanimity of opinion and stability in techniques and behaviour patterns, which are inconceivable in a rapidly changing modern society.

Social organisation is the net result of the interaction of the forces (integration and differentiation) within the social groups. The group is part of social organisation.

Elements

- Society
- Culture
- Personality

Characteristics

1. Unanimity among the members of society
   Unanimity among the members can be maintained only so long as people are prompt and ready to accept their status and respective roles within the Social organisation. The roles of individuals are determined on the basis of this social status. The promptness of people in accepting their own status and role is a feature of social organisation.

2. Control of society on the activities of the individuals
   Society exercises its control through the media of habits, custom, traditions, mores, rituals and institutions. It creates unanimity between the group members. Social disorganisation starts the moment, this control of society is lifted from the members.

SOCIAL DISORGANISATION

Society is a web of organised social relationships. The process whereby social relationships become disorganised is known as 'Social disorganisation'. In Social disorganisation all the processes like habits, institutions and associations will be disorganised.

When individual satisfactorily performs the roles, which attach to his particular status in society, the society retains its organised character. A society becomes disorganised when these roles become disorderly. People forget their duties, social laws diminishes, balance between the various parts of society is disturbed, social ideas become degenerate and the entire social structure will be in a chaotic state.

'Significant discrepancy between social standards and social actuality'.

Social disorganisation is a relative phenomenon and the two, 'Social organisation' and 'Social disorganisation' are the dual aspects of the whole functioning of the social system. When the forces of social change create a threat to social stability and as a result of which gives raise to social problems.

'Social disorganisation implies some breakdown in the Social organisation, i.e. equilibrium of forces, a decay in the social structure, so that old habits and forms of social control no longer function effectively'—*Elliot and Merrill*

Definition

- 'Maladjustment between the various elements in the total cultural configuration as to endanger the survival of the group or as seriously to interfere with the satisfaction of the fundamental desires of its members with the result that social cohesion is destroyed'—*Gillin and Gillin*

- 'Social organisation consists of the coordination of individual responses as a consequence of the operation of conventionalised patterns of consensus and control, any change in the cultural context which impedes or destroys the functioning of the patterns of coordination which constitute the social order represents Social disorganisation'—*Dr Mowrer*

Characteristics of Social Disorganisation

Conflict of Mores and of Institutions

In every society there are some mores and institutions, on the basis of which the life of the members proceeds smoothly and in an organised manner. With the passage of time these mores and institutions become obsolete and fail to satisfy the needs of the members of society. New ideals arise and new institutions are formed out of differences in opinions and ideals. In this way society is broken into numerous groups. Some people want to retain certain mores and institutions while others ask for complete elimination. And yet others wish to achieve a synthesis between the ancient and the modern social mores and institutions. This conflict destroys the consensus in society with the destruction of consensus, organisation is disrupted and disorganisation sets in, e.g.: Differences of opinion in respect of many social institutions and social laws like divorce, untouchability widow remarriage.

Transfer of Functions from One Group to Another

In an organised society, the functions of each group are predetermined. But society is dynamic and hence these functions of the groups cannot remain the same for a long time. As time passes the functions of one group are transferred to another. This disorderliness encourages social disorganisation, e.g.: In the ancient social system the functions of family, state, caste and other groups were determined and definite. As time progressed the state acquired many of the functions traditionally associated with the family, e.g : Many functions of the caste were taken over by class groups.

Personal Individualisation

In the organised society the functions of an individual are determined from the social viewpoint, e.g.: Marriage, occupation were based on some definite patterns in ancient India.

But in modern age of individualism, every person thinks upon all the important matters of life from his viewpoint. In every instant he wants to take an independent decision and does not want to take into consideration the interests of society. In this way modern young men and women want to decide an important matters, e.g: Marriage, family, occupation, travel, moral conduct, are in accordance with or from the viewpoint induced by their personal views without caring for the society. The cause of personal individualisation is the change in and diversification of social values.

Change in Social Values

A change in the social structure means change in the status, roles and functions of its members. In an organised society the status and functions of each individual are well defined and everyone works accordingly. This maintains the society in an organised condition. But as the time passes changes in social values and things are accompanied by changes in these status and roles. This change takes over by the precise definition of an individual's status and functions therefore they do as they please. Due to this social disorganisation sets in, e.g: Disorganisation of family and caste system in India; changes in functions and status of women in Indian society.

Conclusion: Social disorganisation means a lack of system in the mutual relationships of persons in their respective status and functions in social values in mores and in institutions. The relation of all these breaks up and social consensus disappears.

Social Disorganisation is a Process

Since society is a dynamic entity, the Social disorganisation is a process. Status and roles are continually changing in society and concurrently with them the social structure also changes, but it is not essential that the collapse of a specific structure be always disadvantageous or harmful. Sometimes this is the nature of a preparation for a new social structure, which is to evolve in future. Hence, Sociologists regard Social disorganisation as a natural process rather than as a malady. Social disorganisation temporarily disrupts the existing social order so that a new Social organisation may replace it. New social laws come into being according to the values and a new structure of society is created. This novel structure becomes static and inflexible with the passage of time and fails to adapt to the varying social values. Then this structure also breaks down. Social disorganisation is an indication of the existence of diseased or disruptive elements in society.

Causes of Social Disorganisation

Social Change

Human society is dynamic everywhere. Its various elements, mores, institutions, associations etc., are constantly changing. In it, the old mores come into conflict with new situations the result of which is that the unanimity of society is destroyed.

Cultural Factors

Maladjustment in Existing Institutions

Poverty is considered to be the outgrowth of capitalistic system and the institution of private property, which creates in-equalities of wealth.

Cultural Lag Approach

Developed by *Ogburn.* It has been pointed out that changes in the material and non-material culture are not uniform leading to social disorganisation, e.g: Changes in the material culture are readily adopted due to apparent utility of new articles, which bring immediate changes in human relations. On the other hand, the social institutions or mores, which controls social relationships generally rigid with the result that there may arise social disorganisation. Thus social maladjustment is the consequence of delay in the reciprocal changes in the dependent part of culture necessitated by discoveries and inventions in material culture. This may also be called the technological factor of social disorganisation, e.g: Rapid industrialisation and urbanisation bring many problems like poor housing conditions, establishment of slums, industrial accidents, unbalanced ratio of sexes, etc. may lead to social disorganisation.

All the elements of society do not undergo an equal degree of change and modification. Physical elements change rather conveniently, but the non-material elements change at a slow rate and their change lags behind the change in physical elements. Beliefs and thoughts change with great difficulty, but not much time is needed for the adoption of material things.

Cultural Conflicts

The conflicting attitudes or values different groups or individuals, etc. results in social disorganisation. The values are of two kinds:

- Subjective
- Objective

Subjective values: Those which are fixed by individuals or groups according to the situation or circumstances in which they are placed and which are suited to their interests.

Objective values: The consciousness of the society is formed on the basis of collective thinking and for the benefit of the whole society.

War

War introduces confusion and disorder in society. The young men of the community are consumed in war, young women are widowed, soldiers have to live in camps faraway from their families. All these factors tend to weaken sexual ties. Sexual relationships are further influenced by a change in the male-female ratio. Social values are injured by war. The value of human life is reduced.

Crisis

Crisis is an occurrence, which interrupts smooth running habits, by focusing attention upon a conflict situation.

a. *Precipitate crisis:* Which is so sudden as to deprive people of their senses, e.g : Death of a great leader, terrible accident, famine, catastrophe. These crises change the situations and functions of many individuals. New circumstances are created, which necessitate completely new conditions. In order to face this crisis it becomes essential to think of some solution.
b. *Cumulative crisis:* It is not manifested instantaneously but gradually takes root and develops as a result of many successive incidents, e.g : Division of India consequent creation of Pakistan. The mutual hatred and distrust of the Hindus and the Muslims increased by successive steps and exhibited in communal riots.

Change in Social Values

Social organisation derives its strength from social values and it is destroyed when some is inflicted upon them and the process of disorganisation sets in. Changes in social values necessitate new social institutions and associations. This creates disorder in society. The status and roles of people change in accordance with the changes in social values. They take time to adapt and adjust themselves. In this way, disorganisation spreads.

Existing values in Indian society have undergone a major change, which has created a great difference in the status and roles of the two sexes and of people belonging to various castes and classes. As a result, a major conflict between the old and new values has been created. Consequently, one sees the process of social disorganisation working rapidly.

Psychological Factors

The social processes like imitation, conflict, competition, accommodation, assimilation, communication, builts up the dynamic organisation of society. When members of the society live in close proximity there is constant communication takes place among them. The communication can function effectively only when there is common understanding or common consciousness. As complete unanimity of attitudes and values can hardly be reached in modern societies. Communication is generally incomplete and fragmentary.

Symbols used do not mean exactly the same thing to all men who use them. Words, phrases and ideas arouse different trains of thought in different persons and there is some disequilibrium in the society. Thus communication may result in conflict or competition. They are destructive to the organisation of the larger group. These processes operate in all the spheres, e.g: Cultural, economic, political, religious, etc.

Differences between social organisation and social disorganisation

Social organisation	*Social disorganisation*
Consensus of opinion among members regarding status and roles	Disintegration of roles and statuses
All parts are in equilibrium and its members derive satisfaction from organised society	Stability looses and dissatisfaction results among its members
Mutual satisfactory social relationship	Replacement of social relationships which bring disappointment, thwarted wishes (frustration), irritation and unhappiness
Unanimity	Multiplicity of opinions
Homogeneity of population	Heterogeneity of population
Mutual faith/trust	Distrust
Similarity in interests and attitudes	Individuality and varied interests and attitudes
Intelligent rational behaviour	Hedonistic behaviour
Emphasis on duties	Emphasis on rights
Protection of sacred elements	Degeneration of scared elements
Sincerity	Ostentation
Peace and happiness	Disturbance and pain
Synthesis between status, role and functions	Contradiction between status and function
Clarity of situation and activities	Lack of clarity of situation and activities
Synthesis/harmony of mores and institutions	Conflict between mores and institutions
Orderly relationships	Disorder in social relationships
Strong social control	Absence of social control
Harmony between various parts of society and individual	Conflict between society and individual
Respect for social laws	Disregard of social laws

SOCIAL PATHOLOGY

Introduction

Sociology has its branch, social pathology. As in anatomy, we study the structure of body and its function in physiology and in pathology we study the abnormalities and diseases of the body. In sociology we study the functional aspects of society, in social pathology we study the abnormal functions of social relations and deviations of normal social relations.

The social structure is abstract. The relationship between social structure and its sub-structures is neither fixed nor definite. It is dynamic and fluid in which changes are constantly occurring.

Definition

- 'Serious maladjustments between the various elements in the cultural configuration so as to endanger the survival of the group or as seriously to interfere into the satisfactions of the fundamental desires of its members with the result that social cohesion is destroyed'—*John Lewis Gillin and John Philip Gillin*
- 'The study of man's failure to adjust himself and his institutions to the necessities of the existence to the end that he may survive and meet fairly with the felt needs of his nature'—*John Lewis Gillin*

Moaning

There should be harmony among the various parts, components and aspects of culture. All the components of society are interdependent, interactive and affect each other. The absence of disharmony is bound to generate conflicts and tensions. If the disharmony allowed to persist, it gets deep into roots of the tree of culture and ultimately ruins it. Maladjustment of social relationships results in 'social pathology'. The people mistrust each other and leads to disintegration.

Scope

The social interaction and interrelation between various units of social structure, i.e. interpersonal, intercommunal, intergroup, etc. are constantly exist. These interrelations and interactions generate associative and dissociative social processes. The modern sociologist conceives the society as a dynamic process, in society new ideas and inventions affect and disturb the equilibrium. The social adjustments are under constant pressure of change. Unless suitable changes and modifications is not an indication of any disease, the crisis between old and new facts, patterns of ideas and ways of life is symptomatic of progress and a healthy change. Social pathology does a diagnostic activity.

Utility

a. *For social reforms:* The social reformer is a doctor of the society, who has chosen to dedicate himself to the prevention, cure and eradication of the social evils and diseases. For the success of social reformer the knowledge of social pathology is useful.
b. *For government:* To maintain social order and peace.
c. *For common man:* The knowledge of social pathology can be useful for everyone to have successful adjustment in society, whatever the filed it may be.

Scales of Social Pathological Condition

1. *Simple rates:* Observing the incidence of prevailing social problems.
2. *Composition of population:* The number of young people will be affected more than old.
3. *Social distance:* The more the social distance, the more the chances of maladjustment.
4. *Participation:* The greater the participation of individuals in various social activities, the greater is the chance of appropriate adjustment.

SOCIAL PROBLEMS

Social problems are the result of the failure of a society to adapt its social institutions and culture to its growing needs. They are man made and is one of the major sources of social suffering. The lives of all members of a social group are directly or indirectly affected by this suffering. All members of society have to pay and must be made to pay in some form or the other for these social deficits and breaches in the social order. Men from infancy seek security. Irrespective of the cause of social inequality or unequal distribution of opportunity the fact remains that every social group has members whose plight calls for serious public attention and vigorous social action to cement the breaches and overcome the deficits in order to restore a state of social equilibrium within the society. A realisation of this type is possible with a sympathetic attitude supported by scientific understanding of the nature, extent, social diagnosis and therapeutic action to resolve a social problem. Social problems are behaviour pattern or conditions that are considered objectionable or undesirable by many members of a society. With the increase in number of social problems the society cannot work smoothly or social progress is hampered/hindered and social disorganisation exists. When an individual or a group of individuals is disorganised and is not functioning according to the norms laid down by the society, the social problem is said to exist.

Definition

- 'A social problem is any deviant behaviour in a disapproved direction of such a degree that it exceeds the tolerance limit of the community'—*Lundberg*
- 'Significant discrepancy between social standards and social actuality'.
- 'Morally wrong but the majority or substantial minority within the society' —*Green*

Every Social Problem Implies Three Things

1. Something should be done to change the situation, which constitutes a problem.
2. The existing social order has to be changed to solve the problem.
3. The situation regarded a problem is undesirable but is not inevitable.

Nature of Social Problem

The individual who conforms to social norms is socially normal and as a consequence, he considers himself normal. But the individual who is detected for violating the norms is a deviant. Generally it is a group of individually disorganized persons having the same problem, which represents a social problem.

The individual, social disorganisation and social problems are interrelated and dependent.

Individual disorganisation → Social disorganisation → Social problem.

Social disorganisation → Social problem → Individual disorganisation.

Thus social disorganisation is always the resultant of some breakdown in the Social organisation. Social problems are the conditions threatening the well being of society.

Classification of Social Problem

- Economic problems, e.g: Poverty, unemployment, dependency.
- Biological problems, e.g: Physical diseases and defects.
- Psychological problem, e.g: Neurosis, psychosis, epilepsy, feeble mindedness, suicide, alcoholism.
- Cultural problems, e.g: Problems of the aged, the homeless and the widowed, divorce, illegitimacy, crime and juvenile delinquency.

JUVENILE DELINQUENCY

Definition

- 'A juvenile delinquent is a person between the ages of 15 to 17, who indulges in anti-social activity'.
- 'Juvenile delinquent, who breaks the law, is a vagrant, persists in disobeying orders, whose behaviour endangers his own moral life as well as the moral life of other'.

- 'Juvenile delinquent involves wrongdoing by a child or a young person, who is under age specified by the law of the place concerned'—*Dr. Sethna*
- 'A delinquent is a person under age, who is guilty of anti-social act and whose misconduct is an infraction of law'—*Newmeyer*

Causes of Juvenile Delinquency

Social Causes

Defects of the family: In broken families, where family ties and mutual intimate relationships have been destroyed.

Parent-child relationship: When the child is deprived of love and is scolded constantly on every occasion, child develops feeling of revolt and hatred, so that he runs away from the house and falls into a life of criminals. It induces a feeling of insecurity and develops mental complexes. If the parents has negative attitude, hurt the child's feelings and lead to insecurity children's tendency towards crime is aggravated.

Character and conduct of parents at home: The child's personality is considerably influenced by the character and conduct of their parents. Child has been able to mould their behaviour according to socially accepted values and conceptions. If parents are indulged in such behaviour like telling lies, hypocritical behaviour, sexual immorality and stealing will have effect over the childs' development.

Influence of siblings or criminal relatives: Child's personality is susceptible to the influence of his siblings' personality apart from the personality and mutual relationship of the parents. If the siblings in the family manifest criminal tendencies and immoral behaviour the youngsters are invariably influenced by it.

Defects in the School

- Next to the family, the child's personality is influenced by the school.
- Theft and sex crimes.
- Low intelligence level.
- Roaming outside the school (vagrancy)
- Criticism by parents and teachers.
- Gaining membership of a gang and criminals.
- Punishment by teachers.
- Weakness in some subject.
- Level of education is too high.
- Lack of companionship or influence of bad companion.

Influence of Cinemas or Movies

Mass-media activities.

Physical Abnormalities

Like handicapped children have to overcome their insecurity develops deliquescent behaviour.

War and Post-war Condition

While the father is in war zone and mother is in some occupation due to this the children's education is considerably affected. In wartime, wherever there is bombing, the adolescents took the greatest part in looting and smashing the houses.

Social Disorganisation

Disorganisation of society leads to increase in criminal activity. Modern industrial societies where lack of synthesis and equality, creates tension. This tension inspires young men and women to perform delinquent activities.

Displacement

Displacement of thoughts, ideas, attitudes, in a negative manner influence child's conduct and demoralise the child's values.

Psychological Causes

a. Intellectual weakness
b. Mental diseases
c. Psychopathic personality

Is a cause of crime and juvenile delinquency where there is total absence of love, affection and control. The individual is very unsocialised, irritable, cruel, obstinate, suspicious, self-centered, lonely, full of feelings of revenge, backward and hypersexual or uncontrolled sexual behaviour. In extreme cases, the person lacks the ability to sympathize completely devoid of repentance over their own cruel doings and the pain or suffering of others.

Personality Defects

The method of an individual's adaptation to environment. Criminal children resort to illegal modes of such adaptation.

- Degree of freedom
- Irresponsibility
- Revolt
- Homicidal tendency
- Suspicious
- Lack of control
- Sadism
- Emotional and social maladjustment
- Extrovert behaviour
- Immaturity in sentiment
- Lack of emotional balance, unbalanced through lack of love and affection
- Disobedient and unsocial
- Inferiority complex

Economic Causes

- Poverty
- Poor working condition
- Unemployment
- Child labour
- Unfulfilled desires

Control of Juvenile Delinquency

Probation

Juvenile delinquents are kept under the supervision of a probation officer, whose job is to look after the delinquent, to help him in getting established in normal life and to see that the delinquent observes the rules of bail-bond. Thus the delinquent not only gets a chance to reform himself, but also gets advice and concrete help.

Reformatory Institutions

To reform inmate delinquents, the institutions provide an all round personality development by sufficient means of separating the inmates by providing adequate facilities to meet the basic needs such as proper sanitary arrangements, water supply, food clothing and bedding for the inmates and vocational or industrial training. When delinquent becomes sick medical aid will be provided.

Certified Schools (Fit persons institution)

These are established for the treatment of juvenile delinquent. The schools are of two types:

1. Junior school < 12–13 years of age. (Primary education)
2. Intermediate school 13–15 years of age. (Technical education)
3. Senior school between 15 to 17 years of age. (Industrial training)

The children are generally confined there upto a certain age limit and for about 2–3 years, but the school authorities can make an early discharge. After their release they are kept under the charge of a welfare officer or probation officer.

Auxiliary Homes

These are attached to certified schools, here the delinquents are kept for sometime and studied by a social worker and then they are sent to the certified schools according to the nature and aptitude of a young offender.

Foster Homes

These are specially for delinquent children of under 10 years of age, who cannot be sent to approved or certified schools unless the court is satisfied that they cannot be dealt with otherwise. These are generally run by voluntary agencies, aided by government.

Uncared Children Institutions

The children in the pre-delinquent or near delinquent stage, who are mostly found in a state of destitution or neglect, are cared for. All over the country they are situated, managed by private philanthropists.

Reformatory School

These are meant for the education and vocational training of delinquent children with much regard to the type of crime committed. The delinquents are removed from bad environments and placed in the reformatory school for sometime after which they can adapt some vocation learnt in the school. Young offenders, under 15 years are imprisoned for 3–7 years.

Borstal Institutions

It is a system of detaining juvenile delinquents, first correctional purpose of reformatory is at borstal. Special treatment is provided for adolescent offenders between the ages of 15–21 years.

Two types of borstal institutions:

1. Open institutions: Open environment with no surrounding wall.
2. Closed institutions: Converted prison building where maximum security provided.

Industrial training where arduous physical training and education will be given according to the age, record and character of the inmate so as to deter them from committing crime again. The training is different for boys and girls, e.g: Mixed farming, building and engineering, laundry, cooking and housework. 2–3 years is the term of borstal but the date of release is decided by the borstal authorities according to conduct and progress of the inmate. The person is attached to borstal associate or probation officer, whose duties are to see that he is fitted in the trade for which he has been trained.

Psychological Techniques

1. *Play therapy:* The delinquent children are given opportunities to participate in such plays, which give expression to the repressed motives and help in the development of creative energy.
2. *Finger painting:* The child is given plain papers and some colors. Child is allowed to paint in his own way. The purpose is not painting, but expression of repressed motives in the child, which leaves them sensible and healthy.
3. *Psychodrama:* The child is allowed to participate in different roles in group drama and thereby manifest their repressed motives. The Psychologists reform delinquents by creating healthy atmosphere in the family and by providing adequate healthy recreation. Coordinated and concentrated efforts of teachers, guardians, and government are required to organise psychodramas by delinquent children.

4. *Government measures:*
   - Formal education
   - Vocational training in a number of trades is imported to the inmates. Certified, reformatory and borstal schools enable them to settle down in trades learnt in school.
   - Follow up services are given. Training in citizenship of democratic living. The juvenile delinquents are encouraged to take part in extra-curricular activities, e.g.: Sports, debate, dramas, music and scouting.
   - Rehabilitation—guidance and training. Family community based programs has to be organised to improve environment and to reduce the peer group influences.
5. *Behaviour therapy:* Motivate the child by reinforcing good habits, which modify maladaptive behaviour.
6. *Family therapy:* To establish intimate relationship safeguards childs freedom by engaging them in useful activities.

Prevention of juvenile delinquency

1. *Team work of private and public agencies:* These assist parents and guardians in locating difficult children in danger of maladjustment and in recognizing early symptoms of unhappiness, conflict and insecurity.
2. *Training of members and staff of all organisations:* Counsels to recognize the juvenile delinquents and to overcome the difficulties.
3. *Establishment of child guidance clinics:* Diagnostic facilities are established in the schools to treat seriously disturbed and maladjusted children.
4. *Education of the family:* Health professionals should educate the family members about preventive measures and rehabilitation of the clients with juvenile delinquency.
5. *Establishment of recreational agencies:* Provision for sport activities, cultural activities, organisational activities.

6. *Assistance to under privileged children:* Character building agencies like schools, churches should be encouraged to serve under privileged children.
7. *Propaganda:* Through mass media like newspaper, magazines, radio, TV, motion pictures, to encourage the parents for good child rearing practices.

CRIME

Against the social problems, society has got some degree of social disapproval, depending upon the effect of their behaviour over the society.

Definition

- 'An act forbidden by the law of the land and for which penalty is prescribed'—*C. Darrow*
- 'A form of anti-social behaviour that has violated public sentiment to such an extent as to be forbidden by statute'.

Nature of Crime

'The criminal is a person who does an act in violation of the law'. Crime is that 'behaviour which is prohibited by the criminal code'. Crime is generally recognised as transgressions against the traditions and mores of the community. Crime therefore may be regarded as behaviour of individuals, which the group strongly disapproves.

Crime is a anti-social behaviour, which the group rejects and to which it attaches penalties. It is a disturbance in the social relations.

CAUSES OF CRIME

Physical Factors

The physical environment, which includes climate, season, geological condition, affects indirectly upon the density of population, economic development and cultural institution.

Physical defects turn a man into a criminal due to these deformities, he lags behind his fellow beings in many respects and in order to remove this difference he turns to criminal.

Factors concerning for physical development, e.g: Heredity, early sexual maturity, mental defects and nervous instability, e.g: Feeble mindedness was found to be a major cause of crime (Epilepsy attacks and emotional disturbances are more common)

Disease hampers the progress and this social degradation spurs them to engage in anti-social activities, e.g: A person, who, being very ugly fails to win a woman's love tries to gain ascendancy over her by the power of money, which he amasses by illegitimate means or by sheer distinct of physical power, e.g: Rape and sexual crimes increase in murder. In adolescence, the aggressive tendency grows.

Biological Factors

Physiological / Constitutional factor

A born criminal type, which was characterised by irregularities of body and mind. They possess a greater measure of anomalies, e.g: Asymmetry of skull, low retreating forehead, strongly arched brows, large outstanding ears, sparse beard, tattooing, left handedness, relative insensibility to pain, acuteness of vision, obtuseness of the sense of smell or of taste, touch and hearing, lack of moral sense, violent temper, extreme vanity, improvidence.

Hereditary Factor

- Weak mindedness (Physical and mental capacity is limited)
- Dysgenic traits; Alcoholism, Prostitution, Criminality, Insanity, Pauperism were transmitted biologically in family strains.
- The presence of: Mental disease and ailments, Hysteria, Epilepsy, Neurotic traits, Alcoholism, Suicide, Begging in

the familial and ancestral background leads to mental disorder, crime, prostitution, vagabondage, quarrelsomeness, unsociability, homosexuality, perversities and drug addiction.

Glandular Factor

Functioning of the glands determines temperament, intelligence, character, personality as well as of physical and mental pathology. Physical growth, mental deficiency, temperamental types, body build, mental alienations and alternations, emotional balance, neurological and psychological functioning became explainable partially or wholly in terms of abnormal or inadequate functioning of the ductless glands.

Glandular disturbances could account for many disharmony, defective, unstable and inadequate qualities found in the suspected constitutional inferiority of criminals.

Mental and Psychological Factors

- Unable to adopt approved social behaviour
- Motivation to criminal behaviour
- Mental deficiency: Subnormality, feeble/weak mindedness, low-grade mentality
- Mental disorder: Criminal insane
- Mental mechanism: Unconscious motivating forces, fixations, conflicts, frustrations, neuroses, inferiority, regression, guilt feelings, psychic trauma
- Motivation to behaviour: New experience, response, recognition, security

The system of motivation is based on organic needs arising from the body and the external social situations. Individuals either turn directly to delinquency in order to get their wishes satisfied or resort to delinquency as a result of blockages in the satisfaction of wishes in the normal channels, e.g: Delinquency behaviour is 'A response to inner and outer pressure', i.e. a form of self-expression. Interferences with the ordinary satisfaction of wishes by thwarting and deprivation lead to substitute satisfactions as a means of affecting dissatisfaction. Unsatisfactory fulfillment of wishes and associated emotional distress is expected to constitute an important cause of crime.

Environmental Factor

Family Condition

Broken marriage: Most dominant factor in the social causes of crime due to:

- Death of the mother or the father or both
- Divorce or separation
- Defective home conditions
- Family disorganisation
- Degradation in the control of family
- Devoid of love and affection
- No respect to their elders
- Need of a carefree, unrestricted, individual life (Prone for to sex crime)
- Undesirable domestic conditions like adultery, abortion, miscarriages, prostitution, juvenile delinquency.

Size of family: The larger the family, the more difficult to support and to supervise. Consequently, children are neglected and get into trouble—delinquent behaviour.

Sibling position: The surveys revealed the second child in the family—committed the most severe crime. The next to youngest—more likely to commit offence.

Unsatisfactory parent-child relationship: causes behaviour problems.

Democratic homes: The presence of demoralizing conditions in the home, e.g: Alcoholism, immorality.

Lack of supervision or control over children: Is an important cause in juvenile delinquency. It may be in the form of:

- Negligence
- Ignorance of parents

- Temperament or personality of parents
- Absence of parents in the home due to their employment
- Defective home discipline.

The Companionship Factor

- Much case was observed that the delinquency and criminal activity is an affair of association of two or more individuals, e.g: Fights and riots, dacoits, village vendettas.
- Roaming in the streets of city slums—delinquency
- The patterns and traditions of gang life and having more social contact—antisocial behaviour
- The contacts in custody and friendship, e.g: Pick-pocket, cut throat are learnt from the custody.

Community Conditions

Community disorganisation: Due to the weakening of institutional and primary group influence over the lives and conduct of individuals. The influence of existing social rules of behaviour upon individual members of the group decay of social opinion, decay of communal social solidarity.

Density and overloading: Thickly populated areas (urban contacts), children get into difficulty while roaming in the streets because of the inability of parents and neighbours to watch over their conduct. Over crowded in the houses leads to family indiscipline and lack of morality.

Agencies of moral risk: Amusements of low moral tone, cheap dance halls, gambling parlours are responsible for the demoralisation of young children.

Cinemas

Cinemas influence indirectly the male criminals by teaching crime techniques like exhibiting many kinds of crimes, stimulating the desire for wealth and comforts, showing ways and means of appropriating them illegally, arousing the feeling of bravado, toughness and adventure, by arousing profound sexual urges, stimulating day dreams of criminal jobs, it directs or urges many young and inexperienced woman to illegitimate relations and crimes by setting alight the sexual desire. The desire for exhibition, lovemaking, independence and variety, the pictures stimulate sex instincts, the possibilities for the occurrence of bad sex habits under cover of darkness in the theatres.

Economic Conditions

Most of the criminals tend to come from the bad housing conditions, unemployment, child labor, bad company, economic handicaps of bread winner, economic insecurity, which are by products of industrialism are considered as important factors in crime.

Poverty: A hungry man can do literally anything in order to meet his hunger. Poor girls are easily entranced by men who violate them, put them on the market places. Many commit suicide and murder of entire family due to poverty.

Unemployment: Many young men commit suicide when they are frustrated by extreme poverty and continued unemployment. Many turn to stealing, pick-pockets, robbery Some unemployed youth may create disturbance-causing violence. Most gangsters do not work, gangsterism is their only occupation.

Industrialisation: It has destroyed the family life of millions of labourers. They work very hard for 8–10 hours in the day during which they have to suffer many inconveniences and for this, they have to live in towns far away from their families. Continued existence of this type leads them to indulge in alcoholism and prostitution and this encourages other crimes like murder, assault, disturbance, robbery. Housing becomes a problem in an industrial town when the population increases beyond limits. In some towns, thousands of families live in houses having single room, the married members have no privacy, which leads to sex crimes of the other young members of the family. Many men are compelled to live alone and this tends to unbalance the ratio of men to women, which consequently encourages sex crimes. Many girls from rural areas are deceived with promises of employment and brought to towns where they are forced to adopt prostitution.

Urbanisation

In cities, the society fails to exercise control over the individual who loses his identity in the mob after having committed a crime. In towns, there are better opportunities for picking pockets and practicing deception in a crowd. Absence of healthy recreation in the town and hence the cinemas are over-crowded. Gambling indecent theatres and wine shops provide means of spurious recreation. This encourages crime.

Superstition

Superstition exists in illiterate, ignorant masses and more among scheduled tribes. Murders are committed in the belief that human sacrifice would reveal hidden treasure. A strong belief in spells and sacrifice to obtain material wealth is a frequent cause of crime.

Factions and Feuds

The unfortunate legacy of the caste system tends to create narrow channels of though and a tendency to think and act in terms of little groups is the main factor in the creation of tensions. Blood feuds have been carried on between two branches of a single family.

Exploitation of Children by Adults

Exploitation of children for the purpose of stealing by bad elements of society engaged in anti-social activities is very common in big cities. The smugglers make use of juveniles and females for transporting the illicit liquors and food grains as in case of their detection punishment is corrective measure. The employer sometimes exploits the children, who then take to stealing with a feeling of revenge.

Absence of Social Control

Previously, the caste Panchayat in the village kept control over the behaviour and conduct of the members of the caste. Punishments such as exterminating the guilty person from the caste, tends to control and check crime effectively. Today, Social organisations have been deprived of all their authority. With better facilities of transport being available, the criminal can commit the crime and abscond from the village to the town or to the villages from the towns.

In cities the social relations became impersonal, an individual may commit a crime and conceal his identity in the city mob. The disappearance of the control of caste organisation is another cause of crime in India.

Defective Education

Illiteracy and lack of education are considered as important causes of crime. Modern education does not develop the character of students in right direction.

Modern education increases the selfishness, disorderliness and impertinence. Ethical and religious education has no place in the modern educational system. Even after completing the education, an individual is not capable of earning his livelihood and many well-educated people remain unemployed for many years. Late employment leads to late marriage all these tend to criminal activities.

Literature (Newspaper)

It increases criminal activity by publishing methods of crime through news items. By printing news of major crimes and showing their advantages and circulating the name of criminals, highlighting the causes which tends to increase the crime, by warning and alerting criminals by publishing police methods.

Use of Alcohol

People with low standard of life, cultivate the habit of alcoholism, commits crimes. Drinking affects not only the drinker and makes them a criminal, but it also has a deleterious influence on their entire family and inclines men, women and children towards crime both directly as well as indirectly.

Prohibition of Widow Remarriage

Many young widows do not remarry for the rest of their lives, such a decision, however, do not annihilate their sexual passions and these rather lie dormant in a corner of the mind and wait or a suitable opportunity. Even if the religious, she is pursued by men and is lured to the path of evil and sin by many threat, which leads to adultery, miscarriage, abortion, infanticide. When these sinful practices are made public many women commits suicide.

Defects of the Marriage and Dowry System

Dowry system urges the parents of the girls to earn money through illegitimate means for their daughter's marriage, it leads to suicide by many girls who cannot bear to see the degraded condition of their parents. The dowry system further encouraged late marriage. Lack of wealth compels a girl to remain unmarried throughout her life or utmost she is married to an old man for to an unsuitable partner. All these also tend to increase sex crimes in the society.

Very often the parents do not care to ask the girl or boy or opinion and sometimes even proceed against the opinion of the girl/boy. Thus results in suicide and other crimes.

Religion

Religion encourages the difference of opinion between people on matters of religion and hatred for the other religion. Communal riots and crimes, e.g: Looting, murder perpetrated in order to increase the followers of one's own religion and to injure another religion. Crimes are committed during communal riots, helpless women were nuded and taken in procession in the name of religion.

Change in Social Values

Materialism, individualism, rationalism, craze for women, absence of sex restrictions has led to a disregard of ancient social values, new values have been restated. It inspires crime because any individual can manage to produce an argument to justify it when they are improper.

Geographical Causes

Crimes of rape are more common in plains than in the mountains or plateaus.

Political Causes

Now-a-days many criminals go scot free with proper legal advice because there is opportunity to prove truth false and falsehood true. This encourages them to engage in further criminal activity. On the other hand, innocent persons who are prosecuted and convicted in their place also become criminals as a reaction. The ill treatment to which the prison inmates are subjected also hardens the softest criminals. Crimes are further encouraged by the inefficiency, immorality and corruption of police department. People connected with political groups unobtrusively assist criminals and make use of them to inflict injury upon and to defame members of opposing groups.

Methods of Crime Detection

Free Association Test

A list of words is provided, the list containing some words that are quite ordinary, while others associations with the experiences of the pseudo-criminal student. There are some others words that have no reasonable connection with the criminal experience. Single words are individually read out to the individual present in the room, and the individual is required to record the word that immediately springs into their mind in response to the word as well as the time taken to react to it. The list is then repeated in the reverse order and on the basis of their reactions the criminal is distinguished. The criminal's associative reactions to certain important words are more peculiar than the normal individual. Criminal takes a lot of time to react to certain words. When the list of words is repeated in reverse order the criminal's reactions to the important or significant words will change that has to be recorded.

Blood Pressure Test

The change in BP is indicative of the occasion at which the individual under test has attempted to deceive. A person trying to deceive is normally assailed by the emotions of fear and anger with the result that systolic BP increases. The need to deceive caused changes in BP as well as constriction in the normal respiratory activity. Cardio-pneumo-psychograph can be taken to discover attempts at criminal activities.

Psychogalvanic Reflex Test

It records and exhibits changes in glandular secretion under conditions of abnormal stimulation and excitation. Sweat gland excretion changes under emotional stress. When a person is asked questions regarding a crime he is assailed by fear and anger with the result he perspires freely. The changes can be measured in terms of psychogalvanic reflex and a shrewd guess can be made whether he is criminal or not.

Brain Wave Pattern Test (EEG)

When a person is transferred from a state of relaxation to one of excitation or stimulation the brain wave pattern changes.

Control of Crime

Probation

The postponement on certain conditions laid down by the prosecuting authority of the punishment due to a criminal by law. These individuals are kept under the guardianship of a probation officer instead of being imprisoned. Ways of life, conduct, physical and mental condition are taken into account before placing the criminal under probation.

Probation officer performs certain functions for treating the criminal problems:

- To keep criminals in his personal care
- Try to improve and reform criminals
- To compile the life histories of criminals and try to trace these tendencies through them
- To supply relevant information to courts regarding the criminals
- To render assistance to criminals in getting employment
- Advices for solutions to problems
- To prepare them as a good citizens of the nation
- If no sign of improvement, try to put them on the right track by convincing and cautioning them.

Parole

It is a means of reforming criminals. The criminal is given over to the protection of the probation officer, without being punished, but a criminal is placed on parole, after he has served a short prison sentence, placed under the parole officer. He maintains contact with the criminal keeps an eye on him and tries to reform him.

III. Reformatory homes

When criminals commit a crime in ignorance and compelled by circumstances or where this criminal tendency is attributable to a mental or psychic defect will be kept in reformatory homes but the reform of a criminal who willfully violates moral laws, prone for punishment.

a. Juvenile reformatories, to reform criminals by means of educating them and to implement rehabilitative activities in order to prepare them as a responsible citizens. Before placing criminals in reformatory homes, the IQ levels are assessed based on IQ the activities will be planned. The lifetime imprisonment and short-term vacancy also placed in reformatory homes.
b. Adult reformatories, adults will receive education in military discipline, physical exercise, religion, the principles of citizenship etc. The JD are educated and efforts are made to turn them into good citizens by providing adequate care.

Prison

A model prison is set up, the inmates are provided with all the opportunities to develop their personalities and effort is made to make them able citizens.

In Varanasi district, India, dam across Chandra prabha, a model prison was setup. There were no police to look after them, facilities such as canteen, hospital, reading room, radio, library, cinema etc were provided. The welfare officers and teachers will educate the prisoners. They were paid wages, a part of which is retained to be given to them on release in order to enable them to start some business.

Psychoanalysis

Crimes are caused due to repressed complexes and tendencies of sex and jealousy causes desires and frustrated sexual passions. Thus, education and psychoanalytic treatment is needed for preventing crimes instead of punishment.

Crime is a mental or neural disease, which can be eliminated by searching out repressed unconscious complexes transporting them to the conscious level, finding their causes by effecting their sublimation through means acceptable to the society.

Difference between juvenile delinquency and crime

Crime	*Juvenile delinquency*
Age: above 20 years	Below 20 years
Activities: performing antisocial activities	Persistent law breakers with truant behaviour
Intention to gain something	Acts will not benefit them, sometimes even unaware of the objective of their actions
Does not find a suitable mode of manifesting his sense of humour	Commits a crime with the intention to enjoy and indulge a sense of humour
Preplanned and well organised basis the activities will be performed	Not planned

WHITE-COLLAR CRIME

It induces criminal behaviour in ordinary citizens and or which they are considered to be criminals by the dominant political group in a country. It is harmful to the well being of the society as a whole.

Definition

- 'It is a crime committed by a person of respectability and high social status in the course of his occupation'.
- 'Desire to gratify their economic wants'.
- 'The rewards for unethical behaviour afford many temptations, e.g : Build homes, merchandise, illegal operations and legal assistance to criminals'.

- 'Confusiòn in values with white-collar crime'
- 'Certain offences are condemned irrespective of the individual who commits them'.
- 'The illegal economic activities of the upper social class'.

WAR

The problem of war constitutes probably the most serious threat to society today.

Causes

- Clash of economic interests
- Psychological in nature—man is aggressive by nature
- Unbridled sovereignty of states
- Power politics
- Empire system, desire for power, glory, sense of modern economic life, insecurity in life
- Denial of freedom to certain nations
- Racial inequality
- Absence of even handed justice to all alike
- Non-existence of machinery for peaceful change

Effects of War

- Modern wars are physical conflicts between politically discrete
- It causes mental derangement in the armed services by creating strains on the minds of the soldiers
- Social institutions like family, school, church become subordinated to the state
- The traditional functions of institutions neglected
- War separates many husbands and wives, encourages hasty and often ill-considered marriages and prevents many parents from providing the parental supervision that they would otherwise give to their children
- A relaxation of sex morality occurs in a nation at war

- Loss of human dignity
- Reduces the productivity of nation
- Disrupts international economy, trade, breaks up the old system of trade relationships and brings about new forms of international economic disequilibria
- Upsets the international financial structure and results in a host of unpayable and trade discouraging international debts
- The aftermath of every war has been stagnation in international trade.

UNEMPLOYMENT

Definition

- 'Non-availability of work even though there is a desire to do it'.
- 'The able-bodied persons of working age, who are willing to work, are not able to find work at the current wage levels'.
- 'Unemployment is forced and involuntary separation from remunerative work on the part of the normal working force during normal working time, normal wages and under normal conditions'—*Fair Child*

Forms (Types)

Cyclical Unemployment

It results from trade cycles, profit, loss, fluctuations in the present level, e.g : Depression in trade, thousands of people are thrown out of work. It may be caused due to cyclic functions of the industry, e.g : The course of business shows alternating periods of booms and depressions.

Sudden Unemployment

Results from business, which engages workers periodically, e.g : Workers are turned out from time to time when the work in factories decreases.

Arising from Failure in Industry or Business

Many factories close down as they are unable to compete with others or varied reasons after a short period of existence and their workers are left without work.

Arising from Seasonal Business

People engaged in seasonal business work, are engaged in it are thrown out of work. Sudden fluctuation of activities in a particular period of the year. At one time activity is very brisk and the employer requires a large labour force to deal with the rest of work. At other times, the work is comparatively slack, labour force becomes unemployed, e.g : Crops in agriculture, labourers in building constructions.

Frictional Unemployment

It is caused by changes in industrial structure, which are constantly occurring. Modern businesses are essentially dynamic, throwing some workers out of employment for the time being. Demand is constantly shifting from one product to another leaving behind a trail of unemployment.

Technical Unemployment

The increase in technology means a displacement of human labour with advance in technology some manufacturing processes have become so perfect as to be virtually automatic. Some may be absorb the displaced labour in the production of new commodities, but it is a fact that advance technology reduces the demand for labourers.

Temporary Unemployment

When young people have completed their education and training they remain unemployed for a few days. Experienced persons will have some advantage in the competitive market.

Voluntary Unemployment

It results from the refusal of labour to accept a cut in the rate of real wages. But such unemployment cannot exist under full equilibrium conditions, when there is free competition.

Arising from Shortage of Capital, Equipment or Other Complementary Resources

This type of unemployment was found in under-developed countries. Production is carried on with insufficient amount of real capital per head of the population. Shortage of goods and services has insufficient employment opportunity resulting in a surplus labour force.

Involuntary Unemployment

Is not getting suitable compensation for their qualification and capabilities, become unemployed for a short period of time.

Subjective Unemployment

It is caused by physical or mental shortcomings of the individual.

Objective Unemployment

It is caused by factors beyond the control of individual and is related to objective circumstances, e.g: Seasonal unemployment, structural unemployment.

Causes

Personal Factors

- Defects in character
- Physical disability, deformity
- Mental and moral deficiency of the labourers
- Mental illness

- Accidents
- Defective education and training
- Throwing responsibility on wrong shoulders.

Age Factor

Young men after completion of their education and training at this age find difficulty in getting jobs because of their inexperience. Older people are more prone to accidents and are less adaptable. They will be candidates for pensions.

Vocational Unfitness

Too many young people have no understanding of their own abilities or interests and no particular task in mind when they get training. Willingness to do anything may seem to indicate a working desire on the part of the person seeking work. Employers, on the other hand may seek qualified and competent trained workers. More people trained in a particular profession than required. The demand is less than the supply and hence unemployment will result.

Illness / Physical Disabilities

Many workers are temporarily or permanently unemployed because of illness or other physical disabilities. Industrial accidents are often fatal and sometimes make the workers permanently disabled.

Technological Factor

Advances in technical skills and highly specialized division of labour, able-bodied and capable men are unable to secure jobs.

Economic Factor

Unemployment complex may be ascribed to dislocations in industries and to disorganisation of economic structure.

Excessive Increase in the Population

Increased pressure upon the land and an increase in the number of the unemployment.

Limited Land

The population is increasing while the land is limited.

Lack of Subsidiary Industries

The landless farmer or with less land or infertile land, remains unemployed.

Agriculture Depends Upon Rain

In India, agriculture is a gamble with the rain. If the rain arrives at the right time and are neither excessive nor scare, the harvest is good. But if the rain comes at the wrong time or insufficient quantity, they spell disaster for agriculture. In the absence of rain famines occur and thousands of people become unemployed.

Unscientific and Absolute Methods of Cultivation

In India the old unscientific method of farming is still being pursued, consequently, the farmer can not feed properly and many people what they produce from their farm is unable to meet the needs of the children, e.g: Could not able to provide proper education, or cannot engage them is suitable profession.

Subdivision of Land

The land is subdivided into small portions, fragmentation of land falls very low and sometimes the land becomes an uneconomic holding.

Main Reasons given for Unemployment Among the Educated were

A. Rightly or wrongly there is an impression among the public that investment in education by an individual should yield for him a return in terms of a remunerative job.

B. An educated person naturally looks for a job suited to his particular type of education. He has received with the result that there has been an abundance of supply in regard to certain occupations and professions and shortage in others, depending upon the development of education in the country.
C. The regional preferences shown by the educated which complicate the problem.
D. General disinclination among the educated to look for employment other than office jobs.

Disorganisation of Agriculture

Extreme unorganized and diversified land of agriculture leads to unemployment.

Evil effect of Unemployment

Unemployment has many bad consequences not only for the worker himself but also for the worker's family and the community at large. He suffers from personal disorganisation, his health is affected, his family and the community are also affected.

Unemployment and Personal Disorganisation

Unemployment, whether of a seasonal or permanent nature undermines the life organisation of a worker. The unemployed person faces a discouraging outlook.

Unsteady employment:

- Undermines the worker's physique
- Deadens the mind
- Weakens the ambition
- Moral value of the group are distorted or lose their significance

- Destroys his capacity for continuous sustained endeavor
- Induces a liking for idleness and self-indulgence
- Lacks self-respect and the sense of responsibility
- Prevents hope of family advancement
- Destroys a workman's feeling that he is taking good care of his family.

New Entrants

Young persons who have just finished their education and training have entered in the labour market with full of enthusiasm and vigour. When they cannot get employment they become disillusioned and cynics. Having no outlet for creative energy they become delinquents and commit robbery or bank hold-ups. The anti-social activities offer the only chance to the undisciplined youth. They become disappointed when they find no market for their services.

The plight of the experienced unemployed person, discouraged and depressed may become cynical, irritable and disagreeable in his home. The unemployed often unable to do steady work, unreliable, inefficient and 'good for nothing'. Moral values of the group are distorted or lose their significance. Savings exhausted and credit denied he might become a rebel. He may steal because his children need the basic meal for a day. Because of their inability to face economic insecurity and loss of status for themselves and their family, some may end in suicide. Full of bitterness, loss of self-respect as economic insecurity observed during old age. Migratory casual workers are most maladjusted men, being mobile they have no permanent community interest or family ties to act as a stabilizing force. Unemployment frustrates hopes and brings loss of status.

Unemployment and Low Health

Those who are unemployed have insufficient resources to maintain their own health or their family members' health.

For example: Limited diet, low consumption of essential food elements, and the inability to pay for ordinary medical care. Inability to meet the needs of dependents results in worries and anxiety, which further affects their health. The stress and strain of worry, the restlessness, lack of usual activity, the new obligations for wife and children,etc. will affect his health.

Unemployment and Family Disorganisation

In addition to the physical and mental deprivation and the havoc of unemployment wrecks on the personality of the breadwinner, as well his family. When the regular income fails, the families' fall back upon their own savings, however, low they may be. After the meager savings are exhausted the inevitable borrowing either in cash or in goods starts. Valuable articles are sold and ornaments are mortgaged.

Families suffer starvation by resorting to unbelievable economy in food. Bodies sapped through such undernourishment become prey for ill health. Thus, there is an almost universal failure among the unemployed and under paid labourers to take adequate care of their family members' health.

In desperation, the children may be induced to industry earlier, their education may be stopped and the wife seek employment knowing fully well that her husband can secure nothing. She, thus, assumes a double load (working area and household work). Her energy is soon exhausted and she becomes irritable with a nervous break down in the office. If she is not working, her anxiety concerning the husbands' unemployment may affect her mind, the children may become irritable and the whole family organisation may be threatened. The family may often break up to secure help from relatives or friends. The father can seldom cook or intelligently care the children.

Unemployment and Community Disorganisation

Owing to unemployment in the country its resources are not utilized to the full extent and production is less than the maximum, which affects the standard of living of the people. Owing to illness, crime and mental illness many social problems arise leading to social disorganisation. Those unemployed are not only a problem to themselves but are a charge on the society, like hospitalisation, emergency relief, increase in police strength, scene of family disputes, costs the public.

REMEDIAL MEASURES FOR UNEMPLOYMENT

Removal of Personal Disabilities

The personal disabilities of a person include illness, physical handicaps, old age, inexperience. The suggested measures are:

Provision of Socialised Health Services

To place the worker back to work in the shortest possible time so that he and his family may not suffer from lack of income. It is necessary to provide him medical facilities free of cost or at a nominal cost. Under ESI Act, many of the factory workers are provided medical facilities and cash benefits under the sickness insurance scheme. Adequate wages are provided with medical care, which is their first line of defense for the health of the workers. Large numbers of people are underfed owing to poor income and are susceptible to many diseases. Maximum wage act was passed in 1951. Rise in wages through increase in productivity and proper economic development reneeded.

Vocational Education and Educational Planning

Educators generally think that they are preparing young people for life and not for making a living. Many technical institutes are developed for training of young men. To remove unemployment among the educated, educational planning and emphasis on vocational training is necessary. There is no life without a good living and educators must recognise the importance of preparation for a life work as a part of educational process.

Remedial Measures for Unemployment Among Educated

- By advancing loans for establishing small-scale industries requiring capital amount
- Providing vocational training facilities
- Assist in procuring raw material and the disposal of the finished goods
- Expansion of education closely linked with future requirement has to be planned
- Discovering vocational aptitude and provide vocational counselling, development of cooperative sector, reorganize system of education, expansion of rural economy,
- Development of university employment bureau to remove the hardship felt by educated youth
- Start industrial estates which provide factory sites with facilities as transport, supply of electricity, water and gas.
- Apprenticeship training by employers
- Strengthening of cooperative organisation in the sphere of production and distribution, e.g : Manufacturing industries like hand tools, small tools, sports goods, and furniture. Feeder industries like forge shops, automobile shops, machinery parts, electroplating, galvanising.
- Orientation camps have to be organised to remove the disinclination on the part of the educated to undertake manual work to discover the vocational aptitude of the youth.
- The expansion of education and training facilities should be closely linked to the future requirements of the economy

- Small scale and medium industries will often provide growing opportunity for absorbing educated persons in gainful and productive work
- Expansion in agriculture, industries and transport will provide a large and increasing demand for persons with skill and vocational or technical training. Short period of training for specific jobs will be provided.
- Development of cooperatives for credit, marketing and farming, growth of processing industries, development of scientific agriculture and establishment of democratic institutions at the district, village level.

Rural programming, planning rural industries should be organised on cooperative basis as far as possible to provide financial, technical, marketing facilities easily, the development of such lines will keep the educated leadership in the rural areas.

Economic Development to Remove Poverty and Unemployment

To create employment opportunities in all economic sectors (agriculture and industry) through proper planning is essential. In rural areas, starting of major and minor irrigation works, land reclamation schemes. The revival and development of rural industries, old handicrafts, the extent of mixed farming. Undertaking of public work programmes in slack agricultural seasons may be planned.

In urban areas, expansion of large-scale industries and the starting of new ones, to save the existing small-scale industries and encourage starting of similar new industries.

The development of agriculture, industries, roads, major and minor irrigation works, building and construction activities will indirectly leads to development of territory sector, it means that there will be more demand for transport, storage, banking and other services. Additional employment in the non-agricultural sector has to be generated. Provision of more irrigation facilities would provide opportunities of work on full-time basis. Reclamation of land, expansion and development, schemes of plantations, horticulture are developed.

Development of Agriculture

The employment opportunities in the agriculture sector may be increased through:

- The construction of major and minor irrigation projects
- Land reclamation
- Expansion and development of plantation
- Intensive cultivation and horticulture
- Development of fisheries and forest.
- Development of industries like small—scale, large-scale, village and cottage industries including handicrafts.
- Building construction activities—houses for labourers and middle class people.
- Development of territory sector in the fields of education, health, social services and official by expansion of these services.

Removal of Seasonal Unemployment

The manufacturers can take up the production of some other commodities in the slack season. Special rural work programmes like irrigation, forestation, soil conservation, land reclamation, improvement of communication can be organised.

Unemployment Owing to Difficulties in the Migration of Labour and Change in Technology

- Location of projects in the public sectors
- Providing loans to local business and industrialists at relatively favourable terms
- Reserving certain percentage of contract in the public sector for persons belonging to those areas

- Adoption of other fiscal measures to induce inflow of private capital.

Remedies for Agriculture Unemployment

Improvement in the agricultural system.

- Prevent further sub-division of land into even smaller pieces
- Creation of economic holdings as well as increase in the output
- Intensive cultivation do not exploit the natural resources to the fullest extent of their potentiality
- Proper rotation of crops is followed
- Good seeds, tools, manure, animals has to be arranged for better production
- Proper arrangement of irrigation through minor and major projects to avoid dependence of cultivation upon the rains. Development of subsidiary industries like dairy farm, poultry, furniture making, weaving. Public construction like road building, drain digging.

PROSTITUTION

It is a burning social problem around the globe. Combinations of factors are enhancing the prostitution. It is a crime associated with sex.

Definition

- 'Promiscuous (indiscriminate) intercourse for hire whether in money or in kind'.
- 'The practice of habitual or intermittent sexual union, more or less promiscuous, for mercenary inducement with accompanying emotional indifference'—*Geoffrey*
- 'A prostitute is a person who agrees to have sexual intercourse with any person, who offers money for such an act'.

Constituents

- Illicit (illegal) and promiscuous sexual intercourse
- Mercenary basis whether in cash or in kind
- Lack of affection or personal interest.

Elements

- Barter (exchange)
- Promiscuity
- Emotional indifference
- Brings personal disorganisation and also it affects the life organisation of the family and the community at large.

Causes

- Poverty leads the women to prostitution
- Uneducated women who cannot earn their livelihood by any other means get into prostitution
- Premarital/extra marital relationships
- Biological cause—defective sex organs, sex urge in human beings
- Socio-economic factors
  - Poverty
  - Modern industrialisation
  - Rapid urbanisation
  - Lack of family and social control
  - Lack of moral teaching
  - More contacts between men and women during employment
  - Over-crowding
  - Commercialised recreation including cinemas and dancing hall
  - Alcoholism
  - Late marriage
  - High standard of living
  - Destitution
  - Bad working condition

- Corruption
- Immoral traffic in women and children
- Under-age employment of girls
- Lack of privacy
- Inability to get married
- Bad neighbourhood
- Illegitimate motherhood
- Neglected by husband

- Psychological causes
  - Mental deficiency
  - Impotency in male
  - Nymphomania
  - Sexually not satisfying with one partner
  - Ignorance
  - Desire for easy money, easy life
  - Low moral values
  - Vested interests
- Religious factor
  - Devadasi system
- Cultural: Polygamy and Polyandry
  - Chastity—unchastity
  - Pimps

Causes of Prostitution in Unmarried Person

- Unfulfillment of their sexual urges
- Social barrier to their satisfaction
- Double standards of morality
- Women are stigmatized for illicit intercourse
- Postponement of marriage due to economic necessity
- Sex stimulating literature
- Lack of social disapproval in men
- Indecent shows
- Lustful conversation
- Lack of moral teaching
- Curiosity for sex experience.

Among Married Persons

- Unsatisfactory marital relationship
- To escape from emotional tensions, which arised in their marriage and exists because of temperamental or cultural differences between couples
- Monotony of marital relationship.

Among Widowers

- Loneliness
- Fulfillment of sexual desire.

For Women

Economic causes
- Poverty
- Destitution
- No other visible means of support
- Immoral environment
- Early employment
- Under privileged economic groups
- Poor working environment
- Social values against unchastity
- A girl who had illicit relationship because of some reasons if often made to feel that she had nothing left to lose because she had already lost all. Social values with respect to chastity tend to make it difficult for such a girl to regain her social status and confirm to the accepted standards.

Temperamental Traits

- Young sex offenders with low IQ values
- Lack of temperamental make up traits
- Excessive restlessness
- Lack of affection
- Defiance of authority and irascibility (resistance).

Ignorance

- Exploiting girls from rural communities by offering employment
- Alcoholism
- Vested interests
- Highly profitable nature of business
- Deception
- Kidnapping
- Being forced into the profession.

Social Factors

- Restrictions on widow remarriage
- Devadasi system.

Among Males

- Forced bachelorhood
- Separation from families
- Widowers
- Unsatisfactory marital relationship
- Interested in variety means.

Type

The Overt Prostitute

Professional registered, unregistered prostitute who live in brothel houses. Act as entertainers, supplement to their legitimate earnings.

Clandestine Group

- Variety of women, who enter into sex relationships for mercenary (heir) considerations.
- Occasional prostitute: Alternate periods of reforms with period of active prostitution
- Incidental prostitute: Scanty legitimate income, by the role of sex favour increased income

- Married women resort to mercenary and adulterous practices serving a restricted clientele
- Concubine system under which the mistress or her guardians (if she is a young girl) enters into agreement with a male member for a minimum stipulated period.

Evil Effects of Prostitution

Personal Disorganisation

Chastity and faithfulness have been held up as the primary virtues for women, while men have been overlooked in the sexual disorder. Prostitution is a necessary counterpart to the socially sanctioned license for men. So long as this double standard remains this evil is bound to remain. Women suffer great personal deterioration than men due to the existing double standard.

Two stages of maladjustment as an aftermath of unsocial sex activities:

1. The dual person may not suffer a complete moral collapse and personal efficiency is generally by the mental conflict and physical strain on their marginal existence.
2. The demoralised person: Results in complete personal demoralisation. Repeated violations of the code are almost certain to bring about irremediable loss of status. Eventually the individual man or woman may lose all contact with the respectable elements of the community and may resign him or herself to a life on the fringe of society. This complete change in basic attitudes towards society and social values has taken place, which results in complete demoralisation.

Family Disorganisation

Greatest stigma is attached to the prostitute. It wrecks personality and affects marital relationships. It affects family life by transmitting disease like STD/VD thus brings social disorganisation. Prostitution brings not only personal disorganisation of the persons concerned, but also affects the life organisation of the family and the community at large. The married men may get some venereal disease from the prostitute, which may affect his wife and children. Similarly, a married woman who resorts to clandestine prostitution may get the disease from her other client.

Prostitution does not exact its full price in social ostracism (excluding out from the group), shame and stigma. Through promiscuous sex relationship venereal disease have acquired to the half of the victim, the other half are innocent victims like wives and children of men who acquired the disease in premarital or extra-marital contacts. Sex relations of the wife or husband may also be the cause of friction in the family and divorce may be the ultimate result.

Community Disorganisation

Prostitution also brings widespread disorganisation of the community in which it operates. It has two aspects:

Commercial Aspect

Commercial exploitation becomes institutionalized, deeply rooted in the deteriorated local community of the larger city. This means due to its relatively permanent position in the city, it becomes still more accessible to the public and results more profitable. It in turn strengthens the hands of the persons engaged in the business. It includes brothels, call flats, disorderly hotels, restaurants and tenements, which are devoted exclusively to prostitution. Alcoholism, gambling are added as an additional attraction but solely for the purpose of increase in customers for the primary business.

Health Point of View

Venereal diseases, e.g: Syphilis, gonorrhea, AIDS are of vital concern. They are devastating diseases but also they are factors in other social problems like crimes, insanity.

Legislation and Prostitution

The East India Company made certain regulations dealing with sexual offences. Later on in Indian penal code provisions were made

- To protect the modesty
- To protect women against forced illicit sexual intercourse
- Imprisonment upto one year or fine or both for insulting the modesty of any woman by any word, sound, gesture or exhibition of any object or intruding on her privacy
- Buying and selling minor girls for immoral purposes and imparting in sex offence
- Imprisonment or fine or both for 10 years for kidnapping, abducting any person, forced to marry or illicit contact
- 10 years of imprisonment for selling, letting for hire, buying, possession of girl under 18 years or age for any unlawful or immoral purpose, rape.

Social Control of Prostitution

- Social rejection of the profession by acquainting young people with the dangers of venereal diseases.
- Literature has to prepare to create awareness of public about the consequences of prostitution.
- Establishment of VD/STD clinics.
- Segregation of diseased patients—handle them in the same way any other person suffering from common diseases.
- Poverty should be alleviated and women who had gone astray are treated with sympathy and good educations are provided.
- State should provide alternate jobs to make them live with honour and dignity in society.

Prevention of Prostitution

Prevention of Prostitution (Act 1923)

The sex offences under this Act are:

- Living on the earnings of prostitution of another
- Soliciting in a public place

- Procuring, keeping or managing a brothel
  - UP Naik Girls Protection Act 1929
  - The Bombay Devadasi Protection Act 1934
  - Prevention of Dedication Act 1934
  - Madras Devadasi Act 1947

Any Act intended to dedicate a woman as a Devadasi with or without her consent was made illegal.

- Suppression of Immoral Traffic Act 1956

Detention of girls in protective homes established by private social welfare agencies.

Sex Education

Dangers of venereal diseases, gravity of the consequences of the evils of prostitution both to the individual and to the society as a whole. Value of self-control (at homes and at schools). Decent family life.

Employment Opportunities

For women who are forced to prostitution under economic stress.

Removal of Certain Social Customs

Widow remarriage, dowry system avoidance, double standards to be discouraged.

Publicity and Propaganda

Public should be enlightened about the law and to report any nuisance in their surrounding areas. Discouraging the sex stimulating literature. Spread of information about the hazards of prostitution and laws.

Social Aspects of Sexually Transmitted Diseases

- Social stigma associated with STD will make the individual not to reveal to others including to family members

- Like to suffer with the problem rather than obtaining health services
- The society will not permit the diseased individual to lead comfortable societal life
- The members of the society will prohibit the diseased individual from taking part in any social activities
- The off-springs of the affected individual will also suffer from the stigma.

POVERTY

Definition

- 'A condition in which a person either because of inadequate income or unwise expenditures, does not maintain a scale of living high enough to provide for his mental and physical efficiency and to enable him and his natural dependents to function usually according to the standards of a society of which he is a member'—*John L Gillin and Gillin*
- Poverty exists when one is not able to get sufficient food and other necessities of life.
- 'Poverty is the insufficient supply of those things, which are requisite for an individual to maintain himself and those dependent upon him in health and vigour'—*Goddard JG*
- 'A man is called poor when he is unable to gather the means to keep himself and his family in health'.
- 'Poverty is a relative concept, its increase or decrease can be ascertained by the more or less proportion of the necessary things of life for the individual and his family'.
- 'Man is considered as rich or poor according to the degree in which he can afford to enjoy the necessaries, the conveniences and the amusements of life'—*Adam Smith*

Poverty and unemployment are the two major social problems causing sickness, personal, family and community disorganisation. Another term used parallel to poverty is dependency, the condition of life in which one depends for his subsistence either in whole or in part upon some other agencies than his natural supporters. Poverty and richness are relative terms.

Poverty line: It is determined by the customs and mode of living. It is relative to the scale of living and conditions of others in a given group culture, or status. Further, the scale of living may be different in different social groups in the same culture and each group tends to formulate a standard of living, which is considered necessary for a decent living. The actual scale of living compared with the standard of living measures the extent of poverty.

Types

1. *Absolute poverty:* Individual is not able to maintain a minimum decent standard of living to maintain himself and his family.
2. *Relative poverty:* A person may be relatively poor among the persons of his own group who are relatively rich.

Measurement of Poverty

Measuring richness or poverty of a country is the availability of goods and services for consumption in a particular year. This is known as, National income or Dividend of a country. To measure national income expert economists are needed. It has some utility in measuring the standard of living of any country. Income is the result of productive activity. Payment of compensation received by a factor of production for its productive use. An aggregate of all the income of the people in a community or country earns is called **National income.** It is the total annual value of all goods and services produced by a country measured in terms of money.

Net National Product: It is the aggregate of economic activity during a specified period together with the net income from abroad.

Economic Welfare: The amount of national income accrued in a particular period.

Gross National Product: The value of output or the sum of gross income shares. The market value of the output of goods and services produced by nation's economy during a stated period of time is equal to personal consumption plus gross private investment plus government purchases of goods and services.

GNP is also considered as the sum of the shares of gross nation income accruing to the different members of the community. From GNP if we subtract the value of capital goods produced we get Net National Product.

NNP = GNP–Depreciation

Per Capita Income

It refers to the average income per head in a country. Divide the national income by the population. As population increases the national income increases substantially but the per capita income does not increase. High population growth of India is reflected by the low per capita income of the country.

Causes of Poverty

According to Gillin and Gillin

1. Incapacity of the individual
   - Hereditary weakness of an individual
   - Depressing aptitudes and attitudes towards work as a result of early conditioning
   - Physical handicaps because of accident or disease
2. Adverse physical environment
   - Poor natural resources
   - Adverse climate and weather
   - Insects, pests
   - Natural disasters
3. Economic factors
   - Shortage of capital

- Uneven distribution of wealth
- Business depression
- Technological changes which may replace labour

4. Defects in social organisation
   - Rapid technological changes (when it is difficult to make economic and social arrangement to cope with new situations
   - Educational shortcomings
   - Inadequate health machinery for the protection of new occupational diseases
   - Bad housing
   - Employment of husband and wife outside home leaving little time for socialisation of children and difficulties of youth to find employment because of inexperience
5. War: Most active and strong are skilled some are disabled, many women become widowed, inflation affects standard of living
6. Personal factors.

Physical Weakness, Sickness (Hereditary or accidental)

'Poverty and sickness form a vicious partnership each helping the other to add to the miseries of the most unfortunate of mankind'—*Hunter*

Due to sickness, a man is unable to work and his income decreases, a major portion of his income is also spent on the cure of the disease. Thus sickness increases poverty; poverty also increases sickness since hard labour in the absence of sufficient nutrition increases many diseases among the labourers.

Mental Diseases

With mental disease a person becomes incapable of doing anything. This decreases his income and increases poverty. On the other hand, poverty also increases mental disease since it is difficult to maintain the balance of the mind in a state of poverty.

'Poverty alone directly produces insanity among the indigent poor'.

Accidents

They make the person entirely incapable of work or it reduces his capacity for it, e.g : If the earning member of a family is involved in some serious accident the whole family becomes poor.

Illiteracy

It increases poverty since the capacity to earn of a illiterate person is very low, on the other hand, many persons are compelled to remain illiterate because of poverty. Thus poverty and illiteracy together from a vicious circle to increase the troubles of the poor people.

Idleness

Many persons, inspite of sufficient opportunity to work do not work because of idleness and hence remain poor.

Extravagance

An extravagance person can waste any amount of money in no time. In fact the cause of poverty is not a lower income but excess of expenditure over income. In India, extravagance on the festivals and marriages can be easily observed every where, with the result, that sufficient money is not available for education, sanitation, light, medicine, and other necessities of life.

Demoralisation

Demoralisation or the lowering of character and morale leads to personal disorganisation and finally to poverty, e.g:

Alcoholism, prostitution, gambling, evil habits will affect even the persons of sufficiently high economic status, reduces the capacity and cause escapism thus leading to poverty.

Large Family

Too many children to bring up, the standard of living is definitely lowered and the leads to poor quality of life.

Geographical Causes

Unfavourable Climate and Weather

Favourable climate and weather is very much necessary for work as well as for production of agriculture and industries. Hence in the extremely cold climates the amount of work and production is considerably lowered thus leading to poverty.

Absence of Natural Resources

Natural resources like fertile land, sufficient water, minerals and other natural products. In deserts, high mountains and extremely cold countries remain poor.

Natural Calamity

Absence of timely rains, excessive or deficient rains in India will lead to poverty.

Economic Causes

- *Agricultural:* Absence of sufficient manure, absence of improved tools and machines, absences of means of irrigation and cattle of highbred, sufficient means to protect the fields from pests and animals.
- *Unequal distribution:* Even the production is sufficient, unequal distribution of goods and things results in poverty.
- *Economic depression:* Decrease in trade and commerce, lock out of mills and factories, unemployment of millions of labourers and small traders, low standard of living.

- *Unproductive hoarding:* If a major portion of the wealth of the country is hoarded in unproductive forms, the economic development of the country is seriously handicapped.
- *Unwise economic policy:* Sometimes in spite of the presence of sufficient resources and manpower in a country, the people remain poor because of the unwise economic policy of the government.

Social Factors

- *Joint family system:* Discourages young persons to go out and strive for new ventures due to minimum security provided by the family, people become lethargic and develops the stay-at-home-habit.
- *Caste system:* Is a hindrance to the development of new industries and it discouraged some persons to leave their traditional occupation lest they may be out-casted.
- *Religious belief:* Karma theory confined to ignorant and illiterate people. (some believed as we could not change our fate, there was no use of much effort and the results were preordained).

  Concept of *maya*, some may feel this world was illusionary and there was no use in acquiring much wealth.
- *Faulty educational system:* Due to faulty educational system, the youths' were not given proper guidance/counselling in choosing their profession, leads to unemployment, which generates poverty.
- *Absence of training in home science:* Mismanagement of household is a serious cause of poverty everywhere. It is due to lack of sufficient training to woman in home science, without such training many middle class families remain poor.
- *Evil customs and traditions:* Dowry system: It compels many families to remain poor inspite of all the efforts of their men folk to earn.
- *Insufficient provision of medical aid:* Causes delayed cure, prolonged illness, permanent displacement, untimely death.

- *War:* It devastates prospering lands in rich countries, with heavy loss of poverty and manpower. It upsets the balance of society by disrupting moral standard and socio-economic system. Gives a serious blow to trade and commerce both national and international. Epidemics spreads, adds to the misery of the people.

Political Factor

Due to political subordination of the country, the British Government exploited the situation for their interest. The government did not render any assistance to the cultivation to use new techniques of agriculture.

Biological Factor

Over population, occurrences of famine decreased, decrease in death rate and increase in birth rate.

Poverty and Disorganisation

Low income of a family is unstable to meet the total needs of its members, e.g: Food for children, poor clothing, illness, and such people become discouraged and cannot perform their functions properly.

Under the above conditions, the community cannot have healthy children, educated children, socialised men. Children are forced to work at an early age to supplement the family income. Women are compelled to work, even when there is nobody to look after the children at home.

Remedial Measures for Poverty

Agricultural development

1. Better farming facilities
2. Redistribution of land
3. Development of animal husbandry, poultry
4. Establishment of small cottage industries

Supporting occupations has to be improved like handicrafts, weaving, and pottery.

Educate the public to broaden the total outlook of the people thereby standard of living will be enhanced. Intensified family welfare programmes have to be organised at remote corners of the country to reduce the problems of over population. Minimum wages has to be fixed for the agriculture labourers. Improve marketing facilities. Redistribution of land. Electrification facilities in rural areas have to be increased for irrigation and house lighting. Implementation of social security schemes, like old age pension, sickness benefit or assistance schemes.

Anti-poverty Programmes

The fifth five-year plan (1974–79) accepted 'Removal of poverty' as its main goal. In seventh five-year plan poverty alleviation programmes have to be viewed in the wider perspective of socio-economic transformation taking place in the country.

Aims

- Overall economic growth in terms of generating productive assets and skills as well as income for the poor
- Needed resources and the capabilities for running programmes
- Demand for goods and services produced by the poorer household enterprises significantly in response to the overall increase in incomes in the country so that the visibility of household enterprises depends critically on the sustained increase in national income
- To ensure the pattern of overall economic growth itself to generate adequate income for poorer sections through its greater impact on employment generation and on the development of the less developed regions

- Social transformation involving structural changes, educational development, growth in awareness and change in outlook, motivation and attitudes, providing health for the people.

The poverty alleviation programmes launched by Indian government are:

1. Integrated Rural development programme (IRDP)—1978-79
2. Training of rural youth for self-employment (TRYSEM)—1979
3. Development of women and children in rural areas (DWACRA)—1979
4. National rural employment programme (NREP)
5. Rural landless employment guarantee programme (RLEGP)
6. Jawahar Rozgar Yojana
7. Drought prone areas programme—1973

Socio-economic Programmes (1958)

To provide work and wages to the economically backward, physically handicapped and socially maladjusted families. It provides financial assistance to voluntary bodies that want to organise income-generating activities. Voluntary bodies will give grants and loans up to Rs. 20,000/- to 3 lakhs for setting up production units of small industries, dairies, animal husbandry projects, self-employment units like vegetable vending, supply of sewing machines, assistance to handlooms, etc.

Drought Prone Area Programme (DPAP 1972–73)

The midterm appraisal of the fourth plan, the rural works programme was re-designated as the 'Drought Prone Area Programme'. In this orientation is towards area development. Criteria to select the areas is: Low extent of irrigated areas, low level of rainfall, erratic distribution of rainfall, and high periodicity of drought, etc. it is entrusted to the DRDA.

Objectives of DPAP are:
- Reducing the severity of the impact of drought
- Stabilizing the income of the people particularly the weaker sections of society
- Restoration of ecological balance.

Training of Rural Youth for Self-employment (TRYSEM 15th Aug, 1979)

To equip the rural youth in 18–35 years of age group, who are below the poverty line with necessary skills and technology to enable them to seek self employment.

Objective

Wage employment. Special provisions in the scheme are:
- 50% of the trained youths should be from scheduled castes and scheduled tribe
- 40% of youth trained should be women
- In case of widows, 5 years upper age limit will be relaxed, 3% for physically handicapped
- Training will be conducted in: Polytechnics, Krishi Vigyan Kendras, Nehru Yuvak Kendras, Khadi and Village industries boards, State institute of rural development, Extension training centre,
- Duration of training is flexible
- Every TRYSEM trainee is potential IRDP beneficiary
- Trainees will receive stipends during their training
- Tool kits at free of cost is supplied
- Payment is given for purchase of raw materials
- Honorarium is paid to training personnel for augmenting training infrastructure, financial assistance will be given.

Integrated Rural Development Programme (1980, Oct 2nd)

This programme is intended to the all round development of the entire rural population through development of all sectors of rural society. A strategy designed to liberate the rural poor from the age-old bondage of degraded life and to awaken and activate the entire rural population in the process of achieving and sharing higher levels of production. Rural development involves several categories of integration between different categories or sectors like rural economy, agriculture, off-farm activities, industries, etc. with forward and backward linkages, economic and social development, total area and target group approach, credit with technical services, human resource development with human resource needs by intense education and training programmes with anticipated income generating schemes with the minimum needs programmes of education, rural health, water supply, nutrition, etc.

IRDP was launched in all the blocks of the country linked self-employment programme for poverty alleviations as a centrally sponsored scheme funded on 50:50 basis by the centre and state. Assistance will be given in the form of subsidiary and credit from banks for households living below the poverty line in order to enable them to acquire assets or skill for taking self employment venture. Fourty percent of the total assistance is reserved for the women. IRDP is being implemented by the district rural development agency (DRDA).

Objective

To eradicate poverty from rural areas by providing income generating assets. The ministry of rural development, Government of India is responsible for the release of central share of funds, policy formulation, overall guidance, monitoring and evaluation of the programme.

Employment Guarantee Scheme (EGS 1981)

To generate employment among villagers and create assets in the rural areas. Villages are selected from dry and drought prone areas where the agriculture labourers are without any job due to failure in rainfall.

Development of Women and Children in Rural Areas (DWCRA 1982–83)

It is a sub-scheme of IRDP. As a pilot basis in 1982 it has started in 50 districts, later in 1994–95 extended to all districts of the country.

Aims

- To improve the living conditions, socio and economic status of women and children
- Provision of opportunities for self-employment and access to basic social services
- To provide income generating skills and activities for poor women
- To encourage the habit of thrift and credit among women to make them self-reliant
- Enhances the welfare and quality of life of family and community
- To improve the access of rural women to health, education, safe drinking water, sanitation and nutrition
- To create employment opportunities for rural women, who are below poverty line
- To organise the beneficiaries according to group activities
- To enhance production among rural poor
- To establish crèche, balwadies, etc. facilities for children of working women.

DWACRA group consists of 10-15 women to take up economic activities suited to their skills, aptitude and local conditions. A revolving fund of Rs. 25,000/- per group is given to meet their working capital requirements. It creates more awareness among communities to enable them to demand social services provided by the state and also share responsibilities in the management and in implementation of services at community level.

Employment and Income Generating Training Cum Employment Cum Production Units (1982–83)

Trains the people in trades, electronics, printing, binding, watch manufacturing, handlooms, computer programming etc., for the weaker section of the society and provide them employment on a sustained basis. It is carried out through public sector undertaking/corporations/voluntary organisations. Norwegian agency for International development will assist the activities like stipend for trainees Rs 250/- per month, cost of equipment, salary of instructors, rent of the building.

Self Employment to Educated Unemployment Youth (SEEUY 1983–84)

Objective

- To provide opportunities of employment and income through creating productive assets to educated unemployed youth
- To encourage educated unemployed youth to undertake self-employment ventures in industry, service, business by providing package of financial assistance.

Target Group

- Youth who studies matriculation and above
- 18–35 years of age
- Family annual income should not be more than Rs 15,000
- Women and technically trained persons are given due consideration.

Self Employment Programme for Urban Poor (SEPUP 1986)

In consultation with the Reserve Bank of India this scheme was formulated.

Aims

To provide self-employment to the urban poor, living in metropolitan/urban/semi-urban centres covering 10,000 people. Assistance will be given in the form of bank credit and subsidiaries for families below the subsistence level. It promotes activities like bookbinding, shoe/cycle/stove/pressure cooker repairing, paper/polythene bag vendors, new paper shops, tailoring, ready-made garment shops. Composite loan of Rs 5000/- is sanctioned.

Support to Training Cum Employment Programmes for Women (STEP 1986)

To improve and strengthen the component of women in the sectors of agriculture, animal husbandry, dairying, fisheries, handlooms, handicrafts, Khadi, village industries and sericulture.

Women will be given special training on health, literacy. Training will be given in new technical skills, management and basic accounting. Ninety percent of assistance will be given by the implementing agency for the project.

Jawahar Rozgar Yojana (JRY 1989)

- Generates additional employment for the unemployed and under employed men and women in the rural areas
- Strengthens rural economic infrastructure by sustaining employment
- Creates community and social assets for their direct and continuing benefits
- For positive impact on wage levels
- Promotes quality of life among rural population.

Features

- Expenditure is shared by centre and state in 80 : 20 ratio

- Preference in employment to SC, ST and freed bonded labourers and women (30%)
- 60% of the resources have to be spent on wage component
- 2 kgs of food grains/day; 50 paise/kg will be given to the workers in revamped blocks of the nation
- Work preferably will be taken up during the lean agriculture season and continued in busy agricultural period also
- DRDA/Zilla Parishad may spend maximum of Rs 50,000/- on training of officials involved in implementation of JRY at district/block/village panchayat level.

Employment Assurance Scheme (EAS 1993)

- To provide assured gainful employment during the lean agriculture seasons of 100 days of unskilled manual work to the rural poor, who are in need of employment and seeking it
- To create economic infrastructure and community assets for sustained employment and development
- Beneficiaries are 18–60 years of age, a maximum of 2 adults per family are provided employment under the scheme.

Swarnjayanti Gram Swarozgar Yojana (SGSY April, 1999)

Holistic programme covering all aspects of self-employment, e.g: Organisation of the poor women into self-help groups, training credit, technology, infrastructure, and marketing. Funded by centre and state with a ratio of 75:25.

Objective

- To bring every assisted family above the poverty line within 3 years through provision of micro-enterprise
- The beneficiaries are known as, 'swarozgaris'.

Features

- To establish a large number of micro enterprises in the rural areas

- To bring every assisted family above the poverty line in 3 years
- To focus on group approach
- To promote multiple credit on skill development through well designed training courses
- Focused on vulnerable groups among the poor.

Self help Groups (SHGS)

'All for all' is the basic concept. Mainly concerned with poor (weaker sections concerning to women) and it is for the people, by the people and of the people. It is working under micro level, and generates self-confidence, self-security, self-reliance and social defence. It encourages the women volunteers to organise themselves in a group for eradication of poverty of its members. Every month each member of the group should save a minimum of Rs. 10 to 15/- or more till six months and thus become eligible to apply for a loan to start income generating activities like dairy farming, agriculture, sericulture, poultry, goat and sheep rearing.

Objectives

- To inculcate the habit of saving and banking among rural women
- To improve moral thrust and confidence between bankers and rural women
- To develop team spirit, active participation of group members in welfare activities.

Principles

- Social homogeneity
- Social support
- Internality
- Experimental learning
- Social movement

- Self determination
- Active participation.

Advantages

- Total group members involvement is organisation of activities
- Possible for close monitoring of the activities
- Positive social processes will be activated
- Access to and efficient use of common pool resources
- Activation of democratic process where group interaction, reciprocity and decision-making process will be maintained
- Regulated by mutually accepted group rules.

Development of Women and Children in Urban Areas (DWCUA)

- It provides revolving fund of Rs 25,000/- to the group (10–15 women) belonging to poverty group for undertaking economic group activities and ancillary services, e.g: Nutrition, health, childcare, family welfare, immunisation, literacy, adult education facilities
- Establishes crèche, balwadies, etc. facilities for working women
- Fosters a collective approach to their problems
- Enhances their power and to resist exploitation
- Generates income for the urban poor by inculcating productive activities.

Salient Features

- Group approach
- Participatory approach
- Revolving fund
- Thrift and credit
- No target driven
- Fosters income generating activities

- Training and awareness.

Grants in Aid for Assistance

To provide financial assistance for building construction, equipment, furniture, postage, stationary, telephone, etc.

BEGGARY

Beggary is a form of personal disorganisation as it indicates the failure of the individual to adjust himself with his social milieu. It is a symptom of social disorganisation as the beggar in the street at once reminds us of the ill-organised society, which is not able to adjust him properly.

Definition

- 'A beggar is one who asks for alms or charity or performs such actions, which derive sympathy from others and who give something in return'
- 'A person without means of subsistence and wandering about or found in public places or allowing himself to be used as an exhibit for the purpose of begging'.

Causes

Beggary is a result of multiple factors and several situations favour the institution of beggary, e.g: Sickness or disease, physical inability, mental derangement, old age all these comes under biological cause, personal or social maladjustment, poverty, unemployment, disruption of joint family, family disorganisation.

Family is an integral part of our social relationship, which influences our patterns of behaviour and activities. Any disturbance in our home condition especially in the case of a poor one leads to broken family, which in return gives to beggary. The other causes are:

- Death of parent or husband or bread winner

- Step-parental treatment
- Maltreatment
- Desertion by husband
- No support for female and children
- Community disorganisation
- Social customs like sain, bhatt, tribes like Nats and Beriyas
- Religious causes like *Sadhu* or *fakir*
- Indiscriminate alms giving by the public
- Social customs, which forces the individual to give something to the beggars, orphans.

Types

1. *Able-bodied adult beggar:* Who beg either because they are unemployed or under employed or have no other sources to fall back upon or they do not prefer to work. They encourage honest workers to take up beggary.
2. *Able-bodied child beggar:* When parents are unable to support the children, they encourage the child for begging. Family disorganisation like death of parents, maltreatment, neglects by parents, etc. will leads the child to leave the home and resorts its own end.
3. *Hereditary beggar:* Nats, Jugglers, Bajiars, Sains, Bhats, Kanjars. They do not attach any social stigma to this profession and take it from their very childhood. To some of them, their children are an asset who can excite more pity in human heart and can earn more and support their parents.
4. *Sick or diseased beggar:* Who suffers from chronic diseases like leprosy, sexually transmitted diseases, tuberculosis, skin infections.
5. *Infirm or old:* Like Faqirs, Sadhus, Guardians of temple, mosque.

Techniques Employed

Ordinary Technique

- Appeal to human sentiments
- Arouse sympathy on one hand
- Adjust himself to varying situations
- Desire to make oneself comfortable in this life
- Blessings that the beggar showers on the giver of alms has direct reference to fulfillment of their desire predicting the future in positive means.

Techniques to Attract Attention

- Intonation
- Facial expressions
- General bodily postures
- Under go alteration as they do for people in grief and agony
- Use of stereo types appeals to emotion
- Impress upon the mind of his patrons.

Technique Employed by Religious Mendicants

- Organising some religious feast
- Removing natural calamity or disease or to bring rains
- Making pilgrims to all the religious centres
- Giving blessings to people and an assurance of a happy life
- Constructing a temple or mosque.

Use of Coercive Methods

- Beggar may force a man by turning himself as a nuisance to him by holding or touching the feet
- By coming nearer to people
- By showing wounds or abnormalities.

Use of Tricks

- Snake charmers

- Cow charmers
- Palmists.

Remedial Measures

Special homes for the insane and disabled, provision of workhouses, child-care institute has to be developed. Provision of family welfare services for the needy population. Rehabilitation homes, comprehensive social security measures, licensing of religious mendicants, economic resources and discouraging the beggary aspect.

NEGLECT OF ELDERS

In Indian society, elderly people are facing problems at some levels. The recognition of elderly problems is an important aspect of behaviour that needs attention, it directs the outcome of the changes age pyramid, value system and withdrawal of support from the family. It will have a profound effect on the moral fibre of the society.

Abuse of elders in the social institutions i.e., family is emerging as a burning issue. As aging population becomes more and more pronounced, concern for the quality of life and well being of elder people is also increasing parallel to this concern.

In traditional period in our Indian society elderly people are treated with a position, like higher social status, respect, privilege and power. They are able to do productive work for a longer period with much care from the family members. In the fast changing Indian scenario, the position of respect of the aged in society is inversely proportional to 'social progress' or 'development' of the human society, the resultant burden causes elderly abuse. It is less common where family ties are very strong.

Definition

- The infliction of physical, emotional or psychological harm on an older adult (usually over 65 years)

- Level of elderly abuse (According to Bennett, Baring Stoke, Kingston and Penhale 1997).

Macro Abuse

Issues at the societal level, e.g: Lack of access to health care, poor social security and institutional abuse.

Mezzo Abuse

The injustice heaped on older people at the community level, e.g: Ageism, anti-social activities against older people and marginalising them.

Micro Abuse

It deals with the conflicts and interactions between two people, i.e. an adult family member or a caregiver in an institution and older person.

Dimensions of Elderly Abuse

Wolf and Pillemer (1989) and the National elder abuse incidence survey (US 1998) stated

- Physical abuse, e.g: Slapping or shoving, severe beating, restraining
- Emotional or psychological abuse, e.g: Name calling, verbal assault, silent treatment like insulting and threatening
- Sexual abuse, e.g: Sexual exhibition to rape
- Financial or material exploitation, e.g: Misuse of an elder's funds
- Failure/neglect of elders to provide appropriate assistance by caregivers. It may be unnoticed of caregivers that they are failing to meet the needs or with intention alone harming the elders
- Unsatisfactory living environment including hazardous living condition
- Violation of rights, e.g: Reduction of personal freedom or autonomy, involuntary commitment, guardianship, etc.

Causes

Socio-cultural Factors

- Maltreatment of the elderly in the family context
- Degeneration of the joint family system
- Dislocation of cultural and familial bonds
- Failure on the part of the sons to look after the aged
- Lack of support for family members
- Intergenerational transmission of violence—growing up in an abusive home as an antecedent to violence.

Psychopathology

- Personality problem
- Mental illness like psychosis
- Alcoholism
- Unable to control aggression, older family members
- Senile dementia
- Feeling of burden.

Dependency Related to Social Change

1. Dependency of the victim on the perpetrator of abuse usually on adult child
2. Dependency of the perpetrator on the target of abuse for housing and financial assistance

   Dependency creates an imbalance in exchange processes increases the risk of elder maltreatment.

- Retirement
- Familial stress—individual needs of some family members frequently come into conflict with the needs of other family members leading to stress and instability
- Deprived of active participation and decision making in both occupational and family settings
- The vulnerability of older women to violence, advanced age, widowed, roleless, functionally impaired and living with their children

- Urban set-up is more favourable to develop urban psychosis
- The physical and mental dependency of the elderly in performing daily activities of living
- Deprivation of dignity, responsibility and a feeling of importance
- Dysfunctional parent-child relationships
- Cerebral arteriosclerosis
- Career stress
- Financial vulnerability, reduced income
- Issues related to one's residence
- Irresponsible children
- Pathology of the abuse
- Environmental stress
- Social isolation, invalidism.

Characteristics of the Abused

- Women of 65 years or more
- Cognitive impairment
- Total mood disturbance
- Low level of social support
- Inadequate in income level
- Socially, psychologically and economically dependent on others
- Intolerance of change, heightened irritability, suspiciousness
- Impoverished
- Feeling of delusion, hallucinations
- Spousal abuse
- Depression or agitation
- Elders who are neglected, are a source of extreme stress to the caregivers (e.g: Frail, disabled, dependent)
- Severe mental clouding.

Strategies/Nursing Interventions to overcome the Problems of Elderly Abuse

- Family ties has to be strengthened as major care provider in the society is family social network

- Promote social services and social support to reduce stress in family with dependent elders
- IEC programs has to be conducted to create awareness both elderly and the public about elder abuse and legal right of elderly people
- Involving elders in social programs to prevent social isolation
- Promote availability of facilities to long-term carers in social institutions
- Forms and promote self help group activities
- Mobilize voluntary organisations to meet the needs of elderly to get emotional, social support and self-efficacy
- Provide long-term care and facilities for elders
- Emphasis empowerment and independence of elderly women
- Ensure that elders have sufficient assets and income to manage through one's life
- Give priority to the research on elderly abuse
- Early_identification of elder abuse at social institution level
- Arrange mass media programs to sensitize elderly towards protection from abuse
- Enhance the empowerment of professionals in knowledge and skills who are rendering care to the elders
- Encourage counselling and treatment to cope with personal and family problems that contribute to abuse
- Mobilize Government and Non-Government organisations to strengthen the ongoing welfare services to the elderly in order to maintain their interest
- Ensure better quality of life to elders
- Encourage the primary caregivers, i.e. family members to provide warmth and support to the elders
- Provision for economic security by means of old age allowance, pension, accident benefits, free medical aid, part-time jobs like counselors, guides
- For effective functioning of the family, modify their social environment, where their mental capacities will be utilised

- Flexibility approach in meeting the needs of the client
- Provide conducive environment to live peaceful life up to their end.

ALCOHOLISM

Introduction

Alcoholism is not only determental to the health and welfare of the individual, family, community and society at large. The word 'alcoholism' was first coined by 'magnus huss'. It was derived from Arabic word, 'alkuhl' means 'essence'.

Definition

- The use of alcoholic beverages to the point of causing damage to the individual, society or both.
- 'To designate heavy drinkers of all kinds'—*Alphonse Jacob*
- 'It is a chronic disease manifested by repeated drinking that produces injuring to the drinker's health or to his social or economic functioning'—*S Nambi*

Properties of Alcohol

Alcohol is a clear liquid with a strong burning taste. Rapid absorption of the alcohol is more into the blood stream rather than its elimination. Slow absorption takes place when food is there in the stomach. Elimination of alcohol is through urine and by exhalation.

A concentration of:

- 80–100 mg of alcohol/100 ml blood is intoxication
- 200–250 mg of alcohol/100 ml of blood is loss of consciousness
- 500 mg of alcohol/100 ml of blood is fatal.

All the symptoms can change according to the tolerance.

Process of Alcoholism

Alcoholism is the excessive consumption of alcohol and become addicted to it. It starts with:

- *Experimental:* Due to peer pressure and curiosity individuals starts to consume alcohol.
- *Recreational:* Gradually the frequency of alcohol consumption will increase during cultural meets as an enjoyment.
- *Relaxational:* During weekends or on holidays individuals start enjoying and continue it. If consumed small quantities may not cause problem. It may work out to release the tension, relaxes the mind and sedates the brain from painful emotions and promotes a sense of well-being and pleasure.
- *Compulsive:* Once used to drinking, tendency to develop as compulsive and becomes as an addicts to overcome the discomfort of withdrawal symptoms.

Types of Drinkers

1. *Moderate drinkers*: Moderately consuming alcohol and does not cause much problem.
2. *Problem-drinkers*: As a result of drinking the health will be impaired, affects peace of mind, family disrupted, loss of reputation and drinking will become as a routine.

Causes of Drinking

- To forget miseries and problems of life
- Physical exhaustion
- Hard physical labour
- Certain occupations such as heavy vehicle drivers, labourers, manual workers
- Unhealthy environment
- Ignorance
- Sudden loss in property or close ones
- New ethics: Suddenly if a person become rich, consumes alcohol to show the status

- Chronic stage: Even for small amounts of alcohol a person will start begging, borrowing, stealing. Alcohol takes priority over family or job
- Common in cyclothymiacs personalities
- Disorders like depression, anxiety, phobia are prone to consume as an escape
- Biochemical factors: Role of dopamine and nor epinephrine affects neurotransmitter mechanism
- Psychological factors: Like injustice, inferiority, low self-esteem, poor impulse control. Poor stress management skills, loneliness, desire to escape from reality, a sense of adventure, pleasure seeking etc.
- Sexual immaturity
- Social factors like over-crowding, influence of bad company, cinemas, literature, peer pressure, urbanisation, religious reasons, unemployment, poor social support, fashion—a sign of modernity, social inadequacy, isolation.

Pathogenesis in Alcoholism

- *Pre-alcoholic symptomatic phase:* In conventional social situations an individual starts drinking alcohol but soon experiences tension relief, gradually tolerance for tension decreases such as extent he resorts to alcohol almost daily
- *Prodromal phase:* Sudden onset blackouts, signs of intoxication, loss of memory or events
- *Crucial phase:* Loss of control over drinking, increased isolation, decrease in sexual drive, centering the behaviour around alcohol
- *Chronic phase:* Marked impairment in thinking process leading to alcoholic psychosis, delirium tremor occurs. Develops rationalisation and amenable to treatment
- *Casual to habitual drinker:* Elliott and Merrill has described five stages through which a person has to pass till he becomes complete disorganisation of personality.

1. Morning drinking: Person starts drinking of alcohol in the morning and he feels it is necessary to push him throughout the day
2. Escape drinking: It starts, when a person is not able to face reality of problems without the help of alcohol
3. Increasing consumption: Consumption of alcohol increase in amount leading to personal disorganisation and decreased social values and feels without alcohol he cannot survive
4. Drinking and social function: Absolute necessity in social gatherings
5. Extreme behaviour: Drinks excessively and behaves indiscriminately, e.g: Fighting, abusing, throwing away things, beating wife and children, absurd and dangerous behaviour.

Clinical Features

- Blackout—amnesia of events
- Indigestion—anorexia
- Loss of self-control
- Out bursts of aggressive behaviour
- Sweating
- Unsteady gait, lusterless eyes and haggard look
- Malaise, tremors
- Weakness in feet and legs
- Pain in upper abdomen
- Insomnia.

Evil Effects of Alcoholism

Alcoholism is a social evil and as far as possible every individual should avoid it. Continuous use of alcohol adversely affects the brain and its efficiency. Alcoholism is a main cause of family unhappiness, tensions and total disorganisation. Individual will waste lot of money on alcohol and economic life of family also suffers. Poverty, quarrels, violence and abusive behaviour develop. Children may become delinquents; alcoholic may commit crimes, anti-social activities. It may also associate with gambling, prostitution and at least one-forth of the income are wasted on alcoholism.

Complication of Alcohol Dependence

Medical

Gastrointestinal tract

- Gastritis
- Dyspepsia
- Vomiting
- Peptic ulcer
- Cancer
- Reflex oesophagitis
- Carcinoma of stomach and oesophagus
- Fatty degeneration of the liver
- Cirrhosis of liver
- Hepatitis
- Liver cell carcinoma
- Acute and chronic pancreatitis
- Malabsorption syndrome.

Cardiovascular system

- Cardiomyopathy
- High risk for myocardial infarction.

Blood

- Folic acid deficiency anemia
- Decreased WBC production
- Central nervous system
- Peripheral neuropathy
- Epilepsy
- Head injury
- Cerebellar degeneration
- Wernicke's encephalopathy.

Muscle
- Peripheral muscle weakness
- Wasting of muscles.

Skin
- Spider angioma
- Acne.

Nutrition
- Protein deficiency
- Pellagra
- Beriberi.

Reproductive system
- Sexual dysfunction in male
- Failure of ovulation in female.

Pregnancy
- Foetal abnormalities
- Mental retardation
- Growth retardation
- Low birth weight
- Stillbirths.

Psychiatric Disorders

Acute Intoxication

During or shortly after alcohol ingestion characterised by maladaptive behaviour, e.g: Aggressive behaviour, inappropriate sexual behaviour, mood lability, poor judgment, slurred speech, unsteady gait, and nystagmus.

Withdrawal Syndrome

Any rapid decrease in the amount of alcohol content in the blood will produce withdrawal symptoms.

1. Simple withdrawal syndrome
   - Mild tremors
   - Nausea and vomiting

- Weakness
- Irritability
- Insomnia
- Anxiety
- Tachycardia
- Hypertension
- Impaired attention.

2. *Delirium tremors:* • It occurs within 2–4 days of complete or significant abstinence from heavy alcohol drinking characteristics
   - Disordered mental activity
   - Clouding of consciousness
   - Disorientation in time and place
   - Poor attention span
   - Hallucination
   - Psychomotor agitation
   - Shouting
   - Fear
   - Tremors in hand
   - Truncal ataxia
   - Autonomic disturbances like sweating, fever, Tachycardia, dilated pupils, hypertension
   - Insomnia
   - Fear
   - Convulsions
   - Dehydration
   - Leucocytosis
   - Impaired liver function.

Alcoholic Seizures

Tonic-clonic seizures occur 12–48 hours after a heavy bout of drinking; status epilepticus may result.

Alcoholic Hallucinations

Auditory hallucinations during abstinence.

Alcoholic Psychosis

- Behavioural problems
- Thought disturbances
- Delusion
- Hallucination
- Impairment of mental functions
- Morbid jealousy

Depression: Suicide and attempt to suicide are more common

Criminality: Reduces inhibition and increases hostile behaviour, violence and anti-social behaviour.

Social problem
- Marital disharmony

Occupational problems
- Reduced work performance
- Reduced productivity.

Treatment

A through assessment includes:
- An appraisal of current medial, psychological and social problems
- History taking: Drinking pattern, work spot, family pattern, environmental conditions
- Diagnose the extent of habit formation and effects of alcohol over the body
- Formulate nursing diagnosis.

Goal Setting

Short-term goals related to:
- Health
- Marital relationship
- Efficiency in job performance
- Social adjustment

- Healthy family pattern

Long-term goals such as changing the factors that precipitate or maintain excessive drinking.

Therapeutic Modalities

a. Psychotherapy

1. *Motivational interviewing*
   - Explaining the complications and personal risks of consuming the alcohol.
   - Availability of treatment options to change their behaviour related to alcohol consumption.
2. *Individual psychotherapy:* Educate each affected individual the detrimental effects of alcohol consumptions and the coping strategies to overcome the habit; precautionary measures, diversional activities to prevent the occurrence of complications with alcohol consumption.
3. *Group therapy:* Observe the problems of alcoholic, provide an opportunity to observe others problems and discuss with each other and explain them to workout in better ways of coping with these problems.
4. *Counselling:* The therapist has to counsel the client to find out the problem and shows the ways to solve the same. And also guides the individual the various methods to relax the mind and engaging themselves in productive activities.
5. *Aversive conditioning:* It is based on the principle of classical conditioning. The therapist has to explain the behaviour patterns which are pleasurable, pros and cons of alcoholism, maladaptive behaviour, show the clients who are with the complications of alcoholism, and their family problems. The client is exposed to adverse effects of excessive alcohol consumption like chemical induced vomiting, shock, etc. thereby develops aversion towards the evil habits.
6. *Cognitive therapy:* Help the client to identify the maladaptive thinking patterns; evil effects of alcoholism

and guide the individual to slowly reduce the dose of alcohol intake and by understanding the evil effects of alcohol.

7. *Relapse prevention technique:* It helps the client to:
   - Identify high-risk relapse factors and develop strategies to deal with them.
   - Learn the methods to cope with cognitive distortions.

Cue Exposure Technique

Repeated exposures to desensitize the clients to the effects of alcohol and thus improve their ability to remain abstinent.

Supportive Psychotherapy

Symptomatic treatment along with educating the individual about preventive measures against complications.

Behaviour Modification Techniques

Systematic desensitisation, relaxation techniques, operant-conditioning techniques can be used.

Family Therapy

If the head of the family develops alcoholism the total members of the family will be affected with economic crisis, maladjustment, children are prone to develop this bad habit thus family disorganisation occurs hence it is necessary and responsibility of health personnel to educate the social evil effects of alcoholism, care of the clients and preventive measures to adopt.

Treatment of the Client with Withdrawal Effects

Detoxification

It is the process by which an alcohol dependent person recovers from the intoxication effects in a supervised manner.

Benzodiazepines–Chlordiazepoxide 80–200 mg/day
Diazepam 40–80 mg/day to control anxiety, insomnia, agitation and tremors.
Thiamine 100 mg intramuscular for 3–5 days followed by vitamin-B administration 100 mg o.d. for alleast 6 months.

If necessary anti-convulsants, close observation for 5 days, maintenance of intake and output chart. Strict monitoring of vital signs, observation of level of consciousness and orientation, assess fluid and electrolyte balance, if necessary administer IV fluids. High protein diet (if the liver is not damaged) provision of calm and safe environment.

Alcohol Deterrent Therapy

Deterrent agents like disulfiram are given to desentize the individual from alcohol effects and to maintain abstinence.

DRUG ABUSE/DRUG ADDICTION

Introduction

Substances have deleterious effects over the individual. Substance abuse includes alcoholism and drug abuse. People will opt substance abuse for varied reasons like tensions release, solvation of problems, to fulfill their needs like to overcome anxiety, pressure or fatigue, experimental use, recreational use or circumstantial phase. No single factor can be identified as a cause for drug addiction.

Progressive Changes in a Drug Addict

Drug Use

People will use drugs to relieve physical and psychological problems and for mood alteration effects.

Tolerance

When a person uses drug for first time, even for a small dose, drug is very effective, whereas on repeated use increasing doses are required as the individual lost his sensitivity to a particular drug.

Drug Dependence

Person may be dependent up on one or more drugs. Craving for the drug becomes more and more. To experience drugs psychic effects and to avoid discomfort, compulsion to take the drug on a continuous or intermittent basis.

'It is a maladjustive pattern of substances use leading to significant impairment or distress'—*S Nambi*

'Drug dependence is a detrimental factor for individual and society, due to tolerance, compulsion to take the drug in increase doses'.

Habituation

It results from the repeated consumption of the drug, a desire to continue taking the drug for the sense of improved well being; it will have some degree of psychic dependence on the drug effect, but absence of physical dependence. It will have detrimental effect over the individual.

Drug Abuse

Taking a drug for other than medical reasons, in increased frequency, dose or manner that damages the physical or mental functioning.

Drug Addiction

The risk of addiction is more in mentally ill persons than physically ill. It is 'a state of periodic or chronic intoxication produced by the repeated consumption of a drug'.

Characteristics

- An overpowering desire or need (compulsion) to continue taking the drug and to obtain it by any means

- A tendency to increase the dose
- A psychic and physical dependence on the effects of the drug
- A detrimental effect both on the individual and on the society—WHO 1957.

Withdrawal Syndrome

If drug use is suddenly stopped, client will develop a group of clinical manifestations.

Incidence of Drug Abuse

It is commonly seen in the age group of 16–30 years; unmarried people and the individuals belonging to low socio-economic strata.

Causes for Drug Addiction

Social environment

- To gain acceptance in a group to belong
- Peer group pressure or influence of bad company
- Too many pocket money/loose availability of money
- Escape from social, economic pressures
- Defiant gesture against authority
- Broken families, unhappy home conditions
- Lack of parental control
- Homelessness
- Industrialisation
- Unemployment
- Low socio-economic conditions
- To get relief from strenuous activities
- Relaxed legal systems
- Social prestige
- Social pressures, insisting on consumption of drugs to achieve status
- Low religiosity

- Social deprivation
- Problems within the family
- Lack of recreational facilities
- Easy availability of drugs
- Iatrogenic (Doctor induced)—medical officers in their practice prescribing over dosage, high frequency of drugs.

Individuals with vulnerable personality

- Emotional immaturity
- Sensation seeking
- Impulsivity
- Emotional frustrations
- To overcome depression, anxiety
- Psychopath personality
- Suffering with psychiatric disorders like anxiety, neurosis, schizophrenia
- Low frustration tolerance
- Inability to cope up with tension or difficult situations
- Low self-esteem
- Excessive freedom
- Anti-social personality traits
- Psychological traumatic experiences during early childhood
- Feeling boredom, loneliness
- To express hostility
- Reaction to neglect
- To get thrill or pleasure seek
- Escape from problematic situations
- Deep psychological need
- For curiosity purpose.

Clinical Manifestations

- Euphoria (A sense of well-being)
- Deterioration in moral and ethical sense
- Moodiness
- Dull
- Physiological depression

- Irritability
- Purposefully avoids interaction and communication with family members
- Withdrawal from family activities
- Lethargy
- Lack of motivation, curiosity, enthusiasm, energy and vitality
- Stealing money and valuable items
- Erratic behaviour, confused thoughts.

Physical Symptoms

- Reddening of eyes
- Glazed dull eyes
- Pin-point pupils
- Puffiness under the eyes
- Slurring of speech
- Ataxic gait
- Anorexia
- Weight loss
- Presence of pricks and injection marks all over the body
- Sleep disturbances.

Long-term Effect of Drugs

Tolerance

User needs more and more of the drug to experience the same effect.

Psychological Dependence

Drug becomes central to the user's thoughts, emotions and activities.

Physical Dependence

The body functions normally only if the drug is present and if it stopped suddenly withdrawal symptoms will appear.

Social Cost

Alienation from family, friends, user becomes withdrawn and uncommunicative with the societal members.

Personal Cost

User needs money to support the habit and is caught in a vicious circle, goes to any length to procure money by borrowing, stealing and telling lies.

Physical Cost

- Loss of weight
- Loss of physical stamina
- Unkempt appearance.

Diagnosis of Drug Misuse

In early stages, we have to diagnose drug use by the following:

Physical Signs

Needle tracks, vein thrombosis especially in the anti-cubital fossa, wearing garments with long sleeves in hot weather also, scars.

History of Behavioural Manifestations

- Absence from school or work
- Occupational decline
- Neglect in personal appearance
- Loneliness
- Minor criminal offenses

Medical Presentation

Drug addicts will declare different types like.

- Some may present that they are dependent on drugs

- Some may conceal their dependency and ask for drugs to control or for relief of pain, e.g: Renal colic or dysmenorrhoea
- Some may present with drug related complications like cellulites, pneumonia, serum hepatitis, accidents.

Laboratory Tests

- Raised gamma-glutamy transpeptidase
- Raised mean corpuscular volume
- Urine test for drug concentration.

Management

- Hospitalisation
- Create realistic goals with the client, incorporate positive attitude
- Detoxification
- Supplementation of vitamins, minerals
- Supportive psychotherapy
- Counseling
- Family therapy
- Rehabilitation facilitated through day-care centres.

Rehabilitation

- To enable the drug dependents to leave the drug sub-culture
- To develop new social contracts
- Provide social support when the person makes the transition to normal work and living
- Inculcate responsibility in protecting themselves.

Facilities for Rehabilitating Drug Abusers by Government and Other Voluntary Organisations

Counselling Centre

- Clients are screened for residential treatment and motivating them for withdrawal of drugs

- Extended care after discharge
- Family therapy
- Supportive psychotherapy.

De-addiction Centre

- Keep all lives of communication open
- Medical care—detoxification, primary care
- Educational measures for healthful living, discipline and value of time
- Speak to addicts' friends, teachers, family members in supportive measures.

After-care Centre

Plan for long-term therapeutic community programme (6–9 months) depending up on individual's progress. It consists of structured environment to encourage the members to develop positive peer pressure and to establish healthy relationships, sound values and a productive life style in drug free environment.

Day-care Centres for Women

Provides support to women narcotics and alcoholics who has completed detoxification treatment. In day-care centres, one-year course is offered in which *yoga, sadhana*, meditation, work therapy, individual and group sessions etc., activities will be performed.

Out-reach Services

Family Therapy

- Conducting family association meetings
- Domiciliary visits
- Joint sessions with addicts and family members for holistic approach in therapeutic modalities

- Awareness campaigns in form of seminars, workshops, exhibition will be organizes to improve the knowledge of public about drug addiction.

Relapse in Drug Addiction

In few cases, drug addicts will resume their habit within six months. It is due to poor follow-up and rehabilitative services, easily availability of drugs, persistent pressure from peer group.

Preventive Measures in Drug Addiction

Primary Prevention

- Provide healthy and happy family environment
- Loving, tender-care, establish healthy child-parent relationship
- Give mutual respect for the child
- Taking timeout for fun
- Openly talk to the child and communicate love
- Show interest in child's activities
- Share problems of child, talk to the child and teach how to solve the problems and handle the situations
- Counseling, inform career options and motivate the child to set goals in life
- Parents should not be sarcastic, accusatory or blaming of the child for his behaviour
- Avoid influencing factors like companion which promotes the child for bad habits
- Promote mass-media activities and prepare IEC modules, organize awareness campaigns to improve the knowledge of public, special attention to focus group about the dangers associated with drug abuse and coping strategies to over come stressors
- Insist in general meetings, celebrations at college level that students should not misuse the available freedom.

Related to Drugs

- Limit the availability of drugs
- Legislation measures to be formulated to control the production, supply, sale, possession and export of drugs
- Physicians should be careful, not to prescribe drugs of powerful action and if needed they have to advice to take drugs on prescription
- Drug should be made available for genuine use and safeguard to prevent illicit use.

Secondary Prevention

- Observe closely change in the behaviour of the individual and avail medical assistance as early as possible
- Establish de-addiction centres, after-care centres, day-care centres which will assist the individual and their family members in overcoming the problem of drug addiction
- Early identify the drug abusers
- Treat promptly by specified therapies to prevent the complications of disease.

Tertiary Prevention

- Includes the treatment in the state of severe dependence
- Identify the social agencies which will assist in rehabilitative activities
- Rehabilitation measures has to be planned based on severity of the problem
- Family has to be involved in the restorative and rehabilitative activities.

Nursing Management for Substance Abuse

Assessment

- Observe for at risk factors, physical signs, behavioural
- Find out factual information to confirm the diagnosis
- Assist for laboratory test.

Nursing Diagnosis

- Risk for injury related to intoxification manifestations
- Altered health maintenance related to physical symptoms
- Failure to accept responsibilities
- Ineffective ego processes related to though disturbances
- Inadequate coping strategies due to impairment.

Nursing Interventions

- Close observation of the client is required
- Monitor the level of consciousness, sleeping pattern, health status, behavioural changes
- If needed, use physical restraints to avoid injury
- Reduce environment stimuli
- Use protective devices, take secured precautions against convulsions
- Reorientation of the client if needed
- Use simple, clear, direct language
- Maintain fluid and electrolyte balance
- Meet nutritional needs of the client
- Provide small and frequent feeds
- Assist the client in self-care activities
- Provide psychological support
- Identify maladaptive behaviour
- Don't allow the client to be alone
- Teach the client and family about treatment, rehabilitation and prevention
- Meet the total needs of the client.

Brief Description of Common Drugs used for Drug Addiction Opioids (Narcotics)

For example: Morphine, pethidine, fortwin, tidigesic and Heroin (Brown sugar, Smack)

Route of administration: Injection

Acute intoxication, apathy, bradycardia, hypotension, respiratory depression, sub-normal temperature, pinpointed pupils, thready pulse, coma.

Withdrawal symptoms: Begin within 12 hours of the last dose peak in 24–36 hours, disappear in 5–6 days.

Watery eyes, running nose, anorexia, irritability, tremors, sweating, cramps, nausea, diarrhea, insomnia, fever.

Complications: Parkinsonism, peripheral neuropathy, transverse myelitis.

Treatment

Opoid over-dose can be treated with narcotic antagonists like naloxone, naltrexone.

Maintenance therapy: Behaviour therapy, family therapy.

Morphine

Action

On the cortex, increasing its inhibitory effect on thalamic centres of sensation and raising the pain threshold.

Effected on pain sensation: Depress sensation of all kinds, although itching may be present. If it is taken orally, morphine is quickly absorbed through the intestinal mucosa and is slowly oxidized in the liver. Stimulates parasympathetic nervous system, increased bronchial secretions, respiratory centre failure.

Intoxication effects: Spinal reflex are increased, urinary retention is frequent, constipation and respiratory centre failure.

The tendency of morphine to cause addiction depends on its analgesic and enphorizing effects, also on the fairly rapid tolerance development.

Clinical Picture of an Addict

Miosis, scars or abscesses at the site of carelessly given injections, trophic disturbances of the skin, loss of hair, poor appetite, malnutrition, hepatitis, anxiety, depression, restlessness are banished only to return with the hang-over.

Chronic Abuse

Increasing inactivity, laziness, wasting of time in day-dreams, indecisiveness, paralysis of the ability to make strong and persistent effort. As a secondary consequence, due to need to conceal the habit and to over come social and other barriers in the way of regular supply the client is likely to become fraud, the falsification of prescriptions, embracing insincerity to family, friends, colleagues and doctors, dishonest maneuvers of all kinds and flagrant breaches of the law.

Withdrawal

Abstinence syndrome, euphoria, calm and content give-way to depression, restlessness, physical and mental irritability, habitual constipation changes to diarrhea, anorexia, trembling, malaise and sleeplessness.

Diagnosis

- Papillary changes when the client is under the influence of a dose
- Small injection scars in the skin at accessible sites
- When the client is trying to conceal the addiction a change in mood, debility, tremour, apathy, depression at one time followed, after an absence from the room, at a short interval by alertness and a cheerful humour.

Treatment

Pre-hospital Phase

When the patient is persuaded to enter the hospital; avoid over-prescription of drugs.

Hospitalisation

- *Withdrawal phase:* Total abstinence by substituting drugs, Lethidrone-N ally is the most effective antagonist
- *Rehabilitation phase:* Physical and Emotional rehabilitation
- *Transitional phase:* Making the client able to manage his affairs outside hospital
- *Prolonged after-care phase*: Psychotherapy, family therapy, social therapy, guidance and counselling.

Lysergic Acid Di-ethylamide (LSD-25)

After administration of LSD-25 within 15–20 minutes, autonomic effects occur like rise in body temperature, hypoglycemia, mydriasis and piloerection, psychological changes are delayed for 40–60 minutes, most intense after 1 or 2 hours, e.g: Intense mood effects, euphoria, profound depression, anxiety, unmotivated giggling or laughter, sometimes accompanied by tears, sense of oppressive malaise, perceptual disturbances, visual hyper-aesthesia is common, hallucination, some may experience intense somatic discomfort or pain, feeling themselves crushed, twisted or stretched.

Intoxication, depersonalisation, de-realisation, illusions, synesthesia, autonomic hyper-activity, marked anxiety, impaired judgment.

Withdrawal syndrome: Flashbacks.

Compilations

Anxiety, depression, psychosis, visual hallucinations.

Treatment

Symptomatic management by anti-depressants or anti-psychotic agents.

Cannabis Sativa

The flowering tops of the female plant of *cannabis sativa* have a pleasant intoxication effect. It may be eaten, drunk or smoked (ingestion or inhalation). The drug is always taken in company hence the spread of habit.

Intoxication Effects

Mental phenomena arise 2 to 3 hours after ingestion or almost immediately after inhalation of the drug; floating of air sensation; falling on waves; lightness or dizziness in the head; ringing in the ears; heaviness in the limb; euphoria; increased psycho-motor activity; confused lassitude; elevated moods, mental status—hyperactive, apprehensive, loquacious, suspiciousness; lowered educational activities; psychosis; unreality feeling; double personality; though disorder—fragmentation of thought process, memory disturbances, perplexity and immobility, frequent and sudden interruption of the stream of thought.

Withdrawal Symptoms Occur Between 72-96 Hours

Complications

Acute anxiety, paranoid psychosis, hysterical fugue state like hypomania, schizophrenia, memory impairment.

Treatment

Supportive therapy; symptomatic treatment.

Cocaine

Local anesthetic, it acts centrally as an excitant and enphorizing agent, stimulates sympathetic causing pupil dilatation, skin-pallor, raise in pulse rate, sweating, raise in body temperature.

Addicts if cocaine administered subcutaneously or inhale as a snuff, quickly absorbed through the mucus membrane. Immediate elation with mental agility feelings, greater precision of though and action, fatigue, excited, restless, likes to take and mixes well in society. He may make the impression of a brilliant conversationalist, witty and full of ideas, superficial thinking, over-activity, and lacks direction.

Prognosis and Treatment

Physical and mental ruin—treat with *barbiturates;* if the drug is withdrawn immediately and completely delirium and sub-acute paranoid episode pass off.

Intoxication—amylnitrate is antidose, diazepam, and propranolol.

Withdrawal symptoms: Antidepressants like imipramine, psychotherapy.

Barbiturates

- The doctor should be careful in prescribing drugs of powerful action, such as barbiturate as placebos. These are"cortical depressants acts on autonomic nervous system through hypothalamic centres
- To relieve general restlessness and tension
- To mitigate some physical pain
- To procure a deeper sleep and obviate early morning wakening
- To protect the client against an excessive sensitivity to noises and other sensory stimuli.

Acute Intoxication

Depend on the amount of drug and on its nature and speed of action.

Suicidal attempt, drowsiness, ataxia, asynergia, nystagmus, and hypotonia, slow pulse, respiration and peristalsis, fall in body temperature, paresis, disseminated sclerosis or presenile dementia, renal respiratory failure, coma and death.

Withdrawal Symptoms

Delirium tremor, anxiety, terrifying hallucination, tremulous withdrawal psychosis, convulsions, paranoid reaction, impairment of consciousness.

Complications

Intravenous use can lead to skin abscesses, cellulites, infections, embolism, hypersensitivity reactions.

Treatment

An unhurried regime must be pursued, rehabilitation—contact with the family, plan diligent, systematic, social and medical follow-up services, use of activated charcoal can reduce the absorption, symptomatic managements.

Cyanide

When large doses are taken, the client loses consciousness within 10 seconds and dies with convulsion in 5 minutes, with small dose the symptoms are vertigo, headache, palpitations, drowsiness, severe dyspnoea, convulsions, loss of consciousness, death is due to asphyxia and due to paralysis of respiratory centre, medullary centre.

Inhalants or Volatile Solvent Use

For example: Petrol, aerosol, vanish remover, industrial solvents.

Intoxication

Euphoria, excitement, slurring of speech, apathy, impaired judgment

Withdrawal symptoms

Anxiety, depression.

Complication

Peripheral neuropathy, liver, kidney damage, brain damage, perceptual disorders.

Treatment

Reassurance, diazepam.

Carbon Monoxide Poisoning

The symptoms are lowering of efficiency and of self-control without insight, neuritis, disoriented, clouded consciousness, absent-minded, loss of consciousness, sometimes Parkinson syndrome with akinesia, rigidity and a mask-like facial expression, symptoms of aphasia, apraxia and agnosia are more frequent, the focus vascular damage to the cortex is irreversible.

Treatment

Pure oxygen administration, assistance from an efficient mechanical respirator, hypothermia, CPR technique.

Lead Poisoning

Acts on central nervous system, easily absorbed from the mucous membranes of respiratory or alimentary tract. Confusional state with signs of meningeal irritation, focal signs, e.g: Aphasia, transient paresis, convulsions, and coma.

Slow cases, client manifests are: Retarded depression, dullness, failure of concentration and memory, headache, deafness, transient speech defect, visual disturbances.

Amphetamine

Powerful CNS stimulants with peripheral symptomatic effects, e.g: Pemoline, methylphenidate.

It increases verbal and motor activity, elevates the mood and prevents drowsiness in sleep, to combat apathy, tension, fatigue, depression, hunger and it is useful when heightened confidence and decisiveness are needed.

Euphoria state with excitement, which readily erupts into violence. Deterioration in social adjustment, depression, psychosis, attempted suicide after abrupt withdrawal, to enable them to get through work under pressure, to control obesity among female.

Acute Intoxication

Tachycardia, hypertension, cardiac failure, seizures, tremours, hyperpyrexia, papillary dilation, panic, insomnia, restlessness, irritability, psychosis, paranoid hallucinatory syndrome.

Withdrawal Symptoms

Agitation, depression, apathy, fatigue, hyper-somnia or insomnia.

Complication

Seizures, delirium, arrhythmias, aggressive behaviour, coma.

PROBLEMS OF WOMEN IN MODERN INDIA

Introduction

Women are regarded with high respect in our Indian society. Earlier women too faced certain problems like child marriages, practice of *Sati,* exploitation of widows, Devadasi system, *Pardah* system,etc. which are almost disappeared now with technological advancements, universalisation of education, socio-political movements, modernisation and similar social developments changed the approach of people towards women to a certain extent. It increases the morale, status, self-confidence, individuality, personality, self-respect, talent, capacity and efficiency among women. Equal rights, responsibilities and more opportunities for women to experience and exposed for varied environment. Even though our legislations provides equal opportunity and rights to women and they are also positively responding to the changed socio-political situations; but even then they are facing certain problems.

Increasing Crimes Against Women

Crimes such as violence against women, rape, molestation, dowry harassment, wife battering, kidnapping, selling the women to brothel houses, forcible embracement, prostitution and religious conversion, cheating, sexual abuse and harassments, eve teasing and women abuse. Female genital mutilation and exploitation of women were observed in our modern India.

Female Children are Becoming Victims of Discrimination

Male children were preferred by Indian society., if female foetus is observed, they even go to the extent such as female foeticide, female negligence and discrimination related to the matters like food, dress, health, education, domestic work and occupational avenues are narrower.

Health Problems for Women

Women belong to high-risk group and are more prone for infections and other diseases, because of more responsibilities there is a chance for neglecting their own health, no free time, non-availability of medical facilities, lack of transportation facilities, lame excuses, enjoys dependency role, etc.

Problems of Working Women

Now-a-days women are equally competing with men; increased education status makes them to occupy special roles and positions in almost all fields. The illiterate women also coming forward to do the jobs in factories, textiles, small scale industries, building construction purposes as labourers, agriculture fields. Technological advancements affect the job life of women as clerks, typists and accountants. Though our legislations has given equal rights and opportunities for women, a negligible number of women occupied prestigious positions such as in cabinet, governors, secretaries, legal advisers, ambassadors, Indian administrative services, etc.

Women has to fulfill dual responsibilities if they are employed, she has to adjust herself for both domestic and working environment. In family, she has to complete all household responsibilities, if the family members are cooperating with her, adjust themselves and modifies their life styles accordingly, she will be able to concentrate for office work in an efficient manner; otherwise stress will arise; unable to cope up both activities and suffers with mental illness. In performing familial activities such as rearing practices, caring of children, cooking, meeting the needs of total family members, she may neglect her personal care and health. She has to maintain balance between household activities and occupational activities. Especially the spouse and children has to adjust and accommodate themselves, extend total cooperation to her, in such cases it is added asset for family, otherwise it may lead to quarrel, marital maladjustment, strained interpersonal relationship, unhappiness, broken families and divorce.

If colleagues or co-workers are cooperative, healthy relationships and happy environment will exist, otherwise it affects total life and leads to unhealthy comparisons, heavy work-load, cheating, abuse, harassments either psychological or social, too prolonged working hours, uncooperative staff, misunderstanding, communication gaps, etc. leads to fight or flight reaction to adjust and accommodate herself.

Few examples that can enumerate problems of women in employment:

1. Related to family (Family disorganisation)
   - Unable to balance between household responsibility and working responsibilities
   - Tension in working place is carried over to family
   - Unable to concentrate with the familial activities due to tiredness, lead to indifferences between spouse and with other family members.
2. *Stress and personal care:* Women has to adjust for both family and official activities, due to this she may experience severe stress and several times they won't have sufficient time to think about personal issues and have discrepancies and will neglect their personal care and prone for ill-health and other psychiatric problems.

3. *Resistance to misconduct of seniors and officers:* In the male dominant society, woman are more prone for verbal and some times physical harassment; which leads to discomfort and may lead to change the job or stop working.
4. *Economic dependence:* It is observed that both in rural and urban societies the family members of the women will be waiting for her salary and forcing her to do extra work and get extra remuneration for their personal benefits and the women will not be permitted to spend their earning as they wish at least for their personal care also.
5. *Job insecurity:* Many of the women who are working in different fields are not having enough job security inspite of their education, skill, knowledge, hard work, and punctuality. They will work under so many pressures just because of the fear of loosing the jobs and they will be exploited by different manners for the same reason.
6. *Low wages:* Women who are working in rural areas like agricultural, small-scale industries will be paid very low wages and exploited to do more work for less pay.

Solvation of Problems Related to Women:

1. Equal importance, status should be given
2. Family members should provide cooperation, concern, encouragement, moral support for the women to face any situation courageously.
3. In working area, conducive environment has to be provided to perform their job effectively without any worries or conflicts. Promote team spirit group cohesion among the employees.

THE PROBLEM OF UNDER-PRIVILEGED SECTIONS OF COMMUNITY

Scheduled Castes, Scheduled Tribes and Other Backward Classes

Unprivileged sections are often treated as, 'backward castes' consist of three divisions:

- Scheduled tribes (Girijans)

- Scheduled castes (Harijans)
- Other backward classes

Certain groups are living in hilly areas and villages have suffered isolation and disability. They live in a state of social and economic stagnation. President of India lists these people in pursuance of the relevant provisions of the constitution. *Harijans* in rural area regarded as, 'untouchables'. Majority of the scheduled castes have been regarded as untouchables. In 1928, Simon Commission has used the term for the first time; untouchable castes'. In 1935 and 1950 the Government of India Act designated as. 'Scheduled castes'. But Mahatma Gandhiji addressed them as, 'Harijans'—the people of God.

'The untouchables castes are those who suffer from various social and political disabilities many of which are traditionally prescribed and socially enforced by higher caste'—*Dr DN Majumdar*

'Untouchables are those people who are economically socially, educationally, religiously and politically backward castes which are kept at a distance by other castes'.

'Scheduled castes are an integral part of the village life, performs essential tasks in agriculture, etc'. —*MN Srinivas*

Problems of Schedules Castes

Untouchables/*Varna* system in Vedic period was degenerated into the caste system, since then the scheduled castes are known as untouchables. They have been suffering from social, religious, legal, political, economic, educational and other disabilities. They are deprived of representation, legal rights, civic facilities, educational privileges and economic opportunities.

- *Lower status:* Scheduled castes are called as, 'unholy' 'low' inferior, looked down, social stigma, servants of other caste people, kept at distance.
- *Educational disabilities:* Harijans were forbidden from entering schools and other educational institutions

previously; but now to encourage them in studies, the Government of India introduced reservation system for education and in employment.

- *Civic disabilities—prevention from the sue of public places:* Harijans were not allowed public places like wells, hotels, temples, ponds, schools, hospitals, dharmasahalas, choultries, etc. they were forced to live in, out skirts of the town and villages and were prohibited from certain public activities.
- Religious disabilities
- Harijans were not allowed to place of worship and perform pooja, prohibited from Vedic chants
- *Economic disabilities:* No right to property ownership; selection of limited occupations; landless labourers.
- *Political disabilities:* Earlier, Harijans were given any place in politics, administration and the general governance of India, they were not allowed in public places. After independence, equal opportunities and rights have been praised, yet, they have to become an organised force.

UNTOUCHABILITY

Untouchability is a stigma attached to Hindu religion, Gandhiji regarded this as a, 'leper wound in the whole body of Hindus politics', considered as, 'the hate fullest expression of caste'. It is a mass phenomenon of group prejudices and discrimination affecting majority population in India.

Definition

'Social inhibition of touch, emerging from the characteristics of Indian caste system'

'It is a practice in which lower caste people are kept at a distance and denied of social equality for their touch by the forward caste'.

Laws

Article 17 of the Indian constitution states that, 'untouchability is abolished and its act is forbidden'.

The offences of untouchability includes the following:

- Committing any kind of social injustice like denying access to any public place
- Preventing a person from prayers
- Refusal to sell goods
- Punishable with imprisonment for 6 months or a fine of Rs. 500/- or both. Enforcing occupations, professional enjoyment of any benefit under a charitable trust.

Eradication of Untouchability

From the times of *Buddha* and *Mahaveera* attempts have been made to remove the social disabilities of the backward castes including untouchability. Various social reformers and thinkers have worked related to this and Gandhiji's sincere efforts to abolish untouchability; it was declared illegal under the Indian constitution provision:

An opportunity was given to leader of backward caste, to join the central cabinet and to be the chief architect of the Indian constitution. He worked in promoting the welfare of S.C and elevating their status and self-esteem.

To promote equity, fraternity, liberty and ensures justice for one and all.

- Article 15–17; 38 and 46 indicated that the state shall not discriminate between persons on account of their religion, caste or class
- Article 15(4) and 29 (2) state can make special provision for advancement of scheduled castes, scheduled tribes and backwards.
- Article 16(4); 320(4) and 335 the Government offices and services same reservation is made for SC and ST
- Article 23, SC and ST are given protection against exploitation

- Article 17-part. III declares that untouchability is abolished and its practices in any form is forbidden and anything observed are punishable
- Article 35, the Untouchability Offences Act, 1955 was passed by parliament to make the practice of untouchability or cognizable offence punishable under law. It was substituted by the Protection of Civil Rights Act, which came into force from 19-11-1976
- Article 46, state will look after the educational, economic interests of the depressed classes
- Article 330, 332 and 334, states are reserved for SC and ST in state legislative assemblies
- Article 338, GOI appointed commissioner and other officials for Harijans welfare to look after the special provision extended to SC and ST
- Welfare activities for Harijans by the government viz., plans, programs, projects, schemes to promote education, e.g: Giving concessions like free tuition, stipends, scholarship, free supply of text books, stationary, midday meals, free boarding-lodging facilities
- Giving provision to start small scale industries
- Community development projects and National extensions service for bringing new ideas and accommodating rural people with Harijans under democratic society
- Harijans farmers will be given new agricultural implements with seeds, fertilizers, pesticides at free of cost
- Technical and vocational trainings to start their industries
- Schools for providing basic education with free hostel
- Provisions of reservations in Government jobs
- Economic assistance like loans for starting small scale industries
- Encouraging interaction between upper caste and backward castes to have common understanding and to maintain equity
- Reform Hindu religion as a whole.

Solvation of Social Problems

In the primitive days, for solution of social problem man employed trail and error methods frequently resorted to magic and supernatural powers. The social reformers did a scientific analysis and find out an effective realistic methods to solve the social problem.

Remedial Methods (Reformatory approach)

It treats symptoms or consequences of a problem instead of tackling the underlying causes.

Preventive and Constructive Method (Planning approach)

Strategies adopted to prevent the occurrence of social problem it provides check at its source. It tries to find out the root cause or occurrence of the problem. Better educational opportunities provided through information, education, communication and mobilisation strategies to impart the knowledge to the community by active community participation and involvement methods adopted. Universal education and dissemination of knowledge are the powerful weapons in attacking the social problem and they must be dealt with, as they come up.

Social Planning

Man must plan, based on facts, analysis, scientific approach to deal effectively with the problem faced by him. Man can control his destiny as the social problems are man made origin and he can adequately treat it.

Definition

'A conscious interactional process combining investigation, discussion, agreement and action in order to achieve those conditions relationships and value that are regarded as desirable'—*Himes*

'It is the development of a program, procedure designed to accomplish predetermined objectives for a society or a segment of it'—*Anderson and Parker*

A plan is in achievement to be made within a fixed period of time. It is based on practical approach and a means of social progress.

Aims

- To check the recurrence of social problems
- To bring about a harmonious adjustment of relationships between the different societal parts
- To win mastery over physical and societal forces which affect human evolution
- To maintain social order
- To produce equivalent of a workable blueprint to serve as a program of action
- To adapt our culture to meet the present needs
- To adjust the institutions for changes in conditions of life
- It closes the gap between material culture and social institutions
- To deal effectively with the other societal problems.

Difficulties in Implementing Social Planning

- Real understanding of human society is a problem (Emotional raw material)
- Lack of scientific study to investigate thoroughly about the social problem (Planning without adequate scientific knowledge results failure)
- Lack of man power to carry out the work of social planning
- Vested interests of society, who exercise powerful influence over the Government machinery
- Indifference and apathy of the masses: masses has to learn to view social phenomena objectively and cooperate in the formation and administration of social policy.

Social Planning in India

Government of India formulated the planning, commission to promote the social welfare activities and coordinate the welfare services maintained and social welfare organisations developed to strengthen, improve and extending the existing activities of social welfare and develop new programmes and to carry out new projects. Central Bureau of correctional services developed after care homes to provide appropriate training and to meet the needs of persons especially needy population like rescued women, girls, economically deprived group and scheduled caste population.

Previous Years University Questions

1. Write an essay on 'housing problem' in India. (15 m, MP, 2004)
2. Poverty. (5 m, MP, 2000, 04)
3. Define juvenile delinquency and give its causes. (15 m MP, 2003)
4. Write a short essay on personal disorganisation. (15 m, MP, 2000)
5. Write an essay on problem of housing in our country. (15 m, MP, 2000)
6. Personal disorganisation. (5 m, MP, 1997)
7. Problem of housing. (5 m, MP, 1997)
8. Delinquency. (5 m, MP, 1997)
9. Illiteracy. (5 m, MP, 1997)
10. Prostitution. (5 m, MP, 1997)
11. Causes of prostitution. (5 m, RGUHS, 2000)
12. Consequences of poverty. (5 m, RGUHS, 2000)
13. Problems of Indian women. (5 m, RGHUS, 2000)
14. Describe the problems of modern family because of changes in its function. (10 m, RGUHS, 2001)
15. Health effects of alcoholism. (5 m, RGUHS, 1999; 2001)
16. Consequences of beggary. (5 m, RGUHS, 2001)

17. Explain problems of unemployment.
(2 m, RGUHS, 1997, 2001)
18. Mention types of beggary. (2 m, RGUHS, 2002)
19. Suppression of Immoral Traffic Act.(2 m, RGUHS, 2003)
20. Health consequences of poverty. (2 m, RGUHS, 2003)
21. Health problems of commercial sex.(5 m, RGUHS, 2001)
22. Explain individual disorganisation.(2 m, RGUHS, 2002)
23. What are social problems? Describe any one of the social problems arising from socio-cultural sources.
(5 m, RGUHS, 2003)
24. Problems of old age. (5 m, RGUHS, 2003)
25. Poverty line. (2 m, RGUHS, 2003)
26. Social problems. (2 m, RGUHS, 2003)
27. Health effects of unemployment. (5 m, RGUHS, 2000)
28. Dowry Prohibition Act–mention recent amendments.
(2 m, RGUHS, 2000)
29. What are the health problems of untouchables.
(2 m, RGUHS, 2000)
30. Consequences of poverty. (5 m, RGUHS, 1999)
31. Define social problems. Examine the various social problems of urban areas and their remedies.
(5 m, RGUHS, 2001)
32. Problems of working women. (5 m, RGUHS, 2000)
33. List the health consequences of poverty.
(2 m, RGUHS, 2000)
34. Explain the new code of criminal procedure-section 125.
(2 m, RGUHS, 2000)
35. List the common social problems of urban community.
(2 m, RGUHS, 2000)
36. Social disorganisation. (2 m, RGUHS, 2002, 03)
37. Relationship between slum and alcoholism.
(5 m, RGUHS, 2003)
38. List four social problems of urban society and describe delinquency as a problem. (19 m, NTRUHS, 2002)

39. Describe the social status of old people in India. (19 m, NTRUHS, 2002)
40. Discuss the effects of crime and punishment on society. (19 m, NTRUHS, 2002)
41. List any three social problems and describe one in detail. (19 m, NTRUHS, 2001)
42. Describe about the juvenile delinquency and crime. Explain about the steps to be taken to prevent this problem in our country. (19 m, NTRUHS, 1999)
43. What are the major problems of working women? Explain about the various steps to prevent this. (19 m, NTRUHS, 1999)
44. Write short notes on Prostitution.(9 m, NTRUHS, 1998)
45. What is social disorganisation and explain the causes for social disorganisation. (NTRUHS, 1996)
46. What are the social problems that influence the health of the women in India. Suggest measures to improve the situation. (NTRUHS, 1996)
47. Describe briefly the problems of crime and delinquency and give suggestions to prevent. (NTRUHS, 1984, 85, 86, 95)
48. Discuss the concept of poverty and give suggestions to prevent. (NTRUHS, 1995)
49. What do you understand the term social planning. (NTRUHS, 1995)
50. What are the causes of juvenile delinquency? how it can be controlled. (13 m, SVIMS, Tirupati, 2002)
51. Health issues of commercial sex. (6 m, SVIMS, Tirupati, 2002)
52. Explain the social causes of population explosion in India. (9 m, SVIMS, 2003)
53. Problems of working women. (9 m, SVIMS, 2003)
54. Causes of juvenile delinquency. (5 m, SVIMS, 2003)
55. Social effects of alcoholism. (5 m, RGUHS, Nov-04)
56. Juvenile house. (2 m, RGUHS, Nov-04)

MGR University Question Papers

1. Juvenile delinquency. (5 m, MGRU, Nov-03)
2. Unemployment. (5 m, MGRU, Nov-03)
3. Social problem. (2 m, MGRU)
4. Poverty and unemployment. (5 m, MGRU)
5. Crime and juvenile and its achievements. (5 m, MGRU)
6. Problems of Indian women. (5 m, MGRU)
7. Social disorganisation. (5 m, MGRU)
8. Family disorganisation. (5 m, MGRU)
9. Problem of alcoholism. (5 m, MGRU)
10. Problem of unemployment. (5 m, MGRU)
11. Impact of disorganised society. (5 m, MGRU)
12. Alcoholism. (5 m, MGRU)
13. Population explosion. (5 m, MGRU)
14. What do you understand by 'Social Disorganisation'? What factors may be held responsible for it? (15 m, MGRU)
15. Crime and juvenile delinquency. (5 m, MGRU)
16. Write the nature and causes of social disorganisation in India. (15 m, MGRU)
17. Family disorganisation. (5 m, MGRU, Nov-02)
18. Alcoholism. (5 M, MGRU)
19. Family disorganisation. (5 m, MGRU)
20. Inadequacy of legislative measures to tackle social problems. (5 m, MGRU)

CHAPTER THIRTEEN

Population

The total number of inhabitants living in a particular geographical area is called as, 'Population'. Health in the group depends upon the dynamic relationship between the member of people, the space which they occupy and the skill that they have acquired in providing or meeting their needs. Information about population and other social characteristics will be studied through census, sample registration system, etc. The scientific study of human population is called as, 'Demography'. It focuses its attention on three readily observable human phenomena (i) Changes in population size (ii) The composition of the population and (iii) The distribution of population in space. It deals with five demographic processes like fertility, mortality, marriage, migration, and social mobility. These factors will influence the members in the society. Demography is a fundamental approach to the understanding of human society. The birth depends upon fertility. The demographic processes are to a great extent socially determined. The demographer has to understand the societal factors, which influence population at an extent. The growth of population is having great social concern. Demographer studies both area and other characteristics of population (like age, sex, literacy, religion, occupation, marital pattern), which are socially important. Human population exists in the world through socio-cultural interaction. Population trends depend upon societal characteristics. A balance is necessary between various factors and they are interlinked with each other; e.g: Size of the population and food supply; relation between nutrition and health (related to morbidity and mortality pattern).

TERMINOLOGY

Sex ratio

'The number of females per 1000 males'. Sex composition is affected by the differentials in mortality conditions of males and females, sex selective migration and sex ratio at birth.

In India: Sex ratio 93 females per 1000 males (In 2001).

Density of Population

Number of persons living per square kilometer, e.g: In India density of population is 324/sq. km.

Family Size

'The total number of persons in a family', e.g: In India, family size is 3.1. It depends on duration of marriage, education of the couple, number of live births, living children, preference of male children, desired family size.

Dependency Ratio

'The proportion of persons above 65 years of age and children below 15 years of age who are dependent upon the economically productive age group'.

Life Expectancy

'The average number of years, which a person of that age may expect to live'.

World Population Trend

At the beginning of the Christian Era, world population was estimated to be around 250 million.

Year	*Population (million)*	*Average annual growth rate (%)*
1750	791	—
1800	978	0.4
1850	1262	0.5
1900	1650	0.6
1950	2526	1.1
1960	3037	1.79
1975	4066	1.89
1980	4432	1.72
1987	5000	1.63
1991	5385	1.70
1998	5884	1.60
2000	6054	1.40

(Source: J.E. Park, 2002 17th edition; p: 325)

Population Distribution in India

On 12-10-1999 world population became 6 billion. It is expected to reach 8 billion by 2025. Three forths of the world's population lives in the developing countries. USA ranks third in the world population after India. (According to UN projections India's population will reach 1.52 billion by the year 2050 and will be the highest population in the world surpassing China. India is the second most populous country, next to China, with only 2.4% of the world's land area, and supporting about 16.87% of world's population).

It is obvious that we are adding 16 million people every year, equivalent to the combined population of Harayana and Himachal Pradesh. Though India is only two-fifths the size of USA, its population is three times of that country. On May 11th 2000 India's population reached one billion.

Population in India

Year	Population	Average annual exponential growth rate
1901	138.4	—
1911	252.1	0.56
1921	251.3	(-) 0.03
1931	279	1.04
1941	318.7	1.33
1951	361.1	1.25
1961	439.2	1.96
1971	548.2	2.20
1981	683.3	2.22
1991	843.9	2.14
2001	1027.0	1.93

(Source: J.E.Park, 2002 –P; 327)

India's population has been steadily increasing since 1921 the year, 1921 is called 'big divide'. The crude rate 25, crude death rate 9; growth rate 1.93%. among states, Uttar Pradesh occupies first position with 66.05 million population.

Ranking of most populous states by population size 2001.

State	*Population on 1-3-2001 (million)*	*% of total population*
Uttar Pradesh	166.05	16.17
Maharastra	96.75	9.42
Bihar	82.87	8.07
West Bengal	80.22	7.81
Andhra Pradesh	75.72	7.37
Tamil Nadu	62.11	6.05
Madhya Pradesh	60.38	6.88
Rajasthan	56.47	8.60
Karnataka	52.73	5.14
Gujarat	50.59	4.93

(Source: J.E Park, 2002 P: 328)

The proportion of population below 15 years is showing decline, whereas the elderly population proportion is increasing. The age pyramid of India is typical of under developed countries, with a broad base and a tapering top. Sex ratio is 933 female per 1000 male; Kerala has a sex ratio of 1058 per 1000 male in 2001. The dependency population ratio as per 1995 is 65.5; in that child dependency ratio (0–14 years) is 57.8 and old age (65 and above) is 7.6; density of the population is 324/sq. km. Family size is 3.1. The literacy rate is 65.38% (for male 75.85%, females 54.16%) life expectancy for males 62.80 and 63.80 for female.

Malthusian Theory of Population

The theory of population as enunciated by *T R Malthus*, clergyman may be regarded as the starting point of all modern speculations. *Malthus* in his book, 'An essay on the principles of population as it affects the future improvements of society', it is a still living influence and has been engaging the attention of people in all ages. We should have a general idea of the intellectual, social, political and economic conditions in which he lived.

Industrial Revolution

Malthus witnessed the upsurge of industrial revolution where industries prospered at the expenses of agriculture leading to top sided development. Beside the evils of the capitalism like economic inequality, widespread unemployment, poverty, starvation, exploitation, business fluctuations reared their ugly heads. The entire nation suffered from acute poverty on account of the imbalance between population and food supply.

Deterioration of the Economic Condition

When *Malthus* lived, the British economy was passing through the worst form of economic crisis. Widespread famine, disease, poverty, squalor and unemployment prevailed all-round. Agriculture was passing through a lean period, agricultural slide down put a heavy burden on the society.

Views of Mercantialists and Physiocrats

Mercantialists regarded that a nation's strength depended on the extent to which it is economically self-sufficient and upon the number of its people. It is to violate the natural order.

Influence of William Godwin

Godwin attributed the root of all human misery is administrative inefficiency, bad laws, corrupt rulers, greedy employers and so forth. Some of the man's institutions were abolished and some reformed, suffering would disappear. As a result man's very nature would undergo a radical change so that he would no longer be his worst enemy. He believed that man's sexual passion and his basic impulses were likely to remain what they had been always.

The Idea of Human Progress

The concept of purely static orders in which man was a plaything of destiny was slowly changing during *Malthus* time. This breeze of dynamic order inspired *Malthus* to visualise the change in a dynamic pattern.

The Discovery of Natural Laws

Some men believed in the productive efficiency of man and his nature due to the discovery of natural laws. It was also felt by some that, these natural laws might also operate to determine human behaviour.

Influence of Contemporary Thinkers

They all accepted the fact that birth rate tends to outstrip death rate, which if unchecked will spell disaster to mankind. The ideal number and the surplus population will die of disease, hunger and war.

Assumptions

- Food is necessary to the existence of man
- Passion between sexes is necessary and will remain nearly in its present state

- There is direct relation between standard of living and child bearing
- Law of diminishing returns standard in agriculture.

Statement of the Theory

Malthus states, 'Population, when unchecked increases in a geometrical ratio. Subsistence increases only in an arithmetic ratio'.

According to him, 'The power of population is indefinitely greater than the power in the earth to produce subsistence for man'.

Disequlibrium Between Population and Food Supply

Since population increases in geometrical progression and the food supply in arithmetical progression, population tends to outrun food supply. As *Malthus* wrote, 'A perfectly happy and virtuous community will double every 25 years, but there can be no similar increase in their food. The best lands are taken up first then the inferior, at last the worst, at each stage the amount of food increases in slow arithmetical ratio, man himself increases in a quick geometrical ratio, unless want and vice stop him'. Thus an imbalance is created which leads to over population.

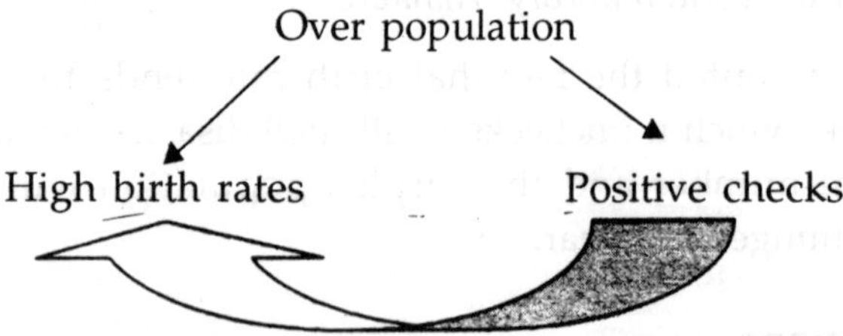

Control of Population

Two kinds of checks to correct the imbalance between population and food supply.

Positive Checks

The checks acts to increase the death rate like, famine, diseases, war, natural calamities, vicious customs with regard to women. *Malthus* felt that, 'The table of nature is laid for limited number of guests and those who come uninvited must starve'. He believed that the positive checks resulted basically from the pressure of population on subsistence. It brings about a short period equilibrium between population and food supply, which is disturbed sooner or later leading to the *Malthusian cycle*.

Over population → Positive checks → High birth rates→ Over population

Preventive Checks

These includes 1) Late marriages 2) Chastity (Pure), these are aimed at checking population growth deliberately.

Moral Restraint

Moral restraint with prudential postponement of early marriage until a family could be supported. According to *Malthus* the struggle for existence is an illustration of the wisdom of nature, which keeps poor people from becoming soft and lazy. He feels that celibacy is the only way out to escape the fury of positive checks. He advised women to remain unmarried till the age of 28.

Artificial Restraints

Malthus treated modern devices of birth control as sin. He believed that checks would never be sufficiently strong to eliminate the operation of the positive checks arising mainly from the pressure of population on subsistence man's sex passions and his material needs were results in essential conflict.

Subsistence Level of Wages

Malthus believed that population always tended to grow to a size, which would yield just barely subsistence, level of wages vice and misery would prevent population from increasing beyond subsistence. Moral restraint can result in restraining the population from growing more rapidly than wages.

Reliance on Diminishing Returns

The art of agriculture do not change, when capital and labour is successively increased by equal amounts of total output increases at a diminishing rate.

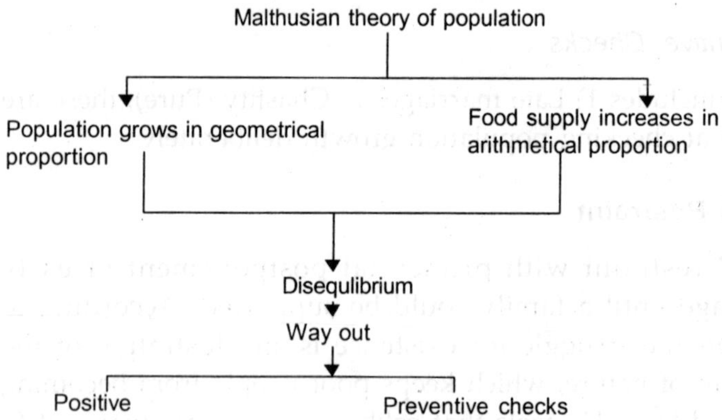

Criticism of the Malthusian Doctrine

1. The basic assumptions of the *Malthusian* theory are not correct.
   - Malthusian notion on food supply is based on a static economic law, i.e. the law of diminishing returns, *Malthus* could foresee the miracles technical progress over a period of time, which have stayed the law of diminishing returns. As a result of which food supply has increased much faster than the arithmetic progression.

- There is no direct relationship between sexual instinct and child bearing. Infact the desire to have children is a noble objective based on social, religious, geographical conditions, while the sex instinct is a base natural desire.
- The postulation that an improvement in standard of living leads to an increase in population is not borne out by facts. The greater the malnutrition, the more the fecundity and frenzy for breeding.
- The sexual urge is not same for all the individuals. It changed according to circumstances and the spread of education, nutrition, entertainment, etc. improved standard of living have resulted in a decline in sexual instinct.

2. The mathematical form of the theory is not correct. Food is produced more than arithmetical progression.
3. *Malthus* could not foresee the opening up of new area rapid improvement in the means of transport acted as a catalyst in the process.
4. History does not support the fear of *Malthus.*
5. Positive checks are not due to over population.
6. Every increase in population is not harmful. Up to the optimum level an increase in population should be welcomed as it will benefit the country to increase its per capita income rapidly.
7. Population is not related to food supply but to total wealth. *Malthusian* theory is based on a weak relationship between population and food supply. As a matter of fact the right relationship is between population and wealth. If a country is materially rich it can feed its millions well by importing food stuffs in exchange for its products or money.
8. Increase in population is the result of a decline in death rate.

Malthusian theory is one-sided. It takes the increase in population as the result of a rising birth rate, whereas population has grown considerably the world over due to decline in death rate. *Malthus* could not foresee the tremendous advancement of medical sciences, which have controlled fatal diseases and made human life longer. In India, *Malthusian* theory is said to operate.

9. Preventive checks do not mean moral restraint. *Malthus* could not imagine the modern duties of contraceptives; moral restraint alone cannot help to control the increase in population, which *Malthus* suggested.
10. *Malthus* failed to recognise the manpower aspect in population. He thought that every baby coming to the world is a burden on society. According to *Cannan*, 'A baby comes to the world not only with a mouth and a stomach but also with a pair of hands. It means that an increase in population means an increase in manpower which may tend to augment production'.
11. *Malthus* held the poor people responsible for their misery. According to *Malthus* the poor people tried to increase their number faster. But *Karl Marx* explained exploitation of labour, unequal distribution, defective Government policies, i.e. are responsible for the poverty of the mass.
12. *Malthus* adopted the inductive method in his principle. Inductive method cannot be of universal application.
13. *Malthus* has forgotten that times can change and when it takes place food production can also increase.
14. *According to Malthus*, every child born is a family will survive, but in communities where birth rate is high, death rate is also high.

Malthusian Theory and Its Application in India

1. *High rate of population growth:* Population increase rate is out stripping the growth in food supply in India every

year, even though food production is increased, it is not meeting the needs of the increased population.

2. Low level of food production in the country.
3. Positive checks are in operation. Thus equilibrium between food supply and birth rate alone does not prove the operation of *Malthus* doctrine. Recurring floods, disease also lends credence to his thesis.
4. Growing emphasis on family planning. Under family schemes, intense efforts are made to popularise the methods of birth control. This is positive proof of the influence of Malthusian doctrine.
5. Enactment of law. Statutory provision of minimum age at marriage and family size is an acceptance of the need to keep the Malthusian ghost at bay.
6. Law of diminishing returns. The traditional way of cultivation. The operation of the law of diminishing returns in many parts of the country is fact supporting the operation of Malthusian theory in India.
7. Rising tide of unemployment, low standard of living, high incidence of birth rate and death rate proves the validity of Malthus in India.
8. India has a very low per capita income. The slow growth in national income was eaten up entirely by the increase in numbers over the plan period.

Neo-Malthusianism

Neo-Malthusians belong to that group of economists and demographers who have blind faith in whatsoever Malthus said about growth of population. Neo-Malthusianism is a movement started by the followers of Malthus views. They believed in checking the growth of population without any restraint on unfettered sexual pleasures propagated their views with spiritual zeal. *Marie Stopes* of Britain and *Margaret Stanger* of America were prominent among the Neo-Malthusians.

Malthus and his followers treated artificial means of birth control as sin. They did not believe that the desire for sex pleasure and the desire for offspring were one and the same. They have adopted the stand that the social, religious and cultural attitudes of the people are rapidly changing and the desire to reduce the number of children in gaining approval everywhere.

The following factors have been cited to suggest their view:

1. Women would like to escape the pangs of births.
2. Many women have come to regard marriage and child bearing and rearing as a hindrance to their freedom.
3. Ladies would not like to have children because it will deform their body shape and make them unattractive.
4. The growing individualistic and happiness-seeking attitude militated against regimentation and family life.
5. The growing importance of state social security measures has provided sufficient guarantee against old age, which prompted many to remain unmarried and lead a care free life,
6. The declining of faith in religion is a positive factor, which reduced the importance of marriage and family life.

Differences Between Malthus and Neo-Malthusian were

1. Malthus did not see any difference between the desire for sex and the desire for children, whereas Neo-Malthusian felt that sex desire is natural whereas desire to procreate is based on religious, social and cultural considerations. The first is mere animal instinct, which arouse the most impetus of passions and is common to all men. The second is frequently social and religious in origin assuming different form according to time and place.
2. Malthus accepted that sex urge is natural, but he has advocated moral restraint, etc. and self-control. Neo-Malthusian believed that the urge of sex is natural, which should not be suppressed. Any attempt to check the sex

desire will create mental agony to the people. This will force people to adopt evil practices.

Malthus firmly believed that artificial means of birth control were wrong and amounted to sin. He observed the restraints recommended by him are pointed out by religion, but they are based upon moral restraints only.

3. Neo-Malthusian encouraged the use of contraceptives as human beings can satisfy their sexual desire without the risk of childbirth. They felt that all sections of the society require birth control. They argued that birth of children by unmarried mothers should be checked, as it will otherwise create evil consequence to society.

   A married woman can maintain her health, if she is not exposed to frequent child bearing. Population growth rate will be checked automatically and the nation will move towards prosperity.
4. Malthus believed that the tendency of population growth to outstrip food supply is a natural phenomenon. Neo-Malthusian held that the use of modern scientific means and methods it is possible to check population growth and increase food production in comparison to population.

Criticism of Neo-Malthusian Views

Critics felt that the use of contraceptives will lead to degeneration of women and create physical, mental and moral suffering. It will have deleterious social consequences, womanhood will be spared at the very source and result in many diseases among women. Extensive use of birth control may lead to the extermination of human race itself.

The Optimum Theory of Population

It is the product of reaction to the Malthusian theory of population. The theory taken into consideration the entire economic aspects related to population, economic conditions and tries to lay down desirable norms regarding population.

Optimum population refers to a state where the population is neither more nor less than the socially desirable level.

Origin and Development of the Theory

The credit for having introduced the term, 'Optimum' in the field of population and presenting the theory goes to *Prof. Edwin Cannan,* who published book 'Wealth' in 1924. The idea was popularised by *Robbins, Dalton and Carr Saunders.* It is concerned with the relation between the size of population and wealth production. It studies the population problem in the light of economic condition.

Assumptions of the Theory

- When the population grows the ratio between total population and working population remains the same
- Production per head of working population and the hours of work remain constant
- When at a point of time, the population of a country increases with that of natural resources, technical knowledge and capital do not change. So the law of diminishing returns begins to operate after some time.
- Population should be treated as labour force and every increase in the labour force affords an opportunity to exploit the material resources available in the country.

Definition

- 'The population at which the standard of life is a maximum is called the optimum population'—*Boulding KE*
- 'The optimum population is that which produces maximum economic welfare. It is same as maximum real income per head, for all practical purposes they may be taken as equivalent'—*Carr Saunders*
- 'At any given time (in a country) there is what may be called a point of maximum return when the amount of labour is such that both an increase and decrease in it would

diminish proportionate returns. On the other hand population is so great that the point has been passed, returns are again less than they might be and remedy is decreased in population'—*Prof Cannan*

Interpretation of the Optimum Population

Population is to be seen as the manpower required for exploitation of the natural resources and promote economic growth. As long as the optimum point is not reached the nation shall not be able to exploit the natural resources properly and fully. On the other hand, when the population crosses that point, then the nation would not get maximum return because the burden on the other resources will tend to be weary and become disproportionate. At the optimum point the resources are fully utilised which gives the ideal combination of factors of production. It also helps in suitable specialisation and division of labour. Consequently the national gross production and per capita income become highest. It is the point at which the external economics are fully utilised and the diseconomies have not set in.

According to *Prof Robbin*, 'the population, which just makes the maximum returns possible is the optimum population. Increase in population is desirable to the extent to which there is increase in production. Every increase in population is welcome according to *Robbins* as long as the people are engaged in some productive work.

Importance of Optimum Population Theory

Despite the difficulties in ascertaining a unique value of the optimum at any given time, the theory is asserted to have value in directing attention to the phenomenon of depressing effect of population growth on per capita income and the desirability of investigating the status of various industries in respect to increase or decrease returns.

The theory is important on the following counts:

1. It stresses the need to control the population and therefore it is useful to support the family planning programmes
2. Emphasis on changing the environment according to time and changing conditions to maintain the equilibrium of society and nation
3. Emphasises the need to increase the per capita income, which can contribute to the welfare of the citizens of a country.
4. Tries to establish earnest connection between population and economic progress.
5. It is an agent of production and points out neither over population nor under population will be beneficial for the country.
6. The theory is based on per capita income, which is scientifically based.
7. Has successfully countered the psychosis that man is a slave of his environment and showed that through judicious combination of factors of production, we can conquer our surroundings.
8. The approach is optimistic. It is devoid of hope and full of misery. In fact, man becomes master of his destiny since he can change the optimum by changing his own efficiency, techniques of production and stock of capital.
9. The theory has a leaning towards welfare economics because when determining the optimum number for a country welfare consideration.
10. There is stress on proper exploitation of natural resources and this approach is growth-oriented.
11. Is based on a forward-looking approach. Production should be increased by increasing the efficiency of the workers and a proper investment programme based on sound planning.
12. It is dynamic, the optimum number will keep on changing.

13. Has significance only in the context of over population. It can describe either type of maladjustment over-population or under-population.

Criticism of the Optimum Theory

It has considerably reduced the practical activity and value of the theory.

1. *There is evidence of optimum level:* It is impossible to measure the optimum level. Optimum population implies qualitative ideal population for the country. The quantitative aspect implies in addition to age, composition, physique, knowledge, intelligence, etc. these variables are subjected to change and are related to environment.
2. *Choice of criteria:* It involves considerations other than scientific also. However, scientific methods are used to clarify them, which is not practical.
3. *Per capita income cannot be correctly measured:* To find out the variation in per head income bristles with insurmountable difficulties. Often per capita income data is inadequate, misleading, unreliable, which make the concept of optimum is of doubtful validity.
4. *Theory ignores the distributional aspect of increase in per capita income:* It is not certain increase in population means increase in per capita income, an increase in wealth often leads to concentration of income in the hands of the few rich, which will create widespread disparity income distribution, which may prove harmful to the economy. Thus the optimum theory of population ignores the distributional aspect of increase in per capita income.
5. *The optimum population is a moving point:* The theory is static. The theory assumes that the stock of capital, natural resources, technique of production, etc. are constant, therefore what is optimum at a point of time may remain so far a period of time. But it is not correct to presume

so. When population varies in the world there is also concomitant variation in technology and organisation. As a result what may be optimum at a point of time might become less or more than the optimum over a period of time.

6. *Theory has no place in state policies:* Employment, output, etc. are sought to be increase with the help of fiscal and monetary policies, but optimum population was not referred to for policy use. Thus the theory has little practical utility.
7. *It is difficult to achieve in practice:* Achieving an optimum population through the exercise of available population policies as well as ascertaining the optimum present formidable difficulties.
8. *Theory neglects social and institutional conditions:* The theory takes into considerations economic factors, while social and institutional conditions in a country also influence the level of population. What is optimum from economic view may not be so from defence consideration of the country. Thus the theory is one-sided.
9. *The theory fails to explain the dynamics of population:* The theory merely helps in finding out the population at a point of time. But the theory does not tell us to why and how the population of the country increases or decreases. So it is not even desirable to call it as a population theory.
10. *The theory is purely materialistic:* It purely adopts materialistic outlook in which progress of society is measured in terms of per capita income. Wealth is not an end in itself, but it is only a means to an end.
11. Is impractical and unscientific
12. *The concept of optimum has been used in different sense:* Various writers have proposed different terms such as 'economic welfare' 'standard of living' 'real income' 'constant output' 'total realised desirability' 'economic optimum'.

Is Optimum Theory an Improvement over the Malthusian Theory?

- *Prof Malthus* has linked population growth with the availability of food or food supplies, whereas the authors of optimum theory linked population growth with natural resources, capital and production techniques
- *Malthus* considered every increase in population is harmful, whereas the optimum theory consider the population harmful only if it exceeds the optimum limit
- *Malthus* was a pessimist with a negative approach
- *Malthus* has concluded that the occurrences of natural calamities like floods, earthquakes. Optimum theory has adopted a realistic stand in this matter
- Optimum criteria have laid down the economically feasible population in the context of natural resources, capital stocks, and technique of production.
- *Malthus* failed to give a scientific assessment of the socially desirable quantities of population
- *Malthusian* theory finds ready application in backward and over populated countries, whereas the optimum theory could be applied to all types of countries whatever be the size of its population
- *Malthus* viewed population from the consumption angle, whereas the optimum theory considers the whole issues from the productive point of view. Every child born was treated as a burden on the available supply of the food. Optimum theory considers the population as addition to labour supply. *Malthus* theory is considered as a static equilibrium theory whereas the optimum theory is more dynamic and volatile
- *Malthus* harps on the theme of moral and religious codes in population theory. While the optimum theory is free from these ethical concepts and adopts a more rationalistic approach

- The optimum theory is more realistic. By taking decline in per capita income as the index of over population it recognises that over-population can exist even when it is not accompanied by the operation of positive checks like wars, epidemics.

Over-Population

'Man is fast becoming the cancer of earth'—*J Huxly*

Growth is a continuous process. Today's growth is a product of the past. It is also heritage of the future. Family of today is the result of the evolution of the desire for group life and satisfaction of basic human needs (companionship, love and sex).

Family is an organised social unit. Infants in it will enjoy, and needs the continuous care of parents. But the family now is not able to provide a conducive atmosphere for health and happiness, due to the increase in number of dependents.

When the crude death rate is subtracted from the crude birth rate the net residual is the current annual growth rate, which excludes migrating population.

It is said that, population growth rate is like trains; trains start slowly and gain momentum, once in motion it is difficult and takes sometime to bring the momentum under control. In the case of train, the limiting factors are mass and inertia, in the population limiting factors are:

- Age distribution
- Marriage customs, traditions
- Cultural activities
- Social and economic factors

The world population growth rate has shown a slight decline 1.7% (1991) from 1.92% (1970).

Growth rate is not uniform in the world, e.g: European countries less than 0.5% every year, Africa 3%, Latin America 2.3%, Asia 2.2%. These differences are due to fertility and mortality rate. Ninety five percent of population growth is occurring in developing countries. One-third of world population is under age of 15 and will soon enter the reproductive span giving more potential for population growth. The expected number of births per women at current fertility rates is:

Africa 6.1, Asia 3.2, Latin America 3.4, North America 2.0, Europe 1.6, India 2.3.

World population is currently growing at the following rates:

176 per minute, 10,564 per hour, 253, 542 per day, 92, 543,000 per year. Every 2 seconds a baby is born in India.

Rapid population growth is the major facts of the era. Its relationship with poverty, malnutrition, illiteracy and political instability are well known.

Population problems has many facets.

- Those of numbers
- Those which relate to the biological quality
- Those of individual community.

Can this finite Globe with the unlimited population growth and a limited possibility of food supplies is the problem of the day.

Rapid Population Growth and Its Impact

Rapid population growth is a major fact of our era, its association in poverty, malnutrition, illiteracy and political instability are well known. The rapid rates of population growth are leading to rapid increase in number of the ill fed with poor houses. This population problem is one of the most fundamental of all human relations. It affects every aspect of human life, individual, national and international health and happiness of individual, families and social progress of nation and international peace.

Population problems have many facets, e.g: Those of numbers and those which relate to biological quality and those of the individual and community.

This is a finite Globe on which men has to satisfy his two universal demands for standing room and food which are positively limited, i.e. today on this finite Globe, the unlimited potentialities of reproduction and limited possibilities of food supplies is the main problem. Over population means too many people in relation to which set of facts or sum of resources of all kinds.

The reason for the growth of population are:

1. Decline in the death rate due to control on infant mortality rate.
2. Control of famine, improved medicine and health facilities and advancement of science and technology.
3. High birth rate is due to universality of marriages, the average age of is as low as 15 years and results in high fertility.
4. Dependency ratio, 42% below 15 years and 8% above 55 years of age, influences rate of savings and investment. Sixty percent of births are from 1st, 2nd, 3rd order of birth. About 22 million children are born annually. Forty percent births are of 4th and high order of birth, which is leading to larger families due to high fertility. Hence 50% of population are depending on the working population.
5. There are 110 million couples in the country and every year 5.5 new couples are added up, whereas only 2.5 million of couples die or cross the age of fertility thereby there is an addition of 3 million couples of the existing couples. So unless 3 million couples limit their family with 2 children, the growth of the population cannot be controlled.
6. Indian people are superstitious, fatalistic, prejudiced and ignorant. They think that it is a sin to prevent the birth of a child and that their religion does not permit this practice. Family planning, many people of the opinion that the use of contraceptive is injurious to health.

7. Among the poor people large families imply more working hands and larger family income. The level of literacy among the poor being very low, their children are driven to work at a comparatively large in number. Parents get returns without much investment from these children's earnings. Thus the low wage structure of the parents combined with wide prevalence of child labour contributes to increase in the population.
8. High infant morbidity and mortality rates also induce the parents to produce more children.
9. Poverty or economic backwardness.
10. Ignorance of couple about hazardous effects of over population.
11. Illiteracy.
12. Lack of insufficient opportunity for employment, no other entertainment. The only recreation with out any expenditure is more sexual contact or enjoying in libido leads to more births without leaving gap between pregnancies.
13. Lack of sufficient nutrients in the body.
14. Migration.
15. Political instability.
16. Urbanisation, industrialisation, mechanisation.

In India population is growing at the rate of 16 million per annum, adding population of Australia every year. That means one Australia is added to India and size of Australia is 3 times bigger than India. If it goes on, it crosses the Soviet Union population, which has an area six times that of India.

India is the first country to adapt family planning as an official programme in 1952. Our five-year plans were structured to meet the challenge of growing of numbers. The task of enlightening people in ways of utilisation of family planning has taken up by government and made available the public at cheap rates. Despite these efforts, however no appreciable decrease in the birth rate is observed.

Evil effects/Consequences of Over Population

Population Growth and National Income

An excessively rapid growth of population in India imposes a heavy strain on our economy, it calls for large investments in new means of production and in social and economic infrastructure and tends to aggregate the existing scarcity of capital for development projects.

The development process becomes all the more strenuous when a country's resources—natural and mineral become increasingly scarce relative to the size of population and its consumption requirements.

The national income of India since independence has been growing at an average rate of 3.5% per annum. But the per capita income during the same period has crept up by only 1.5% per annum. What ever is achieved, in terms of economic growth is neutralised by rising number of population. In 1985, the world development report rightly observes that, 'A war on poverty would simply have to be a war on population'. If the growth in population is not checked we shall soon be faced with slums with underfed and under clothed children dwelling in these slums. Low standard of living due to increase in population and no commensurate increase in national income, every one receives poor share of income.

Changes in the Environment

Soil

Population pressure on means of subsistence. Due to deforestation there is less rain, soil erosion, lack of green pastures. The continued increase of population without any corresponding outlet in employment has only intensified the pressure on the land. The density of population in India is 324 per sq. km. The land-man ratio in general is bad or it is worse when we consider population in relation to agriculture land. The pressure on the land is reflected in steady increase in the number of agricultural labourers. In agriculture we are among the countries with lowest yield per hectare.

Exploration of Coal and Other Minerals

Exploration is going to exhaust all the underground resources within 100 years.

Air Pollution due to Industrialisation

With advanced technology and mechanisation rapid evolution of industrialisation the harmful gases like carbon monoxide and other gases, chemical like nitric acid, fertilizer plants pollutes the environment and thereby leading to more respiratory diseases.

Use of motorcars, machines as petroleum products resulting in liberation of carbon dioxide and carbon monoxide due to which longevity of life is reduced.

Water Pollution

Effluents from various factories is liberated into the rivers, which will have poisonous substances subsequently consumed by the fish, which in turn affect the human beings when they consumed. Presence of oil facts in the water is leading to lack of oxygen and thereby no life in the riverbeds. Increase in consumption of water due to over population may lead to scarcity of water.

Educational Facilities

We are not in a position to meet the demand of population even though ample number of school and colleges are increased. Qualities of educational standards are going down.

Food Problem

There is a big gap between supply and demand. In India each person consumes about 800 grams of food grains and for 1 billion of population the production of grains is not meeting the demand. In the process of economic development income elasticity of demand for food goes up. According to *Malthus theory* of population, 'population increase in geometrical progression and food production increases in arithmetical progression'. Therefore population will always tend to out run available subsistence.

In some countries (Japan) both the density of population and the rate of population growth are high but food production is also very high. The main reason is that the development of science and technology enabled the people to raise food output commensurate with the increase in the population.

The problem of food storage is faced by under developed countries, as they failed to improve agricultural technology fast enough to respond for the challenge of rapidly growing population. Indian government faced high food drain economy, we are importing food from other countries, which has been a constant strain on our slender foreign exchange resource base. Our rising population has kept the per capita availability of cereals almost stable imports of food grains have increased steadily, and productivity indices presents a sad tale.

Twenty to twenty five percent of population within Asian region exists in diets deficient in proteins and calories; more communicable diseases due to over crowding, poor sanitation, unequal distribution of health services.

Population and Unemployment

Rapid population growth without corresponding increases in the level of economic development lead to a large-scale unemployment in urban areas and disguised unemployment in rural areas.

In underdeveloped countries, jobs do not increase the complementary resources particularly capital are not available.

Low income, reduced savings, retarded investment hamper capital formation and increasing job avenues for the raising population are not available. New employment opportunities are essentially problems of capital accumulation and growth. This would generate a high level of economic activity and create new employment potential.

The existence of population pressures makes it extremely difficult for underdeveloped country to absorb the increase in labour force in gainful employment. The existence of population pressures makes it extremely difficult to absorb the increase in labour force in gainful employment; it is Herculean task for underdeveloped countries. Employment is a part of growth process so step by step with growth and development the country has to be taken from the low level of employment to a higher level. Unemployment problem leads to low standard of living and prevents economic growth.

Inflation

Scarcity of commodities leads to increase in price. Production is inproportionate demand hence there are no savings.

Population and the Burden of Unproductive Consumers

The existence of a relatively larger proportion of population in the lower age group and low expectancy in under developed countries, constitutes a drag on the productive effect of the economy.

Need for Population Control

In the world, the economic, social, cultural patterns are changing day-by-day. To maintain quality-of-life criteria, to raise the standard of living, to provide basic consumption, i.e. food, shelter, clothing, education, medical care, to control anti-social behaviour, to reduce social problems like theft, robberies, to prevent over-crowding, to change the attitude of people towards large family size, to overcome deep rooted religious customs, beliefs, attitudes practices favouring larger families, fatalistic attitude, fear about God, children are assets to the family and dependency hence utilisation of family planning services; to stimulate social change affecting fertility, e.g: Increasing the age at marriage, women status, education, employment opportunities, social security, accelerating economic changes to increase per capita income, economic development is best contraceptive. Intensity of information, education and communication programs has to be increased in order to improve the awareness of people about the need of population control.

- Raise the age at marriage has to be enforced
- Legislative enactment in parliament
- Strong disincentives for family of more than three kids in public and private sector
- Less stringent over abortion law
- Mass-media has to be used extensively to propagate small family norm
- Government has to inspire the professionals by giving awards, incentives for the excellent performance in the family welfare activities
- Religious leaders has to come forward to advice small family norms in the large interest of the nation.

Previous Years University Questions

1. Explain the causes of over population in India. (10 m, RGUHS, 2000)
2. Malthusian theory. (2 m, RGUHS, 1997, 2000, 03)
3. What is meant by population density. (2 m, RGUHS, 2002)
4. Describe the characteristics of Indian population growth. (5 m, RGUHS, 2004)
5. Social consequences of population explosion. (2 m, RGUHS, 2001)

6. Malthusian theory of population. (5 m, RGUHS, 2000)
7. Discuss the social causes of population explosion. What are its effects on health. (10 m, RGUHS, 1999)
8. Malthusian theory. (2 m, RGUHS, 2001)
9. Define Malthusian theory. How is it applicable in the Indian population. (5 m, RGUHS, 2002)
10. Explain the concept 'population explosion'. (2 m, RGUHS, 2003)
11. What is age pyramid. (2 m, RGUHS, 2003)
12. Housing and health. (2 m, RGUHS, 1999)
13. Define population explosion. Describe about the methods to prevent this problem in our country. (19 m, NTRUHS, 1999)

MGR University Question Papers

1. Population explosion. (5 m, MGRU)
2. Culture and civilisation. (5 m, MGRU)

CHAPTER FOURTEEN

Community

INTRODUCTION

Community is an organised social life of a locality. We can observe the social relationships within the community. People develop attachment and sentimental identification with the area in which they live and belongs gives rise 'we feeling', ethnocentrism. It represents the common interests of the group community sometimes refers to entire humanity.

Definition

- 'A social group with 'we feeling' and 'living in a given area'—*Bogardus*
- 'The smallest territorial group that can embrace all aspects of social life'—*Kingsley Devis*
- 'An area of social living marked by some degree of social coherence'—*RM Maciver*
- 'A group or collection of groups that inhabits a locality'—*Ogburn and Nimkoff*
- 'Group of people who live and belong together and share whole set of interests'—*Manheim*
- 'A human population living within a limited geographic area and carrying on a common interdependent life'—*Ludnberg*

Meaning

A group of people inhabiting in a given geographic area, sharing a common way of life, working together for certain ends, aware that they belong to the community as well as the larger society. People will have common interest and activities united together with common living patterns and organised social life.

An individual rarely exists alone, he is linked in many ways to his fellow beings, establishes relationship near to him in a definite part of the territory. They will develop social like-mindedness and will have common social ideas, traditions and the sense of belongingness. The social life of the people is affected by the kind of community in which they live.

Elements of Community (Characteristics)

Locality

A community is a territorial group. It occupies defined geographical area. They reside in that locality. Community is locally limited. People will develop social contacts, provides safety, security and protection. Community promotes the people to fulfill their common interests and needs. People possess a strong bond of social solidarity. Locality is a basic factor for community life. Transport and communication facilities will be concentrated for a specific community. The community includes the physical factors like fertile soil, minerals, forests, fisheries, vegetation, resources, climate, etc. community provides peace, protection, common culture and social system.

Community Sentiment

'A feeling of belonging together/we feeling'. People will stay together, share their common interests and be conscious of their unity. People will be identified by their own group, which promotes sense of awareness, living and sharing; developing bondage among the members. In modern times this community sentiment is slowly going down as people may not have a common interest and a common outlook; hence attachment among the members is gradually changing as they belongs to complex nature of society.

Group of people

Groups of people share the basic conditions of common life. Group members can act collectively in an organised manner.

Permanency

Includes permanent group life in definite place community is relatively stable.

Naturality

Community is established in a normal and natural way, they are not made or created by an act of will or by planned efforts. Individuals become members of the group by birth. Community is spontaneous in their origin but not a sudden or automatic existence. The community life is comprehensive.

Likeness

Language, practices, customs, traditions, folkways, mores are common. People share the common way of life and works through customs and traditions.

Wider Ends

People associate not for the fulfillment of a particular end, they are natural and wider but not an artificial. The membership of community is of wide significance.

Particular Name

Each community will have its own specified name indicating the reality in individuality and describes the total personalities.

Legal Status

Community has no legal status.

Size of Community

The term community is used in a relative sense. There are bigger or wider communities, which includes small community like villages, towns, cities, tribes, etc.

Regulation of Relations

A bundle of rules, regulations, customs, traditions, institutions defines and shapes the members. In the rural community informal means of social control is observed like customs, folkways, rituals, mores and beliefs whereas in urban community formal means of social control (e.g: Laws, police, court, armed forces, etc.) is observed.

Dependency

An individual in community is physically dependent on community for fulfillment and satisfaction of physical needs. Psychologically also he is dependent on community as it save from isolation and solitude.

Types

Three-fold classification which is more or less universally accepted.

Urban Community

People living in towns and cities mainly depending on non-agricultural occupations.

Rural Community

People living in villages mainly depending on agriculture and other allied occupations.

Tribal Community

Living in tribal areas, away from the area of influence of civilisation.

Benefits of Community Life

- Provides the individual needed security and protection
- It strengthens the unity among people
- Provides for cooperation among the members. It encourages collective forces (efforts) for fulfillment of community's needs
- Depends on communication system among the members
- Provides the individual with opportunities for the expression of his talents, abilities and personality development
- Provides sense of belongingness
- Community life has its own conflicts and contradictions for the individual. Certain times community life has tensions, clashes due to anti-social tendency of man.

Differences Between Society and Community

Community	Society
Consists of a group of individuals	Web of relationships
Concrete	Abstract
A well defined geographical area is necessary	May not be necessary to have a defined geographical area
More than one society in a community	More than one community
Community sentiment or unity indispensable	Sentiments is not essential
Common objectives are not so extensive and coordinated	Common objectives are coordinated and extensive
Common agreement of interests and objectives are necessary	Common interest will not pay much attention

RURAL COMMUNITY

Introduction

Major portion (74.28%) of our nation belong to rural area and it is the back-bone of the country. Villages are dominating the

Indian way of life. The basic elements of our social structure are the villages, joint family system and caste system. Study of Indian society invariably leads us to the study of villages.

'Rural' word is derived from 'ruralis' means village or town.

Bogardus says, 'Human society has been cradled in the rural group'. The rural society is synonymously called as 'Agrarian society'.

Definition of Village

'People living in a limited physical area who have common interests and common ways of satisfying them'.

'It is a cluster of people living within a narrow territorial radius who share a common way of life'—*AW Green*

Definition of Rural Community

'A group of people depending on agriculture and allied occupations, permanently residing in a geographic area and participating in common socio-economic and cultural activities'.

'Systematic study of rural social organisation, its structure, function and evolution'.

'People who are staying together and living on dispersed farmsteads and in a village which forms the centre of their common activities'—*Dwight Sanderson*

'Social interaction of people and their institutions in the local area the relationships are primary (intimate) in nature'.

'A group of people permanently residing in a definite geographic area who are having community consciousness, i.e. cultural, social and economic relations feel that they are separate from other communities'—*JH Kolb and Brunner*

Meaning (Village Community)

People who are living in a limited physical area, who have common interests and common ways in dealing and satisfying with them. Physical locality, psychological bonds, proximity, sociability encourages solidarity and are mutuality. Rural localities are often referred as 'country neighbourhood'. Rural life has preceded the urban life. It is well known stated fact that 'God made the village and man built the society'.

Rural Community in India: Characteristics of Village or Rural Community

1. *Agricultural occupation:* The main occupation of the rural community is agriculture and allied activities like animal husbandry, poultry, and small enterprises like bee-keeping and fishing.
2. *Natural environment:* Villages have natural set-up. Animals, birds, river, ponds and all other natural things are found in the village. This natural atmosphere enables the rural people to have simple and natural life style too.
3. *Small size:* The village communities are small in size. There may be a few household or small number of people.
4. *Low density of population:* As the villages have large areas of land for cultivation the number of inhabitants is small.
5. *Homogeneity:* The village life has much homogeneity, people of village have common occupation and common style of life. The people of a village share the same customs, traditions and values.
6. *Low mobility:* Mobility means movement of; transition of; people from one place to another or from one social status to another. That is there are physical as well as social mobility. In village, low social mobility is observed, they don't like to change frequently from one place to other place.
7. *Less social differentiation and stratification:* Stratification is based on caste system. In Indian villages there is much differentiation.
8. *Primary group relation:* The rural communities, especially of smaller types, have primary group relationship. The

village is like a large family. Everyone is known personally and the members of the rural community have familistic relation.

Changes in Indian Rural Life

Today Indian villages are undergoing a fast change. The process of industrialisation, urbanisation, modernisation, universalisation of education, etc., has changed the mode of village life. The gap between rural and urban is now-a-days reducing due to advancement in electricity, science, technology, education, modern medicine, transportation and communication,etc. have reached the villages to a large extent.

The facilities like community centres, public reading rooms, libraries, primary health centres, post offices, study centres, schools were developed. Modern trends are giving villages new opportunities to become more progressive and prosperous.

Factors Responsible for Changes in Rural India

1. Occurrence of natural calamities like floods, famines, earthquake.
2. Population increase, industrialisation and urbanisation, communication, national movement, political parties and leaders, ruralites working in urban can be considered as carriers of social change
3. Planned efforts by the Government.
4. Several voluntary organisations.
5. Poverty, unemployment and other socio-economic problems.

It is rather difficult to point out all that is going on in Indian villages as changes patterns but it may be possible for us to cite a few under:

1. Change in rural marriage and family
   - Although child marriages still prevalent, yet, there are educated who get married after attaining adulthood

- Large joint families are changing into smaller ones or nuclear families
- The authority of the father as the head of the family is changing in families, mainly in educated group
- Status of women also changing because of education.

2. Change in economic life
   - At least some villagers have taken to scientific agriculture. The introduction of electricity in rural areas has facilitated change in the mode of agriculture
   - Traditional occupations solely on the basis of caste are also undergoing change
   - Pattern of housing, the style of dress, the types of food consumed and the types of utensils used in the house are also changing.
3. Social life changes
   - The hold on caste and untouchability is on the decline
   - Though inter-dinning of different castes, especially upper and lower castes is difficult, social interaction is present
   - Rate of literacy is increasing due to the introduction of primary schools in many villages
   - Scheduled castes and tribals are receiving help from the Government in order to improve their socio-economic conditions.
4. Political changes
   - Villagers have greater consciousness and they do take part in elections
   - Party-based election was not known in the villages previously, but now villagers are aware of the same
   - Rural leadership is becoming more and more important, it is through them that we can bring about changes in rural communities.

Hazards of Ruralities (Problems of Villages)

The villages are no longer preserving their self-sufficiency and autonomy. The ruralities are also facing several problems.

- People do not opt for change, the practice of using traditional unscientific system of cultivation. Due to illiteracy and ignorance of advanced agricultural operations results in poor yield in crops
- Lack of irrigation facilities and dependence on nature for water always; inadequate supply of electricity, famines, etc., are unfavourable factors for good crops
- Sub-division and fragmentation of land holdings, heavy load on land
- Burden of loans, Indian farmers take hand-loans, bank loans to meet the agriculture needs
- Landless labourers are migrating to urban areas and going for alternate occupations
- Defective marketing system—farmers are feeling that they are not getting the right value for their products, exploitation of villagers are observed
- Lack of transportation and communication facilities causes extreme difficulty in taking the products to the markets
- Effects of natural disasters like floods, famines; leads to poverty and unemployment
- Extravagancy—non-essential items of expenses such as festivals, marriages, pilgrimages and ceremonies
- Exploitation by the elite groups—villagers often exploited by money-lenders, officials, and rich farmers.

Family System

- Increase in population
- Unemployment
- Low educational standard
- Lack of civic amenities like basic medical facilities, electricity, transportation and communication
- Inefficient functioning of the rural administrative bodies like Panchayat systems
- Evil habits are practiced like smoking, alcoholism, fraud, cheating.

Health Hazards

- The birth rate and death rate are higher in the rural community
- In times of disease or ill-health, people prefer to go to places of worship, witchcraft than to a medical official leading to poor utilisation of health care
- The health-care professionals identified certain reasons commonly for non-utilisation or poor utilisation of health care services were: Related to logistics, socio-cultural causes, ignorance, lack of transportation facilities; illiteracy; negligence.

Remedial Measures to Overcome Rural Problems

The socio-economic progress of the nation depends upon the progress of the villages. Scientific method of investigations has to be conducted to find out the ways of dealing or attacking the problems. Identify the strategies to overcome the problems. Government has undertaken various development and welfare programmes like establishing rural development branch in all universities, conducting systematic studies on activities related to rural welfare. It is essential on the part of the rural sociologists and rural economists to conduct extensive systematic and comprehensive studies on problems of villages and identify the solutions for attacking the problems.

Develop right attitudes among the ruralities towards higher education of children, healthy child rearing practices, promotion of sanitation, health, communal harmony, civil rights and responsibilities.

Agriculture Development

Better farming, re-distribution of land, development of poultry, and cottage industries.

Development of Supportive Occupations

For example: Handicrafts, weaving, and pottery.

Rural Development Programmes

The concept of rural development is based on "Developmentalism' according to which the entire village community must be involved in determining the direction of development and also in the distribution of its benefits—*Haripad, R Subramania Iyer, 1993*.

Rural development programmes can be executed successfully only through the active involvement of local people and various functioning departmental agencies. Coordinating among different agencies is essential for making rural development, a reality one.

Phases in rural development are growth, alleviation of poverty by sound economic planning, equality, rural development helps to liberate the energies of the rural people, especially the poor, it raises their full potential and thus improve their capacity as well as commitments to development, organise and govern themselves and the attainment of qualitative life for the individual and for the entire community—*Raj D Sunder, 2000.*

Goals

- 'Integrated and balanced sectoral, spatial and societal development'.

We need to generate resources for rural development through a self-help development process with equity and justice in order to achieve a decentralised, bottom-up process with wide participation.

- To derive maximum benefits from accelerated socio-economic growth and development efforts
- Community participation in decision-making process, e.g: Planning, formulation, implementation, monitoring, evaluation and sharing are the benefits of rural development
- Five-year plan.

Some of the rural developmental programmes which implementation in our nation are:

- Community development programme
- Minimum needs programme
- National extension services
- National adult education programme
- Integrated rural development programme (IRDP)
- Intensive area agriculture programme
- Training of rural youth for self-employment
- National rural development programme
- Development of women and children in rural areas (DWACRA)
- Rural landless employment guarantee programme
- Rural health education
- Family welfare services
- Fixing minimum wages for the labourers
- Better marketing facilities
- Implementation of Prohibition Act
- Redistribution of land
- Rural electrification
- Implementation of social security schemes.

URBAN COMMUNITY

Introduction

Urban community/City community/Civilised society are the terms which are used synonymously. Man built the city and the city in turn made civilised man. City is the product of man and his achievement. It holds both hope and despair. The phenomenon 'change' is observed in urbanisation, the conceptions of efficiency, increased human and spatial interaction and extraordinary complexities of social relationships.

Urbanisation is the spatial dimension of industrial and technological revolution or economic and social development in general. It is a process of becoming urban moving to cities changing from agriculture to other pursuits common to cities and corresponding basic changes in the thinking and behaviour patterns. Urbanisation involves in bringing changes in their social values. Increasing proportion of the population lives in urban localities.

Definition

- 'City is a limited geographic area, inhabited by a largely and closely settled population having many common interests and institutions under a local Government authorised by the state'—*Howrad Woolston (Metropolis)*
- 'A mere collection of individuals and of social convenience, a body of customs and traditions, a state of mind and the organised attitudes and sentiments'—*Park (The City)*
- 'A phenomenon of specialisation, a population aggregate whose occupations are non-agricultural'—*James A Quinn (Urban Sociology)*
- 'Large, dense and permanent settlement of socially heterogeneous individuals'—*Lowis Wirth (Urbanism as a way of life)*
- 'Ecologically speaking urbanism has a demographic and mechanical, technical base viz., a dense aggregate of individuals whose life, career and labour are oriented to the predetermined rhythm and tempo of machinery and the pressure of vast complicated structure and finance, which control mass standardised production'—*Radhakamal Mukherji*

Features of Urban Community

Namelessness

The inhabitants of a city do not come into primary contact with each other. They meet and speak without knowing each other's name, superficial, mechanical, manners of politeness and mutual convenience evolve in the city.

The city dweller treats the strangers as animated machines, rather than as human beings. A citizen may live for several years in a city and may not know the names of neighbourhood who live in the same city area.

Urban contacts are segmental. Institutional norms are not effective in controlling or regulating their social behaviour. Urbanities do not have a feeling of sense of belongingness to any one group or community.

Homelessness

The house problem in a big city is very acute. Many low class people pass their nights on the road pavements. The middle class people have but insufficient accommodation, a room or two and that too in 6th or 7th floor. The child does not get any play space.

Class Extremes

In a city, richest as well as poorest people will be found, the people rolling in luxury and living in grand mansion as well as the people living on pavements and hardly getting two meals a day. The best form of ethical behaviour and the worst racketeering are to be found in cities. Superior creativeness and chronic unemployment are alike urban features.

Social Heterogeneity

City has brought together people from the ends of the earth because they are different and thus useful to one another, variety of groups, each representing a typical culture. The personal traits, the occupations, the cultural life and the ideas of the members of the urban community. In cities we find multiplicity of cultures.

Social Distance

Social contacts are impersonal, segmented, formal politeness takes the place of genuine friendliness. Urbanites become night dwellers, not neighbours.

Energy and Speed

People with ambition work at a tremendous speed, day and night, which stimulate others also to work similarly. Stimulation and inter-stimulation are endless. People indulge in too many activities and inconceivable efforts which ultimately affects their energies. Urban life produces greater emotional tensions and insecurity than does rural life. Cities may be called as consumers of population.

Secondary Control

In urban areas the individual's behaviour is controlled by police, law, courts, etc. but not by family, caste or religion.

Social Mobility

The social status of an individual is determined not by heredity, but by his works and economic status. In cities, social mobility is allowed, a man can achieve as much progress as he wishes according to his intelligence and efforts. Inter-caste marriages are allowed in cities.

Voluntary Associations

People are very firm and insist about their rights. As education and literacy are widespread in cities, the city dwellers are individualistic and think rationally about political and social matters and form their own opinions. They are not orthodox and traditionalists, therefore new associations are formed.

Individuality

On account of voluntary associations and secondary control the city dwellers develop a personality of their own. They are compelled to fashions. They are individualistic, egoistic and selfish.

Lack of Community Feeling

As the urbanities are bust in their individual matters, they have no time to think about others, I feeling is greater in urbanities.

Lack of Unity in the Family

In cities, each member in the family is so busy with their own programmes that they do not interfere with each other's independence.

Moral Laxity

Since there is no control over the individuals, sex is fairly high in urban area. On account of the lack of community feeling, homogeneous family, western influence and an atmosphere of luxury and comfort prevailing in the cities moral laxity results.

Unbalanced Personality

A combination and mixture of untrue facts, looseness in character, morals, artificial environment and the influence of motion pictures and other means of entertainment, high ambition, lustful desires have resulted in providing unbalanced personality of city dwellers.

Rationalism

People think in rationalised manner, analytically react, exhibit his behaviour.

Dynamism

Norms, occupations, way of life, everything in urban areas are subjected for change, mobility phenomena is observed in urban society which is dynamic.

Segmentation

Division and sharing of work, delegation of authority and segmentation of responsibility because of specialisation.

Bureaucratic Organisation

Prevalence of bureaucratic society in urban areas occupies a ranked status in the nation. The bureaucrats don't know each other.

Interpersonal Relationship

Functional, secondary, impersonal relationship exists. After the work completes they may not pay attention to continue the relationship. Many people may not be knowing even their neighbour particulars; by virtue of its size, the city cannot be a primary group.

Size of Population

Greater ranges of individuals vary in their personal traits occupations, cultural life, ideas and attitudes constitute large size of population.

Density of Population

Increase in size of population over a limited area increases its density and produces differentiation and specialisation as a necessary condition for survival, where increased diversification, competition are observed. No emotional ties foster a spirit of exploitation, tension and frustration, etc. are the causes for occurrence of social problems.

Urban Influence on Rural Societies

In India the influence of urban life can be clearly seen in rural society due to urban contact. The influence is evident in such aspects like;

- Family
- Food habits
- Standard of living
- Dress
- Customs
- Believes
- Traditions
- Changing social life, e.g: Caste system-caste occupations diverting to skill persons. Increased comforts reaching to rural areas like restaurants, milk pockets, etc. Caste system slowly giving a part to class system.
- Change in family organisation like selective marriages, nuclear families.
- Changing agriculture techniques like mechanisation.

Growth in Cities

The cities are represented only relative small proportion of the population. The lives of the majority of population predominantly shaped by the rural community. The massive growth of population shift of significant proportion of population to urban areas is a salient feature in urban areas. Industrial revolution caused a demand for a large number of workers as centralised location. Political factors, the cities are the centres of attraction, the training centres for military, defence production, economic centres which predominate in trade or commerce, industrial towns are places with factories, religious cities are those where people visit on pilgrimage and even though more number of educational centres are growing but, even then they are unable to meet the educational needs of children, where 15% of population constitutes. Cities raised living standards significantly, enhanced productive specialisation, efficient transportation system, job opportunities, decentralisations of activities. Industrial revolution, agricultural revolution, communication facility, political factors, security, municipality facility, favourable climate, cultural centres, means of entertainment, art centres, business centres, etc. are some of the causes of growth and development of cities in India.

City Community in India

Certain peculiar traits of the cities in India is as follows:

1. Relatively smaller proportion of the Indian population is urban. According to the Indian census every 10 years, hardly 1/5 th of the Indian population is urban. Thus India is still rural in nature.
2. There are different types of cities in India on the basis of size there are big metropolitan cities like Mumbai, Kolkatta, Delhi, Chennai. There are some small cities and towns like Ujjain, Gwalior, Truvananthapuram. Besides, there are different types of cities in India on the basis of their function. For instance, we have capital cities like Delhi, Hyderabad, Bhopal, and some religious cities like Banaras, Ujjain, Nasik there are industrial cities Bhilai.
3. Indian cities are problematic; our cities have large number of problems like over-crowding, slums, poverty, crimes, delinquency, beggary, prostitution. These problems make the life of the urban man unhappy.
4. Unplanned nature of cities; most of the Indian cities are developed in an unplanned and haphazard manner. That is why there are problems exist.
5. Scene of cultural lag; the urban man has not yet learned to adjust with the urban environment. This is because of several factors like population explosion, rural-urban migration, lack of education and enlightenment, heterogeneity of the city dwellers, pressure of old customs, traditions, folkways, mores and values.
6. Most of the industries, commercial enterprises, centres of higher education are located in urban cities. Thus the entire population around the city has to come for some work or the other. So, Indian cities need planning, re-planning and reorganisation.

Hazards of Urbanisation

Causes

Migration: Wider opportunities for employment, varied exposures for different courses in education will attract the people to migrate to cities, where they believe that their desires will be fulfilled.

Industrial growth: Rapid industrialisation, additional jobs, overcrowding, poor housing, slums formation and polluted environment.

Apathy of Government: State Governments also put many restrictions on local authorities in raising necessary funds for dealing with specific urban problems.

Defective town planning: Growing sense of helplessness of our planners and administrators.

Vested interest forces: It works against people but enhance commercial interests and profits.

Problems

Family Disharmony

In urban area, chances for the occurrence of family disorganisation are more, as urbanites are individualistic, mechanical in nature. They will be concentrating more for their own development and fulfillment of job responsibilities unable to spare their time for their own family and having materialistic nature leads to family disintegration.

Housing and Slum Formation

Due to majority of population are migrating, attracted towards urbanisation, houselessness is a serious problem. Overcrowding, minimum level of residential accommodation is resulting into the formation of slums, scarcity of health and family welfare services, total absence of minimum level of residential accommodation. Pathetic conditions are observed in slum areas.

Depersonalisation

High density of population, apathy, over-crowding has deleterious effects, deviant behaviours, arising of community riots, indifferent of opinions leads to occurrence of psychiatric disorders, where individuals are more subjected to internal disequilibrium.

Potable Water Supply

Due to increased concrete jungles in the cities, the ground water level depleted leading to severe water crisis.

Drainage

Unplanned growth of urbanisation and improper sanitation leads to poor drainage facilities.

Transport and Traffic

Majority of population uses public transport and due to increase in urban population both public and private transport vehicles increased tremendously, which increases traffic and the road transport has not developed adequately to accommodate the increased vehicular growth, noise pollution also resulted.

Power Shortage

With new technologies coming every day and these require electricity supply to operate and simultaneously the production is able to meet the demands, leading to power crisis.

Psychosocial Aspects of Urbanisation

Rapid influence of urbanisation in big cities, the traditional patterns of life, the cultural uniformity, beliefs, social relations, family behaviour, etc. tend to be broken it accelerated social change. Social, family and personal disorganisation; small family norm is observed. Slowly the traditional joint family system is disintegrating. Urbanism is a social system of superficial, transitory human relations, groups and institutions characterised by high physical and social mobility and interchangeability, isolation of economic and other interests and social alignment is based on power.

Psychologically, urbanisation is a system of ideas, attitudes, ideals marked by formal, objective, specific standards which will fit into technology, rapid tempo of life, little provision for personal, emotional, self expression and hence it accompanies individual and social irritation, excitement and strive, struggle for existence, survival of the fittest phenomena commonly observed.

A city is a system of culturally related institutions, groups, which can persist interaction and interchange among individuals with the quest for knowledge, experiences, entertainment and other satisfaction are the motivational factors in urbanisation.

Caste identity is diminishing in urban areas, urbanites participates in networks which includes persons of several castes. Individual orientation, achievement are significant factors. More incidences of inter-caste and inter-religious marriages are observed.

Women status is high, educated, liberal, working equally on par with men. Sharing economic, social responsibilities at families. Higher age marriage is increased in urban community. Divorce, remarriage are the new phenomena among urban women. Politically also urban women are more active, the women candidates reservations is increased in parliament. Urban women is independent, enjoys greater freedom than the rural women. Employment opportunities, wider opportunities, fulfillment of desires in fulfilling individual's desires, aspirations are more in urban areas. Easy access of public utilities, excellent transportation facilities, well equipped mass-media. Adjustment is a way of life in urbanisation. People are more liberal in their approach. There is a wider changes in the institutions of family and caste Panchayat.

Solutions to Urban Problems

- Systematic development of urban centres
- Efficient town planning
- Well distributed viable urban centres throughout the country
- Emphasis on effective implementation of poverty alleviation, urban developmental programmes which can permit multi-functional activities to sustain people in cities
- Regional planning in a logical manner is necessary
- Motivate the industrialists to plan their industries to backward districts is also helps in linear development of metropolitan and big cities.
- Municipalities should find their own resources by collecting appropriate taxes and spending the amount for the development of the cities
- Encourage private transport facilities to operate services as they will charge little and provide better services
- Community centres has to be established by the innovative planners it will act upon neighbourhood needs
- Modify the urban planning and implement radical measures
- City dwellers has to become politically active and organise themselves to change the existing economic and social systems.

Health Problems Associated with Urbanisation

The common diseases among the urban slum dwellers are: Respiratory diseases, fever, G.I.T disorders, skin infections, eye infections, malnutrition, viral infections, chronic toxicity, STD, accidents, drug abuse, alcoholism, crime, delinquency, suicide, prostitution.

Causes

Industrial pollution, over-crowding, poor hygienic practices, food and water contamination.

Strategies to Improve Urban Health Problems

- Provision of safe drinking water, maintaining housing standards, proper disposal of liquid and solid waste, and conducting health awareness campaigns.

Distinguishing features of urban community and rural community (The Urban-Rural contrast)

Feature	*Urban*	*Rural*
Cost of living	High	Low
Transport and communication facilities	Advanced, sophisticated	Lack of good facility
Social interaction	Man is interacted as a 'number' and 'address'	Interacted as a human being
Social contact	Wider, casual, short-lived, impersonal and secondary in nature	Less contacts, durable, long-lasting, intimate, direct, primary in nature
Social relationship	Secondary, many folded relationships, superficial, artificial, lack of privacy	Primary, simple, sincere, traditional and conservative
Community team spirit	Group will work towards 'aim' oriented until work completes	We feeling, more unity, team spirit
Environment	Lives in congestion, psychological isolation leading to more tensed environment and mental illness	Free from psychological tension, nervous strain, lives close with nature
Self reliance	Greatly interdependent in organisation	More self reliant

Contd...

Contd...

Family	Prevalence of nuclear family, weaker relationship, importance to individual	Joint family system, cohesive in unity, less scope for individuality
Institution of marriage	Freedom of selection, divorce is more common	Arranged, strong marriage bonds
Women status	Intelligent, equal status, career-conscious, independent	Ignorant, suppressed, lack of freedom, low social status, plays subordinate roles, assist men folks in occupation
Economic status	All types of class systems are observed, class conflicts are common in city life	Poor, not class conscious
Educational status	Widespread, formal, advanced	Less formal, less stress on education
Neighbourhood	Less importance, strangers	Greater importance, knows all by names
Faith in religion	Less rigid observance	Believe in spiritualism, fatalism
Caste system	Class system is more prominent, less rigid observance of caste distinctions	Rigid caste system. Endogamous group, mobility is not possible in caste system
Culture	Secular type, cosmopolitan	Sacred, conservative, ethnocentrism
Social mobility	Known for 'boiling water in a kettle'	Stable, conservative in nature, compared with 'calm water in a pail'
Size	Too big, less united, more problematic	Too small, limited population, more unity
Density of population	High	Low
Occupation	Professional like manufacture, trade and commerce, wide spread division of labour	Agriculture is the major occupation, less scope for division of labour
Recreational activities	Varied	Simple, limited
Social processes		
Competition	Greater extent	Not much
Conflict	Indirect	Direct
Toleration	Not so great	More, lead to accommodation

Contd...

Contd...

Assimilation	Greater speed of assimilation	Slow process
Cooperation	Indirect, impersonal, division of labour	Direct, personal, socially cooperative in nature
Self-reliant and self-sufficiency	Greatly interdependent in organisation	Vertical solidarity of castes
Politics	Active, more interest	Not active, less interest
Attitude	Cause and effect relationship	Fatalistic view
Nature	Artificial, corrupt, dishonest, unfaithful	Frank, open, genuine
Social segregation	Functional segregation based on occupation was observed	Segregation is based on religion, caste, customs, traditions

Regional Community

India has various religions, which have geographic, cultural and linguistic significance. People have specified pattern of life in specified regions. Regionalism has some advantages and ill-effects too; some times it may affect national unity and integration. People of the same religion will have association, mutual concern and will help each other for their upliftment. They will work for their own group welfare.

Term 'Region'

'A geographic tract, where society held together for a length of time with common cultural characteristics and linguistic specification'.

Kinds of Socio-cultural Regions

- Those delineated by trained observers
- People in the society perceive and which may command their loyalties, identifications and sections

These two kinds are mutually exclusive regions have interactions between one another.

Regions in India

- Southern region
- Central region
- Western region
- Northern region
- North-eastern region
- Regions will have sub-regions, e.g: In southern region: Telugu, Kannada, Coorg, Konkani, Malayalam, Tamil.
- In 1956 linguistic reorganisation of states has taken place. Each sub-region also again diversified with varied cultural, linguistic specificities, same language form closer affinity with each other
- The geographic barriers like rivers, deserts, mountains made different cultural regions
- Regional political parties create intense regional and linguistic feelings among the people with their vested interests. In Andhra Pradesh Telangana, in M.P Chattisgargh, in Bihar Jarkandh, in U.P Uttaranchal.

Advantages of Regionalism

- Promotes regional development and cultural growth
- Interaction is intimate, closer association among the group people is observed
- Enhancement of group solidarity, we feeling, integrity in its own group.

Evil Effects of Regionalism

Promotes National Disintegrity

With the regional and linguistic feelings the unity and integrity of the nation is affected. National interest is compromised due to regional interests.

Deteriorates Economic Progress of the Nation

Narrow regional feeling will affect nation's well-being. Neighbouring states will not cooperate with each other and affects the national development, like cauvery water dispute between Tamil Nadu and Karnataka, Almati dams issue between Andhra Pradesh and Karnataka.

Administrative Problems

Bigger states with more number of districts will have administrative problems.

Measures to Eradicate the Problems Associated with Regionalism

- Encourage the contacts between one region to other region, one state to other, states to nation by arranging cultural integration programs, youth festivals, tours, goodwill visits, rotary club, inter-country meeting, NSS camps, NCC camps, etc.
- Conduct information, education, communication campaigns to increase the extent of broader outlook in the minds of people, encourage the people to learn different languages and acquaint their culture the people
- Promote the activities related to Nations' development and welfare
- Motivate the people to maintain integrity of nation and explain the advantages associated with it
- Discourage the development of terrorism and conduct mass campaigns and explain the public about evil effects associated with terrorism activities
- Mobilise the people to participate in National integrity activities, promote group welfare and solidarity by increasing the morale and conduct of the people.

Previous Years University Questions

1. Problems of rural community. (5 m, RGUHS, 2000)
2. Health problems of rural community. (5 m, RGUHS, 2000)
3. Characteristics of Indian villages. (2 m, RGUHS, 1997)
4. Characteristics of urban community. (5 m, RGUHS, 2001, 03)
5. Definition of community. (5 m, RGUHS, 1997)
6. Describe the characteristics of rural community. (10 m, RGUHS, 2002,04)
7. Mention two urban problems in India. (2 m, RGUHS, 2002)
8. Features of Indian villages. (5 m, RGUHS, 2003)
9. Rural society. (2 m, RGUHS, 2004)
10. Urbanisation and diseases. (5 m, RGUHS, 2001)
11. Health problems in rural community. (2 m, RGUHS, 2000,01)
12. Describe the differences between rural and urban communities. (10 m, RGUHS, 2002, 03)
13. Urbanisation and health. (5 m, RGUHS, 2003)
14. Health problems in urban community. (5 m, RGUHS, 2000)
15. Community sentiment. (2 m, RGUHS, 2003)
16. Health problems in village community. (5 m, RGUHS, 1999)
17. Tribal community. (2 m, RGUHS, 2001)
18. Indian rural village. (2 m, RGUHS, 2001)
19. Discuss briefly the village community. Examine the merits and demerits. (5 m, RGUHS, 2002)
20. Urban social problems. (2 m, RGUHS, 2002)
21. Factors of urban community. (2 m, RGUHS, 2003)
22. Name the basic elements of community. (2 m, RGUHS, 2002)
23. Differentiate between the characteristics of rural and urban culture. (19 m, NTRUHS, 1999)
24. Discuss the characteristics of town and city. (19 m, NTRUHS, 1998)

25. Bring out the social consequences of rapid urbanisation in India. (NTRUHS, 1986)
26. What are the problems faced by urbanisation, how this influence the health of urban community, suggest remedial measures. (NTRUHS, 1996)
27. Explain the causes of growth of urbanisation. (NTRUHS, 1995)
28. What is community, discuss the characteristics of rural and urban community. (NTRUHS, 1995)
29. What are the characteristics of village community. List the health problems of Indian villages. (13 m, SVIMS, Tirupati, 2002)
30. Distinguish between society and community. (5 m, RGUHS, 2002)
31. Explain the importance of urbanisation. (5 m, 1992, NTRUHS)

MGR University Question Papers

1. Enumerate the health and social problems due to urbanisation in India. (10 m, RGUHS, Nov-04)
2. Characteristics of rural community. (5 m, RGUHS, Nov-04)
3. Two major problems of urban community. (2 m, RGUHS, Nov-04)
4. Urbanisation. (2 m, MGRU, Nov-04)
5. Community. (5 m, MGRU, Apr-98)
6. Secondary groups. (5 m, MGRU, Nov-98)
7. Rural reconstruction. (5 m, MGRU)

CHAPTER FIFTEEN

Leadership

INTRODUCTION

Leadership is a common phenomena seen everywhere in the social organisation in one or other form. Leadership is the process of influencing the behaviour of followers by inspiring and motivating to work willingly and enthusiastically for achieving predetermined goals. It is a continuous process of behaviour, where the followers and leader work together cooperatively leadership deals with insight, effectiveness and results; focuses on top; emphasises transformational; activity oriented. Leader should possess a sense of capacity and comfort with risk and change leads to an understanding of the role, collaborative style, multiple cultures; emotional competence; identifying the follower's strengths and weakness; and greater balance and reflection in life leads to energized work force. Leader has to present model behaviour for others and shows the way of life. The individuals in society are generally divided into leader and followers. Emergence of leadership is the result of social process, a bipolar process or behaviour.

Definition

- 'A behaviour that affects the behaviour of other people more than their behaviour affects that of the leader'—*La-Piere and Fransworth*
- 'A concept applied to personality, environment relation to describe the situation when a personality is so placed in the environment that directs the feeling, insight and controls others in pursuit of the common cause'—*Pigor*
- 'Leader is one who has power and authority'—*HT Mazumdar*
- 'Activity of persuading people to cooperate in the achievement of a common objective'—*Allen*
- 'The activity of influencing people to strive willingly for mutual objectives, it affects the behaviour of followers in a situation'—*Terry*
- 'Influencing and energizing of people to work together in a common effort to achieve the purposes of the enterprise'—*Seckler and Hudson*
- 'It is the interpersonal influence exercised in a situation and directed through communication process, towards the attainment of a specified goals'—*Temenbaum el al.*
- 'It is the process of influencing and supporting others to work enthusiastically toward achieving objectives'.
- 'The art of process influencing people, so that they will strive willingly and enthusiastically towards the achievement of group goals'—*Harold Koontz and Heinz Wechrich*
- 'It is the process of situation or reciprocal reinforcement which by the successful interplay of relevant individual differences controls human energy in the pursuit of a common cause'—*Britt*
- 'To keep, to persuade or to direct man, that comes from personal qualities apart from face'—*Maciver and Page*
- 'Leadership is interms of dominance'—*Kimball Young*

- 'Leadership acts or present which influence other persons in share direction'—*Seeman and Moris*

Meaning

- 'To lead' – to excel, to be in advance, to be prominent
- To be head of an organisation
- To hold command
- Leadership depends on 3 things: The individual, followers and conditions, power/authority
- Leadership is a continuous process
- Leadership may be seen in terms of relationship between a leader and his followers, which arises out of their functioning for common goals
- Leader tries to influence the behaviour to individuals (group members) to achieve common goals
- Followers work willingly and enthusiastically to achieve those goals
- There is no coercive force which induces the followers to work, to shape the groups
- Leaders feel the importance of followers. Gives them recognition and conveys them about the importance of activities performed by them
- Leadership styles may be different under different situations
- The ability to lead effectively the group
- Leaders shows the way to solve the problems in working situation and to overcome the obstacles
- Leaders are concerned with bringing together resource, developing strategies, organising and controlling activities in order to achieve the agreed objectives.

Nature

- Traitist—superior individuals who would lead in whatever situation or time they might find themselves

- Situationist—leadership is specific to each situation. It is a way of behaving exhibited by individuals in differing degrees in different situations
- Leader is necessarily a part of the group and leadership is status and role in that group
- Leadership can occur only in relation to other people, none can be a leader all by himself
- Leader establishes reciprocal relationships with the group members
- Leadership facilitates group life.

Elements in Leadership

- Mutual behaviour between the leader and his followers
- Two-way affair, the followers influences the behaviour of the leader as well as the leader behaviour influences the followers
- Without followers, no leader can exist
- The element of willingness, voluntary obedience by the followers, leadership is based on cooperation and goodwill
- It is specific to specific situation, a person cannot be a leader for all situations
- The ability to use power (to control a person possesses—six types of power—coercive, reward, legitimate, expert, referent and information) effectively and in a responsible manner
- The ability to comprehend that people are motivated by different factors at different times and in different situations
- The ability to inspire
- The ability to act in a manner that will develop a conducive climate to respond and arouse motivation
- Dominance—an attempt to guide the others
- Leader influences the feelings, experiences, behaviours and activities of others
- Process of multi-stimulation; leader is influenced by others, he has to model his behaviour according to the aspirations and desires of the followers

- Authority—the suggestions and the directions as given by the leader are accepted by followers, and they accept the superiority of the leadership.

POWER ORIENTATION

Definition

'The influence of an individual who exercises control over others'—*Goldhamer*

Types

1. Physical force
2. Domination
3. Manipulation
4. Legitimate
5. Illegitimate

Power orientation of leadership style depends upon the degree of authority given to the leaders. Power orientation means the authority given by the top management to the leader in order to exercise power in controlling his followers. With power orientation leaders are able to use their authority in influencing the behaviour of their subordinates. However, the leader do not use their authority to control the followers to the fullest extent due to various factors based on power orientation. The leaders degree of use of power can be classified into three categories:

1. Autocratic leadership
2. Participative leadership
3. Free-run leadership

Principles

The art of war

- Learn to fight
- Show the way
- Do it right

- Know the facts
- Expect the worst
- Seize the day
- Burn the bridges
- Do it better
- Pull together
- Keep them guessing

Sensitive Leadership

- 'Eyes and ears—on; hands-off'
- Enabling, facilitating, catalysing—to develop self-confidence and responsibility to other.

Exemplary Leadership

- Monitor the group's progress against norms and objectives
- Credibility, enduring, competence, courage, effective performance
- Strengthening others and building on their strengths
- Fostering collaboration
- Modeling the way
- Path finding
- Recognises people's contributions
- Sets high expectations for themselves and for others
- Enable others to act effectively, they make things happen
- Reaffirms norms, standards, values
- Keep the team on track
- Logical thinking
- Relies upon conventional wisdom.

Inspirational Leadership

- Exceeds limit
- Demonstrating superiority, pre-eminence in skills
- Achievement or excellence
- Awareness in all the spheres where work has to be completed.

Eccentric

- Creative
- Innovative thinking
- Provocative stimulating
- Challenging
- Effective skills in decision making
- Productive results
- Introduces new ways of doing things
- Holistic thinker
- Uses intuition
- Initiates change.

Supportive Followers

- High functional maturity
- Takes ownership of a role, accountability and performance
- Gives out, demonstrable support to the achievement of the team's goals and needs
- Positive, constructive, collaborative
- Alert to changing demands needs, priorities flexibility and adjusts accordingly.

Origin and Development of Leadership

Psychoanalysis

Good family, healthy psychological traits, desire to succeed, inspirative, enthusiastic in nature are some of the traits required for the development of leadership.

Heredity

Innate qualities are gifts of heredity.

Social Stimulation

Social environment stimulates the individual to acquire certain leadership abilities.

Personality

Individuals with type A personality will have attractive and pleasing in nature.

Emergence of a Leader

A person who emerges as a leader among the group is a very unique task. The emerging of leadership depends upon a number of factors. There are several means and techniques for acquiring the ability to do the special jobs. The following are the most important aspects, which help the person to become group leader.

Leadership Training

Training programmes are offered manages to several leadership situations and teach them how to tackle them. The situations are partly real. The trainers create the situation. Varying the managers under going leadership training are provided opportunities to diagnose the problems and think some ways and means in tackling them, which partly involve testing all various types of leadership against relatives. Leadership training gives deep insight and experiences to managers and an appropriate attitudes and behaviours, which they have to adopt in tackling diverse situations on how to gain initiative and come over to a situation. How to inspire and motivate people and the measures in the development of the leader and the group.

Internal Organisational Exposure

Another important reason, which help the person to emerge as a leader is the internal organisational exposure. The critical situations call for application of leadership abilities by the administrators to overcome the situation to see that a leader emerges from the person they have to be put in charge of committees, task of project implementation, coordination, control over employee, which give an opportunity for the manager or the administrator to develop into a very good leader on emerge as a leader in the group.

Autonomy and Accountability

Administrators may be able to sharpen their leadership abilities and emerge as a leader in the group under conditions of relative freedom. They should be allowed a large amount of freedom to evolve their own methods or tackling situations calling for critical leadership abilities. This is possible only organisational support in the form of authority (position power), status, top management, support and adequate description in dispensing rewards and penalties for their subordinates within the framework of certain norms and rules are given.

Opportunities for Interaction

Administrator should also have opportunities to have interact with their subordinates in a more intense and continuous manner so that they can talk or listen to their subordinates to understand their view points and enable them to acquire qualities like sociability, tolerance, non-provocation, resolution of conflict verbal ability and supporting a truth to guide them successfully and emerge as a leader for the problem solving and growth and development of one and all.

Setting Challenges but Realistic Goals

Administrators have to work very hard to achieve the objectives, the in-born leadership ability to emerge as a leader for the group. If the appropriate goals are set which are challenging but realistic.

Job Rotation

Administrators may also emerge as a leader if they help to develop leadership skills by a process of systematic rotation of their jobs. They should be exposed to a variety of superior subordinate relations and job environments, so that they emerge as a leader by developing the ability of coping with situation, which do not permit them to adopt stereotyped styles on approaches.

Spotting of a Leader

In order to achieve the objectives of the organisation, the organisation has to strive hard consistently and continuously. The growth and development of the organisation entirely depends upon the people in the organisation. If the people or human resources are hard working, talented and able, they will be able to achieve their objectives as well as the objectives of the organisation.

In the organisation people work in groups and every group has its own culture, people in the group are unique and different from one another in some respects. In the management it becomes necessary to manage this groups effectively and efficiently, in order to achieve that they have to depend on the leaders of the group, department, division and organisation. Management has to spot new leaders to enable the organisation to grow at good pace.

Spotting leader is a very difficult task in the context of modern organisations. But it is necessary to do so to survive exist grow and develop. Spotting of leader is a process of identifying the leader from the members of the group. The identification of the leader has to be done by keeping in mind various factors. The following are the important in spotting a leader:

- Some people in the group are somewhat more intelligent than the other members. The person who is more intelligent has to be given preference. Because of his intelligence and capacity which is possible to have a overall view of the problems of the group and the organisation

- Persons who have well rounded from the stand point of interest, aptitude, attitude must be selected and given training to become a good leadership
- The persons who have the ability to express their ideas in clear terms to others and explain their position and gain support of other members can be considered as leader.
- People are mentally and emotionally matured and able to devote their full attention to the affairs of the group in general and not influenced by their own occupations can be a good leader
- Persons with powerful inner drive, which impulse are motivates them to strive hard for accomplishment who are ambitious and willing to work long hours to realise their ambitions can be good leader
- Persons who have the ability to think innovatively, understand the importance and cooperative effort, practice social skills and good human relations are capable of becoming a good leader

Thus, by using above methods the management can identify and spot potential people in the group.

Sequential Activities Related to Leader as Mentor

Agree the topic for development

- Identify specific areas for improvement
- Decide delegation of authority and responsibility for the group members
- Give orientation to the group members towards their job performance and expectations
- Identify short-term, long-term goals and objectives.

Promote Discovery

- Active listener
- Analyses systematically
- Push for options and alternatives

- Share your experiences
- Promote learning and ownership.

Set the Parameters

- Establish deadlines
- Monitor the entire process
- Review progress
- Record the events in dairy
- Identify task boundaries and measures.

Authorise to Empower

- Delegation of authority and responsibility
- Take decisions
- Ensure financial, administrative responsibility and controls.

Recap and Review

- Get feedback
- Note down action points
- Agree to start date
- Key milestones.

Follow-up and follow-through

- Monitor progress with the individual
- Check on target and maintain standard
- Agree remedial and exploitive action
- Judge and plan effectively for modification, if needed
- Fix the review dates and attend it sincerely
- Submit regular reports, update the issues.

Theories Related to Leadership

Leadership styles, which leaders may adopt to influence the followers.

Charismatic Leadership/Great Man Theory

'A leader is born and is not made'. A leader has some 'charisma' which acts as influencer. 'Charisma' is a Greek word in a person, which makes him a leader irrespective of the situations, where he works. They inspire followers and broaden their vision and energy. They catch public consciousness. These leaders have high levels of referent power, self-confidence, dominance ability to convince the followers, and the ability to capture the commitment and energy of followers. Leadership qualities cannot be enhanced through education and training, these are inborn and personal in nature, others cannot share these. Situational factors do not have any influence over the leader.

Limitations:

- If the leadership qualities are inborn, it implies that nothing can be done to develop leaders in the organisation
- Situations will not have influence over the charismatic leader but situational variables play their own role in determining leadership effectiveness.

Trait Theory

Leadership traits are not completely inborn, but cannot be acquired through learning and experience. Trait is 'an enduring quality of an individual'. Trait theory approach seeks to determine,' what makes a successful leader' from the leader's own personal characteristics. The individual was a successful because of his certain qualities or characteristics. The ingredients for effective leaders are:

- Self confidence
- Sociability
- Will (initiative, persistence ambition)
- Dominance
- Surgency (talkative, cheerfulness, enthusiasm, expressiveness, alertness and originality)

- Supervisory ability
- Self actualisation
- Self assurance
- Positive attitude
- Charisma, anticipates opportunity
- Creates shared vision
- Demonstrates personal mastery
- Respects social values
- *Innate qualities*—personality, physical and constitutional factors like height, weight, physique, energy, healthy appearance
- *Acquirable qualities*—emotional stability (free from bias), consistent in action, refrains from anger, well adjusted
- *Human relations*—Initiate voluntary cooperation for achieving work establish good interpersonal relationship, develops conducive family environment in working area
- *Empathy*—Ability to look at things objectively understanding them from others point of view, empathy requires respect for other persons, rights, beliefs, values and feelings
- Objectivity in thinking (without any bias or prejudice)
- Self motivating skills and motivating others for high work performance
- Technical skills
- Communicative skills
- Social skills.

Implications:

- A leader requires some traits and qualities to effective
- Many qualities may be developed through training and education development programmes.

Limitations:

- *Generalisation of traits*—Problems in identification and measuring the traits, which may be relevant for a leader to be effective in all situations

- *Applicability of traits*—Leadership is a process of influence reflects in leader's behaviour and not in his traits. Persons have specified characteristics of a leader but not become effective leaders, as the reason for this phenomenon is that, there are no direct cause effect relationship between a trait of a person and his behaviour. Traits are necessary for shaping the behaviour but other situational factors are also important.

Behaviour Theory

Leadership is shown by a person's acts more than by his traits. Groups need some one to perform 'task related functions or problem solving functions'—to solve problems faced by groups in performing their activities.

Group maintenance functions or social functions—actions related to mediate disputes and ensure the individuals feel valued by the group. An individual who is able to perform both roles successfully (by means of effective leadership styles) would be an effective leader.

Leadership behaviour views in 2 ways:

a. Functional behaviour

   It influences followers positively, e.g: Forming clear goals, motivational employees for effectively work to achieve the goals. Raising the group morale, building team spirit, effective two-way communication.

b. Dysfunctional behaviour

   Is unfavourable to the followers and denotes ineffective leadership, inability to accept employee's ideas, poor human relations, display of emotional immaturity.

Implications:

Leaders can shape the group members' behaviour and discards the dysfunctional behaviour.

Limitations:

- A particular behaviour may be functional at a point of time, but may be dysfunctional at another point of time. Thus, time element will be a decider of the effectiveness of the behaviour and not the behaviour
- Nature of followers and the situations under which the leader's behaviour takes place.

Situational Trait Theory/Contingency Theory

Effectiveness of leadership will be affected by the factors (e.g: Group characteristics, organisational factors) associated with the leaders and the situation. This theory has a dual focus, the leader and the situation in which the leader works. How the leader's traits interact with situational factors in determining team effectiveness in task performance. Effective group performance can be achieved only by matching the leader to the situation or by changing the situation to fit the leader. Leader's behaviour is influences by their characteristics, and hierarchical position.

Situational Factors

Subordinates characteristics, leader's situation, position power, group factors and organisational factors.

Implications:

Effective leadership will vary with situation to situation; leader has to adapt management practices along with situational variable.

Limitations:

Quite complex in practice due to varied contingent factors.

Situational Behaviour Theories

Identifying the specific leader behaviour that are most effective in specific leader situations. The behavioural contingencies of the leader that yield the most effective performance by the followers.

Path-goal Theory

It attempts to explain how leader behaviour can positively influence the motivation and job satisfaction of subordinates. Effectiveness in leadership is dependent on clearly defining the paths for subordinates to goal attainment and the degree to which the leader is able to improve the chances that subordinates will achieve their goals. The leader clarifies and set goals for subordinates, helps them to find the best path for achieving the goals and remove the obstacles.

The Expectancy Theory

Employees' motivation is dependent on leader's behaviour that influences goal paths and the relative attractiveness of the goals involved. A person's perception of achieving or prized reward or goal through effective job performance will motivate the individual. However, the individual must see clearly the relationship between the individual's efforts and effective job performance will lead to the desired objective.

Elements:

- Effort—performance expectancy (successful efforts will leads to better performance)
- Performance—outcome expectancy (successful performance will leads to better results or rewards or outcomes)
- The anticipated value of the outcomes or rewards.

The path-goal theory suggests that 4 leadership styles can be used to affect subordinate perceptions of paths and goals.

Theory of Balance

The leader should possess balanced personality and coordination of contradictory qualities, integrated in nature.

- *Theory of flash insight:* Leader should have flashes of insight, and should be able to see the difficulties that face him and ways to solve the problem. Knowledge, intelligence, experience and hard work are the essential qualities of a leader.
- *Theory of marginal uniqueness:* Leader should possess unique qualities, capabilities, extraordinary qualities. It creates personal magnetism, earns respect.
- *Theory of ability and disability:* Leaders may have limitations, even with that, the abilities he has will make a good leader
- *Group process theory:* To solve the bigger problems, individuals work in a group more efficiently, cooperatively, and by selfless service.

Direct Leadership

Leader should orient the followers about their tasks, expectations, work methods, developing work schedules, identifying work evaluation standards.

Supportive Leadership Behaviour

Concern for the well-being and needs of subordinates, creating a pleasant organisational climate by being friendly, approachable, considerative behaviour. It has great impact on subordinates' performance when they are frustrated and dissatisfied.

Participative Leadership Behaviour

Consulting with subordinates, encouraging them by suggestions and carefully considering their ideas when making decisions, which results in increased motivation. The characteristics of subordinates are: Needs, confidence, abilities, work environment–task, reward system and relationship with co-workers are involved.

Achievement Oriented Behaviour:

Leader sets challenging goals seeks improvement of performance by displaying confidence in the abilities of followers.

The Competencies of Leadership

- Ability to create and sustain excellence
- Capacity for anticipatory thinking, envisioning and action
- Interested in group work and works for group interest and welfare
- Skill to tap the available resources
- Good judgment and decision-making skills
- Transformational competence
- Marked capacity to generate alternative ideas
- Integrative competence: Focus on shared visions, aspirations and legitimate role expectations
- Exemplary behaviour
- Ability to define visions and goals with a clear sense of purpose and direction
- Moral sensitivity
- Shows confidence and with whom they work
- Sympathy and dependability
- Readiness to demonstrate personal sacrifice, resolve, determination
- Delegation of responsibility and authority
- Ability to built effective relationship
- Autonomy
- Intuition
- Enthusiastic
- Social adaptability
- Reflector—reflecting ideas related to past
- Theorist—logically analysing the situations
- Pragmatist—trying out ideas, techniques, tools to see the work in practice

- High social intimacy, sociability, friendliness
- Ability to mediate across disciplines and functions
- Ability to recognise and manage paradox
- Non-interference
- Sympathetic nature, empathy skill.

Coach Style

- Directive
- Delegative
- Participative
- Consultative
- Negotiative
- Confident communicator
- Culture custodian
- Bureaucrat
- Enthusiast

Receiving Style

- Receptive
- Self-reliant
- Empowered
- Collaborative
- Informative
- Reciprocating
- Good listener

Physical Qualities

- Sound health
- Vitality
- Endurance
- Enthusiastic

Intellectual Qualities

- Ability to make sound judgment
- Scientific approach
- Prominence, positive interest

Moral Qualities

- Honesty
- Sincerity
- Integrity
- Fair play
- Moral courage
- Will power
- Purpose oriented/broad vision
- Objectivity
- Achievement drive

Social Qualities

- Initiative
- Trust worthy
- Empathy
- Expressiveness

Guidelines for Effective Leadership

- Leaders and organisation should appreciate the unique attributes, predispositions and talents of each leadership organisational preferences in terms of style—leader should challenge the organisational culture, when necessary without destroying it.
- Participative, considerate leader behaviour—that should concern for the people to enhance the health and well-being of followers in the work environment.

Types of Leadership

1. EB Godwin's
   - Intellectuals, e.g: Scientists, authors, artists, philosophers.
   - Executive, e.g: Corporation, presidents, governors, priests, trade union officials.

2. OL Schwarzs'
   - Men of thought
   - Men of action
3. Sir Martin M Conways'
   - Group originator
   - Crowd representative
   - Crowd compeller
   - Crowd exponent
4. E Jemings'
   - Princes
   - Heroes
   - Superman
5. HD Lasswells'
   - The bureaucrat
   - The boss
   - The agitator
   - The theorist
6. HT Mazumdars'
   - Traditional leader, e.g: Brahmin
   - Bureaucratic, e.g: Elected leader
   - Charismatic, e.g: Creates his own authority viz party leader, religious leader
7. Bogarduss'
   - Direct and indirect leadership
   - Social, executive and mental leadership
   - Partisan and scientific leadership
   - Prophets, saints, experts, boss
   - Autocratic, charismatic, paternal and democratic leadership
8. Bratletts'
   - Institutional
   - Dominant leader
   - Persuasive leader
9. Nafes'
   - State leadership
   - Dynamic leadership

10. Formal leadership
    - Informal leadership

Importance of Leadership

Leadership is essential factor, for success of any organisation to function efficiently and effectively. A leader should function as an executive, planner, policy maker, expert, representative, controller, arbitrator, mediator, exampler, purveyor or reward and punishment, establishes good interpersonal relationships. Leader should have versatile personality. The members' activities in and organisation need to be directed in a certain manner to attain the objectives.

- Motivation of employers for effective work performance
- Creating confidence in his followers by guiding them and getting through good results in the organisation
- Building morale—developing positive attitude of employees towards organisation, management and voluntary cooperation to offer their ability to the organisation. High morale leads to high productivity and organisational stability
- As an executive—guiding, directing the behaviour of followers to discharge their duties effectively
- Policy maker—the objectives, values will be maintained when certain policies have been framed. When the leader imposes his own policies, he has to take his followers into confidence
- Planner—to meet the policies and objectives of organisation, leader has to plan effectively, it reflects his imagination and capability
- Expert—leader should have the knowledge of all the things around him
- Controller of interpersonal relationship—leader has to control, guide and direct internal relationship of the group, he should be aware of the qualities of followers and advocates the group thereby he can direct the internal relationship as a successful manner

- Arbitrator and mediator—to keep social relationship intact, to relieve societal tensions or group problems, leader has to mediate the situation and solve the problem
- Ideologist—leader lays down ideology of the group, which guides the actions of the group
- Parent—leader plays the role of parent for the group, protects the interests of his followers, provides conducive environment for better group performance; listens to the problems, provides efforts and guide the followers to solve the problem whereby the group members feels a sense of responsibility, sharing and security
- Scape goat—when the group, which he leads, does not succeed, all the blame is put on the shoulders of the leader. The leader holds responsible for everything—good or bad.

Functions of Leader

Leadership is a highly complex phenomenon, the functions/ responsibilities of the leader vary from one group to the other or depend upon the nature.

Structure the Situation/Surrogator for Individual Responsibility

Leader creates the working environment to his members such that they work effectively, without any conflict, inhibition or bias. He has formulate and define line of authority, delegation of responsibility and orient the duties, so that every one are aware of their functions and responsibilities.

Controlling Group Behaviour

Leader has to prevent individuals from exploiting the group, and the group from exploiting the individuals. It enforces the rules that have been established.

Speaking for the Group /Group Representative

Leader is responsible for translating the groups feelings into words and actions. Leader is the spokes-person for the group; helping to articulate to the members and interpret outsiders the groups' objectives and desires.

Helping the Group to Achieve the Goals and Potentials

Planning, coordinating, decision-making and mobilising the energy of group members, ensures active participation of all group members and utilisation of their diverse capabilities and resources effectively. Making suggestions for actions, evaluating movement towards goal, preventing activities to the goals. Encouraging the members is relieving tensions, gives chances to explore themselves.

Bernard Described the Functions of the Leader as,

- The determination of objectives
- The manipulation of means
- The control of the instrument of action
- The stimulation of coordinated action.

Autocratic Leadership/Authoritarian Leadership/Directive Leadership Monothetic Style

To meet immediate and temporary crisis situations autocratic leadership may be useful. It reduces initiativeness, potentiality of the group. The leader determines the policy, procedures and activities in the group and sets the group goals, controlled group activities with step-by-step directions. The performance of group members is very good, but motivation was low, group members will work only when the leader is present to direct them. Group members are more dependent, submissive, shows less individuality, less friendly praise to each other; marked inter-member irritability, aggressiveness, insecurity, dissatisfaction among group members is observed.

Categories of Autocratic Leadership

Strict Autocrat

The leader influences subordinate behaviour through negative motivation, i.e. by criticising subordinates, imposing penalty, etc.

Benevolent Autocrat

Centralises decision-making power in him, but his motivation style is positive. He can be effective in getting efficiency in many situations.

Incompetent Autocrat

Superior adopts autocratic leadership style just to hide their incompetence.

Advantages of Autocratic Leadership

- Many subordinates likes to work under centralised authority structure and strict discipline
- Provides strong motivation and reward to a manager exercising this style
- It permits very quick decisions as single person takes it
- Less competent subordinates have scope to work as they do negligible planning, organising and decision-making.

Disadvantages

- People don't like to work, when it is strict and negative motivation or lack of motivation
- Low morale, frustration and conflict develops among employees
- More dependency and less individuality in the organisation observed.

Democratic Leadership/Participative Leadership/Consultative Leadership

Emotional involvement of a person in a group situation, which encourages him to contribute to group goals and share responsibility in them. Leader decentralises his decision-making process. It elicits members' active involvement and places minimum restraints on their initiative and creativity, promoting the adaptability to meet changing conditions and demands. The leader discusses, determines policies and assignments together. Group members' shows more interest in their work and originality and keep on working. Cohesiveness was highest among group members; the leader encourages participation by members in deciding group matters and behaves in a friendly, helpful manner to the members. Giving techniques and suggesting alternative procedures, low dependency on group leader, low incidence of irritability, aggressiveness, high frequency of suggestions is observed; high quality group satisfaction, e.g: Family.

Advantages

- Highly motivating technique to employees as they feel elevated when their ideas and suggestions are given weight in decision-making
- Productivity is high as they are partly involved in decisions, thus implement decisions whole heartedly
- Provides organisational stability by raising morale and attitudes of employees high and favourable.

Limitations

- Complex nature of organisation requirement needs through understanding of its problems, which low level employees may not be able to do. Thus participation does not remain meaningful
- Some people in the organisation wants minimum interaction with their superiors or associates, so this technique is discouraging
- It can be used covertly to manipulate employees.

Laissez-faire Leadership

The leader simply stood by and answered when spoken to the groups were entirely on their own in planning and assigning work. Moral and cohesiveness was lowest among group members. The leader allows complete freedom for decisions and activity keeping his initiative and suggestions to a minimum. Group shows little dependency on the leader, irritability, aggressiveness, suggestions for group action and group policy, etc. observed among group members neighbourhood group.

Decision Making in Leadership

It is the core activity in the process of leadership and management. As a decision maker, the leader's role is to create relevant order, coherence, committed synergy through others. Awareness, integrity, courage and competence are the crucial determinants of the decisions. The traditional leader concerns with power, rank and status, which are common in positional authority.

Decision-making behaviour (Logical/Cognitive responses)

Inquiry: Searching, Examining, Probing, Analysing, Defining, Classifying.

Diagnosis: Assessing, Weighing, Clarifying, Crystallising, Simplifying, Prioritising.

Planning: Foreseeing, Predicting, Preparing, Over-viewing, Progressing, Follow-up.

Decision process (Stages in making decisions)

Awareness: (situational analysis), Concern, Information, Scope.

Direction: Problems and obstacles, Priorities and objectives, Strengths and weakness.

Action: (Execution), Opportunities, Threats, Consequences, Outcomes.

Decision-making behaviour (Emotional/Intuitive responses)

Insight: Intuiting, Generating ideas, Exploring, Synthesising, Scanning, Creating options.

Drive: Insisting, Persisting, Resisting, Being resolute, Building purpose, Being determined.

Pace: Sense of timing, Varying speed, Adjusting response, pre-empting, Recognising the right conditions, Taking appropriate action.

Approaches in Decision-making

- Awareness about a problem and identify the problem
- Define the problem
- Establish goals
- Explanation of possible courses of action and their respective consequences
- Deliberation of decision in course of action
- Follow-up through, with revision if necessary.

Process of Decision-making

How we Obtain Information

Sensing

- Look for specific parts, bits and pieces
- Live in and with the present
- Prefer handling practical and tangible matters
- Define the activities in a measurable manner
- Have a start
- Work incrementally and take one step at a time
- Work 'hands on'
- Set procedures and establish routines.

Intuition

- Look for overall context and patterns
- Concerned with possibilities and the future
- Anticipate and speculate about what might be
- Prefer imagining the possibilities
- Like opportunities to be creative and inventive
- Jump in anywhere – leap around and miss out steps and sequences
- Work out overall plan or design
- Like change and variety.

How we make decisions

Thinking
- Decide with 'head'
- Go by logic
- Work by truth, justice and objectivity
- See the things as an 'on-looker', i.e. detached
- Take the longer-term view
- Automatically find flaws and criticise
- Analyse ideas, plan and strategies.

Feeling
- Decide with 'heart'
- Go by personal convictions (what I feel is ....)
- Work by personal rapport and harmony
- See the things as a participant
- Immediate and personal or subjective view
- Appreciate spontaneously.

Degree of order we need

Judging
- Formulate an organised life style with definite structure and order
- Like to be in control
- Decisive
- Define clear goals, parameters, limits and categories
- Feel comfortable with definite ends and closures
- Plan in advance
- Handle deadlines.

Perceiving
- Prefer a flexible life style
- Enjoy freedom, autonomy, flexibility, curiosity, discovery and surprise
- Prefer freedom to explore with no limits
- Like open endedness and chance
- Meet deadlines with last minute rush.

Leader's Style in Decision-making Process

The extent to which leaders are developed and integrated into the care goals and direction of organisation.

As Custodian: Protects, Preserves, Conserves.

As Operator: Follows instructions, Works 'hands on', Do 'how'.

As Master leader: Transforms, Integrates, Mobilises.

As Maverick: Irritant, Initiator, Changing agent.

Leader is aligned with vision, mission and core goals and is integrated into the organisational structure. Operates appropriate level of competence, confidence and managerial maturity.

Master Leader

Integrated, aligned and functionally mature manager as, 'master leader'. He is capable of envisioning future in realistic, strategic, appropriate and operational terms. Identifies appropriate routes to achieve the associated goals and objectives, generates necessary willing synergy (dynamic, adaptive, organisation, renewal).

Operator

Primarily focused on 'docr', follows instructions, works on 'hands-on' and whose time frame is largely 'here and now'. Perception of leaders' role is based on contribution is governed by 'personal experience, common sense empiricism, uncritical and uninformed observation'.

Custodian (Gentleman's club)

Focuses on preservation of the status quo and is more concerned with conservation than transformation.

Maverick Leader

Highly intelligent, clever people whose restless intellectual energy and sense of dissatisfaction provides the stimulus for their need to change the established order. Powerful change agent and may use both 'vinegar' and 'honey' according to the situation in order to bring about what he considers to have necessary change.

Nurse as an Effective Leader

Nurses are functioning in various set-ups viz., educational institutes, hospitals and community settings. They will play different roles, in varying capacities as a team leader; whatever the settings, nurse have to function as an effective leader, by shoulders responsibility to fulfill organisation policies and goals.

- Team leader should have sound knowledge, efficient administrative skills in the area of working
- Keep efforts to understand thoroughly the policies and objectives of the organisation
- Prepares master plan, in advance, to carry out the activities in a smooth manner within scheduled time
- Develops good interpersonal relationships by establishing adequate rapport with all followers
- Wins the confidence of followers
- Incorporates principles of administration and management (planning, organizing, staffing, decision-making, directing, delegating, coordination, cooperation, command, reporting and budgeting) in implementing the activities
- Formulates the job recruitment policies; selects the candidates for varied positions by following organisations policies
- Prepares job charts/responsibilities for all the cadres
- Delegates the responsibilities, encourages group work, team spirit, inspires the members for cohesiveness
- Coordinates interdepartmental and intradepartmental activities
- Conducts counselling sessions with the affected employees, during problematic situations, helps them to cope up with traumatic experiences

- Motivates the employees to conduct staff developmental programs, in-service training programs, etc. for upgradation of knowledge and attaining higher qualification.

Previous Year Questions

1. Define leadership, its meaning, nature and uses in nursing. (10 m, RGUHS, 2002)
2. Leadership techniques. (5 m, RGUHS, 2002)
3. Power orientation. (5 m, RGUHS, 2002)
4. Leadership styles. (2 m, RGUHS, 2002)
5. Nature of leadership. (2 m, RGUHS, 2002)
6. Spotting a leader in group. (2 m, RGUHS, 2002)
7. What are the important features of leadership? How leaders could be developed. (5 m, RGUHS, 2002)
8. Leaders in groups. (2 m, RGUHS, 1997)
9. Leaders in village. (2 m, RGUHS, 1997)
10. Leaders in nursing profession. (2 m, RGUHS, 1997)
11. Yourself as a leader. (2 m, RGUHS, 1997)
12. What is the essence of leadership? How does one acquire such leadership. (5 m, RGUHS, 1997)
13. Potential qualities of a leader. (5 m, RGUHS, 1997)

MGR University Question Papers

1. Qualities of a leader. (5 m, MGRU)

Bibliography

- Basavanthappa BT: *Textbook of Community Health Nursing.* Jaypee brothers Pvt Ltd. New Delhi. 66-70,1999.
- Chandra : *Women and Empowerment.* Indian Journal of Public Administration. July – Sept **vol XLIII. No.3.** 15-20,1977.
- Correspondence MSc psychology material. Annamalai University. Directorate of distance education. Organizational behaviour. 100-102, 2004.
- Harish: *Economic Development and Role of Indian Women.* Common wealth publication. New Delhi. 1996.
- Indrani TK: *Textbook of Sociology for Nurses.* Jaypee brothers Pvt Ltd. New Delhi. 26-28; 60-65, 1998.
- James C Colcman: *Psychology and Effective behaviour.* DB Taraporevala Sons and Co. Pvt. Ltd. 272-298,1971.
- Kasthuri Sundar Rao: *An Introduction to Community Health Nursing.* BI Publcation Pvt. Ltd. Chennai. 337-346, 2000.
- Micheal Williams and Thorogoog: *Mastering Leadership and Techniques for Managing and Leading a Winning Team.* Viver Books Pvt. Ltd., New Delhi. 2003.
- Mathur SS: *Educational Psychology.* Vinod Pustak Mandir, Agra. 45-68; 565-585, 1979.
- Muktha Gupta: *Economic Participation of Women.* Sarup and Sons, New Delhi. 2000.
- Narayana S: *Rural Development Through Women Programme.* Inter India Publication, New Delhi. 1988.
- Park K: *Textbook of Preventive and Social Medicine.* Banarasidas Bharot Publishers, Jabalpur. 319-322, 2002.
- Paul B Paulus: *Group Dynamics Encyclopedia of Human Behaviour.* Academic press. 68-82, 1994.
- Paul Choudhry: *Women Welfare and Development.* Inter India Publication, New Delhi. 1992.
- Pothen KP and Pothen: *Sociology for Nurses.* NR Brothers, Indore. 80-164,1996.

- Shankar Rao CN: *Sociology—Primary Principles of Sociology with an Introduction to Social Thought*. S Chand and Company Ltd, New Delhi. 1997.
- Sharma RN: *Principles of Sociology*. Media Promoters and Publishers Pvt. Ltd., Bombay. 240-255,1993.
- Singh K: *Advance Sociology*. Prakash Kendra, Lucknow. 310-325,1996.
- Suguna B: *Women's Empowerment: Concept and Frame Work Social Welfare*. New Delhi. **Vol 48 no 9** dec 3-6, 2001.
- Suguna B: *Programmes for Women Development Social Welfare*. New Delhi. **Vol. 64. no. 15.** 8-10, 2003.
- Sunder Raj D: *Our Village, Our Work, Social Welfare*. New Delhi. **Vol 48. no 9**. dec. 35-36, 2001.
- Swaminathan M: *Human Nutrition and Diet*. The Bangalore Printing and Publishing Co. Ltd., Bangalore. 132-136,1992.
- Swaminathan: *Nutrition and Dietetics*. The Bangalore Printing and Publishing Co. Ltd., Bangalore. 282-284, 1993.
- TNAI: *A Community Health Nursing Manual*. New Delhi. 65-70, 1992.
- Tripati RS and RP Tiwari: *Perspectives on Indian Women*. APH Publishing Corp., New Delhi. 1999.
- Tiwari RT and RC Sudha: *Rural Development in India*. Asian Publishing House, New Delhi. 1988.
- Vatsyayan: *Principles of Sociology*. Kedar Nath Ram Nath Co. , New Delhi. 117-120, 1994.
- Vidyabhusham and Sachideva DR: *An Introduction to Sociology*. Century Printers, Allahabad. 1996.

Index

A

B

C

D

E

F

G

H

I

N

O

P

Q

R

T

U

V

W

READER SUGGESTIONS SHEET

Please help us to improve the quality of our publications by completing and returning this sheet to us.

Title/Author: **Textbook of Sociology for Nursing Students by KP Neeraja**

Your name and address:

E-mail address,

Phone and Fax:

How did you hear about this book? [please tick appropriate box (es)].

☐ Direct mail from publisher ☐ Conference ☐ Bookshop

☐ Book review ☐ Lecturer recommendation ☐ Friends

☐ Other (please specify) ☐ Website

Type of purchase: ☐ Direct purchase ☐ Bookshop ☐ Friends

Do you have any brief comments on the book?

Please return this sheet to the name and address given below.

JAYPEE BROTHERS

MEDICAL PUBLISHERS (P) LTD

EMCA House, 23/23B Ansari Road, Daryaganj

New Delhi 110 002, India